STUDY GUIDE FOR

Anatomy & Physiology

NINTH EDITION

KEVIN T. PATTON

GARY A. THIBODEAU

Written by: **LINDA SWISHER, RN, EdD**

ELSEVIER

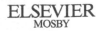

ELSEVIER
MOSBY

3251 Riverport Lane
St. Louis, Missouri 63043

Study Guide for Anatomy & Physiology, Ninth Edition ISBN: 978-0-323-31689-7

Executive Content Strategist: Kellie White
Content Development Manager: Billie Sharp
Content Development Specialist: Joe Gramlich
Content Coordinator: Samantha Taylor
Publishing Services Manager: Deborah Vogel
Project Manager: Divya Krishnakumar
Design Direction: Brian Salisbury

Printed in the United States of America

Last digit is the print number: 9 8 7 6 5

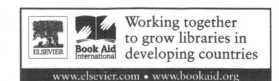

Working together
to grow libraries in
developing countries

www.elsevier.com • www.bookaid.org

Introduction

This study guide to accompany *Anatomy and Physiology*, ninth edition, is designed to help you be successful in learning anatomy and physiology. Before attempting to complete any chapter in the study guide, thoroughly read the corresponding chapter in the textbook, learn the key terms listed at the beginning and end of each textbook chapter, and study your lecture notes. You will then be prepared to complete the questions and exercises that are provided for each chapter.

Each chapter in the study guide begins with a brief overview of the chapter concepts. A variety of questions is offered to help you cover the material effectively. These questions include multiple choice, true or false, matching, short answer, clinical challenges, labeling, and crossword puzzles. After completing the exercises in a chapter, you can check your answers in the back of the book. Each answer is referenced to the appropriate text page. Additionally, questions are grouped into specific topics that correspond to the text. Each major topic of the study guide provides references to specific areas of the text, so if you are having difficulty with a particular grouping of questions, you have a specific reference area to assist you with remedial work. This feature allows you to identify your area of weakness accurately.

MULTIPLE CHOICE

For each multiple choice question, there is only one correct answer out of the choices given. Circle the correct choice.

TRUE OR FALSE

Read each statement carefully and write true or false in the blank provided.

MATCHING

Match each numbered term or statement in the left-hand column with its corresponding lettered term or statement in the right-hand column. Write the correct letters in the blanks provided.

FILL IN THE BLANKS

Fill-in-the-blank questions ask you to recall missing word(s) and insert it (them) into the answer blank(s). These questions may involve sentences or paragraphs.

IDENTIFY THE TERM THAT DOES NOT BELONG

In questions that ask you to identify the incorrect term, three words are given that relate to each other in structure and function, and one more word is included that has no relationship to the other three terms. You are asked to circle the term that does not relate to the others. An example might be: iris, stapes, cornea, and retina. You would circle stapes because all other terms refer to the eye.

APPLICATION QUESTIONS

Application questions ask you to make a judgment based on the information in the chapter. These questions may ask you how you would respond to a situation or to suggest a possible diagnosis for a set of symptoms.

LABELING EXERCISES

Labeling exercises present diagrams with parts that are not identified. According to the directions given, fill in the appropriate labels on the numbered lines or match the numbers with the list of terms provided.

CROSSWORD PUZZLES

Vocabulary words from the *Language of Science* and *Language of Medicine* sections in each chapter of the text have been developed into crossword puzzles. This exercise encourages recall and proper spelling.

ONE LAST QUICK CHECK

This section selects questions from throughout the chapter to provide you with a final review. This mini-test gives you an overview of your knowledge of the chapter after completing all of the other sections. It emphasizes the main concepts of the unit but should not be attempted until the specific topics of the chapter have been mastered.

Acknowledgments

I wish to express my appreciation to the staff at Elsevier, and especially to Tom Wilhelm, Jeff Downing, Kellie White, Billie Sharp, Divya Krishnakumar, Joe Gramlich, and Samantha Taylor for their guidance and support. My continued admiration and thanks to Kevin Patton for another outstanding edition of the text and to Gary Thibodeau who sets the bar for us all to achieve. The time and dedication to science education that you both have given will undoubtedly contribute to the advancement of quality health care for our future and instill in each student a deep appreciation for the wonders of the human body.

Finally, this book is dedicated in memory of my beloved husband Bill—my beautiful connection to the past, and to Sam, Mandi, Billy, Maddie, and Heather—the sunshine of my life and my link to the future.

Linda Swisher, **RN, EdD**

Contents

1

Organization of the Body

The study of anatomy and physiology involves the structure and function of an organism and the relationship of its parts. It starts with a basic organization of the body into different structural levels. Beginning with the smallest level (the cell) and progressing to the largest, most complex level (the system), this chapter familiarizes you with the terminology and the levels of organization needed to facilitate the study of the body in parts or as a whole.

It is also important to be able to identify and describe specific body areas or regions as we progress in this field. The anatomical position is used as a reference when dissecting the body into planes, regions, or cavities. The terminology in this chapter allows you to describe the areas efficiently and accurately. It is important to have a basic understanding of the structural levels of organization—the planes, regions, and cavities of the body—and to be familiar with the terminology used to describe these areas before progressing on to the concept of homeostasis.

I—SCIENCE AND SOCIETY

True or False

1. _____ A hypothesis is a theory with a high degree of confidence.

2. _____ Rigorous experiments that eliminate any influences or biases not being directly tested are called *controlled experiments*.

3. _____ Cadavers are dead bodies.

4. _____ If data proves to be biased in a hypothesis, you may refine the hypothesis.

5. _____ If repeat experiments are consistent, scientists may begin to call a hypothesis, a theory which provides more credibility and confidence.

➡ *If you had difficulty with this section, review page 4.*

II—ANATOMY AND PHYSIOLOGY: LANGUAGE OF SCIENCE AND CHARACTERISTICS OF LIFE

Multiple Choice—select the best answer.

6. *Anatomy* refers to:
   a. using devices to investigate parameters such as heart rate and blood pressure.
   b. investigating human structure via dissection and other methods.
   c. studying the unusual manner in which an organism responds to painful stimuli.
   d. examining the chemistry of life.

7. *Systemic* anatomy refers to anatomical investigation:
   a. at a microscopic level.
   b. that begins in the head and neck and concludes at the feet.
   c. that approaches the study of the body by systems: groups of organs having a common function.
   d. at the cellular level.

8. *Physiology* refers to the:
   a. nature of human function.
   b. structure of the human form.
   c. evolution of human thought.
   d. accuracy of measuring the human physique.

9. The removal of waste products in the body is achieved by a process known as:
   a. secretion.
   b. excretion.
   c. circulation.
   d. conductivity.

10. *Metabolism* is the:
    a. exchange of gases in the blood.
    b. formation of new cells in the body to permit growth.
    c. sum total of all physical and chemical reactions occurring in the body.
    d. production and delivery of specialized substances for diverse body functions.

11. Standardizing terminology avoids:
    a. confusion.
    b. terms that are based on a person's name.
    c. assistance with physiological terms.
    d. misspelling of common terms.

➡ *If you had difficulty with this section, review pages 4-6.*

III—LEVELS OF ORGANIZATION

Multiple Choice—select the best answer.

12. Beginning with the smallest level, the levels of organization of the body are:
    a. cellular, chemical, tissue, organelle, organ, system, organism.
    b. cellular, chemical, organelle, organ, tissue, organism, system.
    c. chemical, cellular, organelle, organ, system, organism.
    d. chemical, organelle, cellular, tissue, organ, system, organism.

13. Molecules are:
    a. combinations of atoms forming larger chemical aggregates.
    b. electrons orbiting a nucleus.
    c. a complex of electrons arranged in orderly shells.
    d. composed of cellular organelles.

14. Mitochondria, Golgi apparatus, and endoplasmic reticulum are examples of:
    a. macromolecules.
    b. cytoplasm.
    c. organelles.
    d. nuclei.

15. Blood production is a function of which system?
    a. circulatory
    b. respiratory
    c. skeletal
    d. urinary

16. Support and movement are functions of which systems?
    a. respiratory, digestive, and urinary systems
    b. reproductive and urinary systems
    c. skeletal and muscular systems
    d. cardiovascular and lymphatic/immune systems

Matching—match the term with the proper selection.

    a. many similar cells that act together to perform a common function
    b. the most complex units that make up the body
    c. a group of several different kinds of tissues arranged to perform a special function
    d. collections of molecules that perform a function
    e. the smallest "living" units of structure and function

17. _____ organelle

18. _____ cells

19. _____ tissue

20. _____ organ

21. _____ systems

Matching—match each system with its corresponding functions.

    a. support and movement
    b. communication, control, and integration
    c. reproduction and development
    d. transportation and defense
    e. respiration, nutrition, and excretion

22. _____ integumentary system

23. _____ skeletal system

24. _____ muscular system

25. _____ nervous system

26. _____ endocrine system

27. _____ digestive system

28. _____ respiratory system

29. _____ cardiovascular system

30. _____ lymphatic system

31. _____ urinary system

32. _____ reproductive system

➲ *If you had difficulty with this section, review pages 7-9.*

IV—ANATOMICAL POSITION, BODY CAVITIES, BODY REGIONS, ANATOMICAL TERMS, BODY PLANES AND SECTIONS

Multiple Choice—select the best answer.

33. In the anatomical position, the subject is:
    a. seated with the head facing forward.
    b. standing with the arms at the sides and palms facing forward.
    c. seated with arms parallel to the ground.
    d. standing with the arms at the sides and palms facing backward.

34. The dorsal body cavity contains the:
    a. brain and spinal cord.
    b. abdominal organs.
    c. pelvic organs.
    d. thoracic organs.

35. The ventral body cavity contains the:
    a. thoracic and abdominopelvic cavities.
    b. thoracic cavity only.
    c. abdominopelvic cavity only.
    d. brain and spinal cord.

36. The axial portion of the body consists of:
    a. arms, neck, and torso.
    b. neck, torso, and legs.
    c. torso, arms, and legs.
    d. head, neck, and torso.

37. The abdominopelvic cavity contains all of the following *except* the:
    a. kidneys.
    b. pancreas.
    c. lungs.
    d. urinary bladder.

38. The mediastinum contains all of the following *except* the:
    a. esophagus.
    b. aorta.
    c. lungs.
    d. trachea.

39. Visceral peritoneum would cover which of the following organs?
    a. heart
    b. liver
    c. lungs
    d. brain

40. A sagittal section would divide the body into:
    a. upper and lower parts.
    b. right and left sides.
    c. front and back portions.
    d. none of the above.

41. A coronal section would divide the body into:
    a. upper and lower parts.
    b. right and left sides.
    c. front and back portions.
    d. none of the above.

42. *Inguinal* is a term referring to which body region?
    a. anterior portion of elbow
    b. armpit
    c. posterior knee
    d. groin

Circle the correct answer.

43. The stomach is (superior or inferior) to the diaphragm.

44. The nose is located on the (anterior or posterior) surface of the body.

45. The lungs lie (medial or lateral) to the heart.

46. The elbow lies (proximal or distal) to the forearm.

47. The skin is (superficial or deep) to the muscles below it.

48. A midsagittal plane divides the body into (equal or unequal) parts.

49. A frontal plane divides the body into (anterior and posterior or superior and inferior) sections.

50. A transverse plane divides the body into (right and left or upper and lower) sections.

51. A coronal plane may also be referred to as a (sagittal or frontal) plane.

Matching—select the correct term from the choices given and insert the letter in the answer blank.

    a. ventral cavity
    b. dorsal cavity

52. _____ thoracic

53. _____ cranial

54. _____ abdominal

55. _____ pelvic

56. _____ mediastinum

57. _____ pleural

Labeling—using the terms provided, label the anatomical directions on the illustration below.

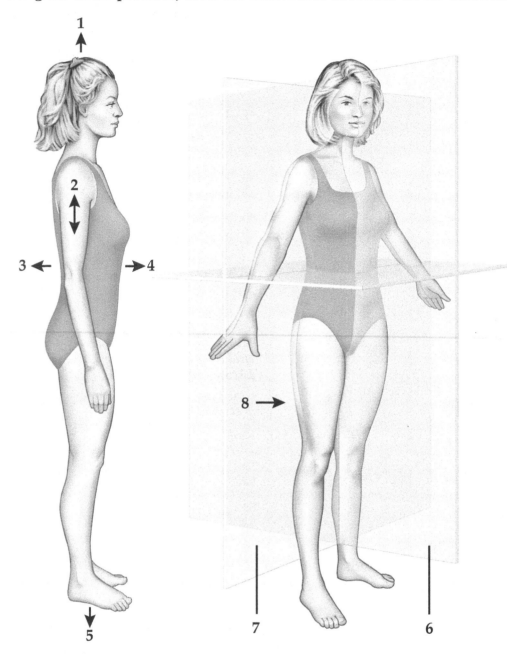

anterior (ventral)
lateral
posterior (dorsal)
proximal

sagittal plane
frontal plane
superior
inferior

1. _____

2. _____

3. _____

4. _____

5. _____

6. _____

7. _____

8. _____

Labeling—label the various body cavities on the diagram below.

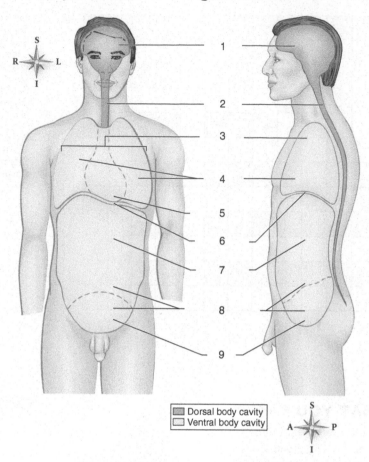

Dorsal body cavity
Ventral body cavity

1. _____
2. _____
3. _____
4. _____
5. _____

6. _____
7. _____
8. _____
9. _____

➜ *If you had difficulty with this section, review pages 9-16.*

CROSSWORD PUZZLE

ACROSS
3. Above; name
6. Side; relating to
7. Internal organ; relating to
8. Instrument; condition
9. Apart; cut; action
10. Back; relating to—hollow; state
11. Organized whole
12. Near; relating to

DOWN
1. Tip; relating to
2. Storeroom
4. Small; life; entire collection
5. Over; throw; action

 APPLYING WHAT YOU KNOW

58. Laurie has had an appendectomy. The nurse is preparing to change the dressing. She knows that the appendix is located in the right iliac inguinal region, the distal portion extending at an angle into the hypogastric region. Place an X on the diagram where the nurse will place the dressing.

59. Penny noticed a lump in her breast. Dr. Reeder noted on her chart that a small mass was located in the left breast medial to the nipple. Place an X where Penny's lump would be located.

60. Madison was injured in a bicycle accident. X-ray films revealed that she had a fracture of the right patella. A cast was applied beginning at the distal femoral region and extending to the pedal region. Place an X where Madison's cast begins and ends.

 DID YOU KNOW?

- Many animals produce tears but only humans weep as a result of emotional stress.
- Men notice subtle signs of sadness in a face only 40% of the time; women pick up on them 90% of the time.

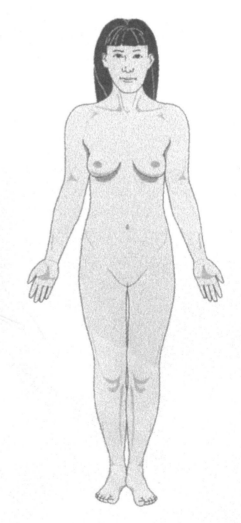

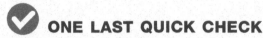

ONE LAST QUICK CHECK

Multiple Choice—select the best answer.

61. The regions frequently used by health professionals to locate pain or tumors divide the abdomen into four basic areas called:
    a. planes.
    b. cavities.
    c. pleural.
    d. quadrants.

62. A lengthwise plane running from front to back that divides the body into right and left sides is called:
    a. transverse.
    b. coronal.
    c. frontal.
    d. sagittal.

63. A study of the functions of living organisms and their parts is called:
    a. physiology.
    b. chemistry.
    c. biology.
    d. none of the above.

64. Which of the following structures does *not* lie within the abdominopelvic cavity?
    a. right iliac region
    b. left antecubital region
    c. left lumbar region
    d. hypogastric region

65. The dorsal body cavity contains components of the:
    a. reproductive system.
    b. digestive system.
    c. respiratory system.
    d. nervous system.

66. If your reference point is "nearest the trunk of the body" versus "farthest from the trunk of the body," where does the elbow lie in relation to the wrist?
    a. anterior
    b. posterior
    c. distal
    d. proximal

67. The buttocks are often used as injection sites. This region can also be called:
    a. sacral.
    b. buccal.
    c. cutaneous.
    d. gluteal.

68. Which of the following is *not* a component of the axial subdivision of the body?
    a. upper extremity
    b. neck
    c. trunk
    d. head

69. A synonym for *medial* is:
    a. toward the side.
    b. in front of.
    c. midline.
    d. anterior.

70. The outer region of an organ may often be referred to as the:
    a. medullary region.
    b. cortical region.
    c. basal region.
    d. apical region.

Fill in the blanks.

71. A principle of standardizing terminology is the avoidance of _____, or terms based upon a person's name.

72. The term _____ _____ means that the right and left sides of humans are mirror images of each other and only one plane can divide the body into left and right sides.

73. _____ refers to an inner region of an organ.

74. The narrow tip of an organ is the _____ portion.

75. Hereditary material called _____ carries the chemical blueprint of the body.

76. _____ is the ability of an organism to sense, monitor, and respond to change in both its external and internal environments.

True or False

77. ____ *Cephalic* is the term used for wrist.

78. ____ Proximal means "away from the trunk."

79. ____ The smallest level of organization is the organelle.

80. ____ The ureters are in the abdominal cavity.

CHAPTER 2

Homeostasis

*H*omeostasis is the term that we use to describe the relatively constant state maintained by the body. A state of relative constancy in the chemical composition of body fluids is necessary for good health. In fact, maintaining the delicate internal fluid environment of the body is critical to survival.

Homeostatic control mechanisms maintain or restore homeostasis by self-regulation through feedback control loops or control systems. Negative feedback control systems are inhibitory, and positive feedback control systems are stimulatory. A feed-forward concept occurs when information flows ahead to another process or feedback loop to trigger a change in anticipation of an event that will follow.

Many diseases are the result of disturbances to homeostasis. The ability of the body to return to normal indicates whether a disease or condition is acute or chronic. If the body returns to homeostasis quickly, the disease is said to be *acute*. If the body is unable to ever return to normal homeostasis, the condition is described as *chronic*.

This chapter reviews homeostasis and the mechanisms involved in maintaining a constant internal environment. It further discusses negative, positive, and feed-forward systems and the effect that they have on homeostasis. The chapter concludes with terminology and principles to consider when reviewing mechanisms of disease and the impact that disturbances to homeostasis have on disease.

I—HOMEOSTASIS AND HOMEOSTATIC CONTROL MECHANISMS

Multiple Choice—*select the best answer.*

1. *Homeostasis* can be defined as the:
   a. relatively constant state maintained by the body.
   b. overall contribution of an organ system.
   c. external stimuli that evoke a disruption to an organism.
   d. lack of cytoplasm within a plasma membrane.

2. Which of the following is *not* a component of a feedback control loop?
   a. sensory mechanism
   b. integrating, or control, center
   c. effector mechanism
   d. stressor stimulator

3. Negative feedback control systems:
   a. oppose a change.
   b. accelerate a change.
   c. ignore a change.
   d. none of the above.

4. Positive feedback control systems:
   a. oppose a change.
   b. accelerate a change.
   c. ignore a change.
   d. none of the above.

5. After food enters the stomach, _____ occurs to increase secretions and assist with digestion in the small intestine.
   a. negative feedback
   b. positive feedback
   c. feed-forward
   d. extrinsic control

True or False

6. _____ Any given physiological parameter will never deviate beyond the set point.

7. _____ In the thermostatically regulated furnace example of negative feedback, the furnace functions as the sensor.

8. _____ Negative feedback systems are inhibitory.

9. _____ The process of childbirth—in which the baby's head causes increased stretching of the reproductive tract, which in turn feeds back to the brain, thus triggering the release of oxytocin—is an example of positive feedback.

10. _____ When cold weather causes the body temperature to decrease, feedback information is relayed through the nerves to the "thermostat" in a part of the brain called the *thalamus*.

➔ *If you had difficulty with this section, review pages 24-31.*

II—MECHANISMS OF DISEASE

Matching—match the term with the proper selection.

a. subjective abnormalities
b. study of disease
c. collection of different signs and symptoms that present a clear picture of a pathological condition
d. study of factors involved in causing a disease
e. objective abnormalities
f. undetermined causes
g. disease native to a local region
h. symptoms appear suddenly and for a short period
i. affects large geographic regions
j. actual pattern of a disease's development

11. _____ pathology

12. _____ signs

13. _____ symptoms

14. _____ etiology

15. _____ syndrome

16. _____ idiopathic

17. _____ acute

18. _____ pandemic

19. _____ endemic

20. _____ pathogenesis

Fill in the blanks.

21. _____ is the organized study of the underlying physiological processes associated with disease.

22. Many diseases are best understood as disturbances of _____.

23. Altered or _____ genes can cause abnormal proteins to be made.

24. An organism that lives in or on another organism to obtain its nutrients is called a _____.

25. Abnormal tissue growths may also be referred to as _____.

➔ *If you had difficulty with this section, review pages 31-33.*

CROSSWORD PUZZLE

ACROSS
1. In; people; relating to
4. Accomplish; agent
5. All; people; relating to
8. Poison
9. Peculiar; disease; relating to
10. Time; relating to
11. Disease; combining form; study of; activity
12. Mushroom

DOWN
2. Common; capacity for
3. Back or again; to send; condition of
6. First; animal
7. Cause; combining form; study; activity

APPLYING WHAT YOU KNOW

26. Sam just finished a big Thanksgiving meal. His blood glucose has elevated sharply after a meal that was heavy in carbohydrates and fats. He is so full that he is uncomfortable. What homeostatic control systems will begin to assist Sam with this temporary stress to his body?

27. Jessica was treated by her doctor for human papillomavirus. He encouraged her to have frequent Pap smears and cautioned her to be vigilant for any uterine pain, bleeding, or other signs of cervical cancer. What is the connection between the virus and cervical cancer?

❓ DID YOU KNOW?

- All living organisms have to have a stable internal environment to function normally.
- The smallest organ, the pineal gland, is the same size as a grain of rice.

✔ ONE LAST QUICK CHECK

Multiple Choice—select the best answer.

28. The body's ability to continuously respond to changes in the environment and maintain consistency in the internal environment is called:
    a. homeostasis.
    b. superficial.
    c. structural levels.
    d. none of the above.

29. When you experience a bacterial infection, your immune system sends chemicals to signal the brain's hypothalamus to "turn up" the _____ temperature, causing your body to shiver.
    a. set point
    b. effector
    c. sensor
    d. feed forward

30. Which of the following is *not* a homeostatic control system?
    a. positive feedback
    b. negative feedback
    c. fast forward
    d. variable feedback

31. The hypothalamus is the body's:
    a. thermostat.
    b. transmitter.
    c. positive feedback control system.
    d. effector.

32. A disease that is native to a local region is referred to as being:
    a. epidemic.
    b. pandemic.
    c. endemic.
    d. idiopathic.

Fill in the blanks.

33. Processes for maintaining or restoring homeostasis are known as _____ _____ _____.

34. _____ _____ is the concept that information may flow ahead to another process to trigger a change in anticipation of an event that will follow.

35. _____ _____ mechanisms operate at the tissue and organ levels.

36. Tiny, primitive cells that lack nuclei and may cause infection are _____.

37. An inherited trait that puts one at greater than normal risk for development of a specific disease is a(n) _____ _____.

True or False

38. _____ If the body's homeostatic system is working properly, an increase in blood glucose will stimulate physiological reactions to cause an opposing effect or a decrease in blood glucose.

39. _____ During the birth of a baby, oxytocin is released to stimulate labor. This is an example of positive feedback.

40. _____ The formation of a blood clot is an example of a negative feedback.

41. _____ Mechanisms that operate at the cell level are known as *intracellular control mechanisms.*

42. _____ A secondary infection, such as pneumonia with an AIDS patient, is referred to as an *opportunistic* infection.

Circle the best answer.

43. The "thermostat" of the brain is the (thalamus or hypothalamus).

44. The hormone that stimulates contractions during labor is (oxytocin or progesterone).

45. Intrinsic control mechanisms are sometimes called (autoregulation or circadian rhythms).

46. (Prions or Protozoa) are proteins that convert proteins of the cell into different proteins.

47. (Infancy or Young adulthood) is the period of greatest homeostatic efficiency.

CHAPTER 3

Chemical Basis of Life

Although anatomy can be studied without knowledge of chemistry, it is hard to imagine an understanding of physiology without a basic comprehension of chemical reactions in the body. Trillions of cells make up the various levels or organization in the body. Our health and survival depend upon the proper chemical maintenance of our cells.

Chemists use the terms *elements* or *compounds* to describe all of the substances (matter) in and around us. Distinguishing these two terms is the fact that an element cannot be broken down. A compound, on the other hand, is made up of two or more elements and has the ability to be broken down into the elements that form it.

Because we cannot see many of the chemical reactions that take place daily in our bodies, it is sometimes difficult to comprehend the principles involved in initiating them. Chemicals are responsible for directing virtually all of our bodily functions. It is therefore important to master the fundamental concepts of chemistry before progressing further in your study of anatomy and physiology.

I—UNITS OF MATTER

Multiple Choice—select the best answer.

1. Which of the following is *not* one of the major elements present in the human body?
   a. oxygen
   b. carbon
   c. iron
   d. hydrogen

2. Which of the following is *not* a subatomic particle?
   a. proton
   b. electron
   c. isotope
   d. neutron

3. The total number of electrons in an atom equals the number of:
   a. neutrons in its nucleus.
   b. electrons in its nucleus.
   c. protons in its nucleus.
   d. ions in its nucleus.

4. An atom can be described as *chemically stable* if its outermost electron shell contains:
   a. three electrons.
   b. five electrons.
   c. six electrons.
   d. eight electrons.

5. Isotopes are atoms of elements that differ in their number of:
   a. protons.
   b. electrons.
   c. neutrons.
   d. nuclei.

6. Ionic bonds are chemical bonds formed by the:
   a. sharing of electrons between atoms.
   b. donation of protons from one atom to another.
   c. transfer of electrons from one atom to another.
   d. acceptance of protons from one atom by another.

7. Chemical bonds formed by the sharing of electrons are called:
   a. ionic.
   b. covalent.
   c. hydrogen.
   d. electronic.

True or False

8. _____ *Matter* is a term used by chemists to describe all the materials or substances around us.

9. _____ *Mass number* refers to the number of protons plus the number of neutrons in the atom's nucleus.

10. _____ Sodium chloride is an example of a covalent bond.

11. _____ Hydrogen bonds form from an equal charge distribution within a molecule.

12. _____ Chemist John Dalton proposed the concept that all matter is composed of atoms.

13. _____ Alpha particles are a type of radiation that travels at a reported speed of 18,000 miles per second.

Identify the following elements:

14. O _____

15. Ca _____

16. K _____

17. Na _____

18. Mg _____

19. Fe _____

20. Se _____

Fill in the blanks.

21. An ionic bond may also be referred to as an

    _____.

22. _____ is anything that has mass and occupies
    space.

23. A bond that results from an unequal charge
    distribution on molecules is a _____ bond.

24. The cloud model concept is called a _____
    _____ and refers to the possibility of
    finding an electron at any specific location outside
    the nucleus.

25. Helium is an _____, or stable element.

➔ *If you had difficulty with this section, review pages 39-44.*

II—CHEMICAL REACTIONS

Fill in the blanks.

26. When two or more substances called *reactants*
    combine to form a different, more complex
    substance, it is known as _____

    _____.

27. _____ _____ result in the
    breakdown of a complex substance into two or more
    simpler substances.

28. _____ _____ proceed in both
    directions.

29. When two different reactants exchange components
    and, as a result, form two new products, they are
    known as _____ _____.

30. The ability of the body to form new tissue in wound
    repair is a good example of _____
    _____.

➔ *If you had difficulty with this section, review pages 45-51.*

III—METABOLISM

Matching—select the best answer.

   a. breaks down larger food molecules into smaller
      units
   b. the form of energy that cells generally use
   c. all the chemical reactions that occur in body cells
   d. joins simple molecules together to form more
      complex ones
   e. key chemical reaction during anabolism

31. _____ catabolism

32. _____ anabolism

33. _____ ATP

34. _____ metabolism

35. _____ dehydration synthesis

➔ *If you had difficulty with this section, review pages 46-47.*

IV—INORGANIC MOLECULES

Multiple Choice—select the best answer.

36. Water plays a key role in such processes as:
    a. cell permeability.
    b. active transport of materials.
    c. secretion.
    d. all of the above.

37. Which of the following is *not* a property of water?
    a. strong polarity
    b. high specific heat
    c. high heat of vaporization
    d. strong acidity

38. Acids:
    a. are proton donors.
    b. dye litmus blue.
    c. release hydrogen ions when in solution.
    d. accept electrons when in an aqueous solution.

39. Substances that accept hydrogen ions are referred to
    as:
    a. acids.
    b. bases.
    c. buffers.
    d. salts.

40. The constancy of the pH homeostatic mechanism is
    caused by the presence of substances called:
    a. salts.
    b. bases.
    c. buffers.
    d. acids.

True or false

41. _____ The pH scale indicates the degree of acidity or alkalinity of a solution.

42. _____ Milk is acid on the pH scale.

43. _____ Litmus will turn red in the presence of an acid.

44. _____ The basic substance of each cell is water.

45. _____ Oxygen and carbon dioxide are examples of organic compounds.

 If you had difficulty with this section, review pages 47-50.

CROSSWORD PUZZLE

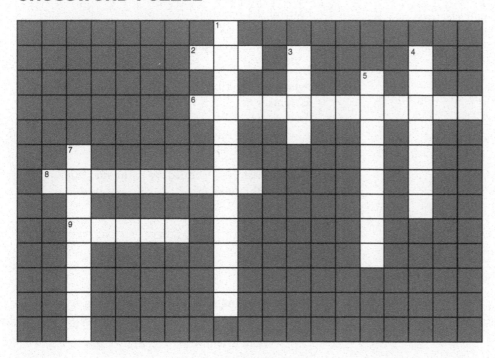

ACROSS
2. To go
6. Send out rays; equal; place
8. To go; band (2 words)
9. Pole; relating to

DOWN
1. With; power; band (2 words)
3. Indivisible
4. Equal; place
5. Mass; small
7. Put together

APPLYING WHAT YOU KNOW

46. Amanda and Steve own a home that was recently discovered to contain very high levels of radon. Where in the house would these levels be greatest? What could be done to eliminate the radon?

47. Mr. Ferber was recently diagnosed with cancer of the prostate. His doctor suggested that they use radioactive isotopes as a treatment regimen. Why might this method be used instead of surgery or chemotherapy?

DID YOU KNOW?

• The only letter not appearing on the Periodic Table is the letter "J."
• Hydrogen is the most abundant element in the universe.

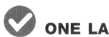

ONE LAST QUICK CHECK

Matching—select the correct answer.

   a. isotopes
   b. element
   c. polar
   d. octet rule
   e. protons

48. _____ this number identifies the element

49. _____ atoms with fewer than eight electrons in the outer energy level will attempt to lose, gain, or share electrons with other atoms to achieve stability.

50. _____ deuterium and tritium

51. _____ hydrogen bond that results from an unequal charge distribution on a molecule.

52. _____ cannot be broken down

Multiple Choice

53. Which one is a major element in the body?
   a. iron
   b. iodine
   c. sulfur
   d. zinc

54. A negatively charged subatomic particle is a (an):
   a. proton
   b. neutron
   c. isotron
   d. electron

55. AB + CD → AD + CB symbolizes a formula for:
   a. synthesis reactions.
   b. decomposition reactions.
   c. exchange reactions.
   d. reversible reaction.

56. Which element is stable?
   a. helium
   b. carbon
   c. oxygen
   d. hydrogen

57. Which of the following bonds is the weakest?
   a. NaCl
   b. H_2
   c. H_2O
   d. CO_2

58. Which one is an example of an element?
   a. Ca
   b. CO_2
   c. H_2O
   d. NaCl

59. This reaction occurs when a complex nutrient is broken down in a cell to release energy for other cellular functions.
   a. decomposition reaction
   b. synthesis reaction
   c. exchange reaction
   d. product reaction

60. When substances are combined to form more complex substances, it is called:
   a. decomposition reaction.
   b. synthesis reactions.
   c. exchange reaction.
   d. reversible reaction.

61. If an atom's outermost shell contains eight electrons, it may be described as:
   a. ionic.
   b. covalent.
   c. chemically stable.
   d. synthesized.

62. Each element is identified by its atomic number, which is the number of _____ in the nucleus.
   a. neutrons
   b. protons
   c. electrons
   d. isotopes

True or False

63. _____ Biochemistry is the field of chemistry that deals with living organisms and life processes.

64. _____ Matter, with the exception of gas, is composed of atoms.

65. _____ The largest naturally occurring atom is uranium.

66. _____ Hydrogen, carbon, and oxygen react chemically because they do not satisfy the octet rule.

67. _____ Protons surround an atom's nucleus in a field or proton cloud that represents different energy levels.

68. _____ Isotopes of an element contain the same number of protons and neutrons.

69. _____ In addition to the chemical symbol for each element on the periodic table, the atomic number and atomic mass are also indicated for each one.

70. _____ The most abundant elements in the body are O, C, H, and N.

71. _____ All carbon atoms, and only carbon atoms, contain six protons and have an atomic number of six.

72. _____ The nature of exchange reactions permits two different reactants to exchange components and form one new product.

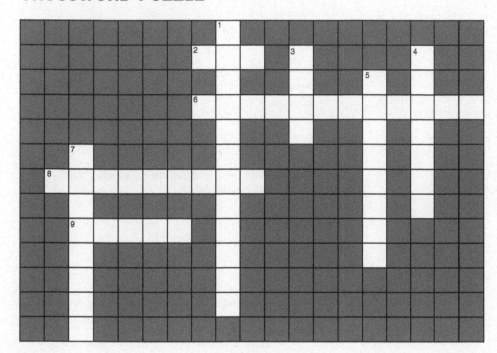

CHAPTER 4

Biomolecules

Most of the structures that make up animals, plants, and microbes are made from a basic class of biomolecules known as *organic molecules*. They are: amino acids (proteins), carbohydrates, lipids (fats), nucleic acids, and related molecules. Without organic compounds, and inorganic compounds such as water, we could not sustain life.

Organic molecules contain carbon. Some contain C-C bonds and others are C-H bonded. Carbon, because of its ability to bond with four other atoms, can form many complex structures. This makes it a perfect molecule for building other compounds. This chapter gives you an appreciation for the biomolecules of the body and for the balance and maintenance required for good health and survival.

I—ORGANIC MOLECULES

Multiple Choice—select the best answer.

1. Which of the following is *not* a type of carbohydrate?
   a. monosaccharides
   b. disaccharides
   c. megasaccharides
   d. polysaccharides

2. Which of the following is *incorrect* in reference to carbohydrates?
   a. They include substances referred to as *sugars*.
   b. They serve critical structural roles in RNA and DNA.
   c. They represent a primary source of chemical energy for body cells.
   d. They are replete with nitrogen atoms.

3. Proteins are composed of ____ commonly occurring amino acids.
   a. 8
   b. 12
   c. 21
   d. 24

4. Amino acids frequently become joined by:
   a. peptide bonds.
   b. phospholipid reactions.
   c. degradation synthesis.
   d. none of the above.

5. Which of the following is *not* an example of proteins?
   a. hormones
   b. antibodies
   c. urine
   d. enzymes

6. A structural lipid found in a cell membrane is a:
   a. triglyceride.
   b. phospholipid.
   c. steroid.
   d. prostaglandin.

7. Which of the following is the correct example of DNA base pairing?
   a. adenine-cytosine
   b. guanine-adenine
   c. adenine-thymine
   d. guanine-thymine

8. A DNA molecule contains each of the following *except*:
   a. sugar.
   b. nitrogenous base.
   c. phosphate.
   d. lipid.

9. DNA differs from RNA in that:
   a. RNA contains ribose instead of deoxyribose.
   b. RNA contains thymine instead of uracil.
   c. RNA contains a double polynucleotide strand.
   d. There is no structural difference between DNA and RNA.

True or False

10. _____ Steroids are poorly distributed throughout the body.

11. _____ High-density lipoprotein (HDL) is also called the "good" cholesterol.

12. _____ Protein compounds have no role in defending the body against harmful agents.

13. _____ The nonessential amino acids can be produced from the other amino acids or from simple organic molecules.

14. _____ Enzymes are functional proteins that bring molecules together or split them apart in chemical reactions.

15. _____ Prostaglandins are "tissue hormones."

Fill in the blanks

16. All proteins have four elements: carbon, oxygen, hydrogen, and _____.

17. The building blocks of all proteins are called _____ _____.

18. The most common type of coil in a polypeptide's secondary structure is called an _____ _____.

19. The final, functioning shape for a protein is often called its _____ _____.

20. The nucleic acid molecule that can act as either an "information molecule" or as a "regulatory molecule" is _____.

➡️ *If you had difficulty with this section, review pages 56-71.*

CROSSWORD PUZZLE

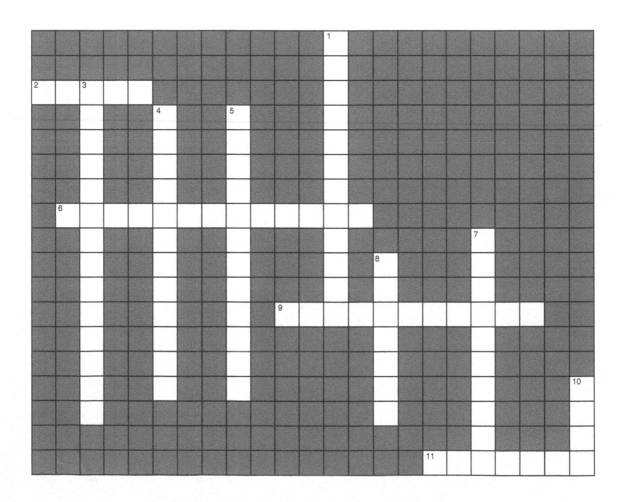

ACROSS
2. Fat; form
6. Large; mass; small
9. Water; loving
11. Sterol; like

DOWN
1. Phosphorus; fat; form
3. Before; stand; acorn; substance
4. Carbon; hydrogen; oxygen
5. Three; sweet; chemical
7. Nut or kernel; chemical
8. Primary; substance
10. Sour

APPLYING WHAT YOU KNOW

21. Shelley just finished preparing a meal of pan-fried hamburgers for her family. While the frying pan was still hot, she poured the liquid grease into a metal container to cool. Later she noticed that the liquid oil had solidified as it cooled. Explain the chemistry of why the now room-temperature fat was solid.

22. Joe recently received his blood report in the mail. His cholesterol was within normal limits, but his triglycerides were elevated. Joe is currently on cholesterol-lowering medication, so he is not concerned as long as his cholesterol is within normal limits. Is this thinking correct? What would you tell Joe?

DID YOU KNOW?

- A protein in semen acts on the female brain to prompt ovulation.
- The lifespan of most proteins totals 2 days or less. However, the recent discovery of extremely long-lived proteins may provide scientists with insight into cell aging and neurodegeneration.
- The protein in eggs is the highest quality of protein found in any food.·
- After a vigorous workout, your triglycerides fall 10%-20% and your HDL increases by the same percentage for 2-3 hours.

ONE LAST QUICK CHECK

Matching—select the best answer.

    a. protein
    b. carbohydrate
    c. lipid

23. _____ ribose

24. _____ steroids

25. _____ amino acid

26. _____ glycerol

27. _____ monosaccharides

28. _____ phospholipids

29. _____ enzymes

Circle the one that doesn't belong.

30. functional group	radicals	R	PKU
31. triglycerides	steroids	prostaglandins	salts
32. glycogen	polysaccharide	macromolecule	calcitriol

Matching—identify each term with its corresponding clue, description, or definition.

   a. antibodies
   b. cholesterol
   c. dehydration synthesis
   d. motif
   e. high-energy bonds
   f. peptide bond
   g. domains
   h. hypertriglyceridemia
   i. nonessential amino acids
   j. denatures

33. _____ Produced from amino acids readily available to the body cells

34. _____ Binds the carboxyl group of one amino acid to the amino group of another amino acid

35. _____ The formation of glycogen from simple sugar "building blocks" is an example.

36. _____ A pattern of alpha helices and/or beta sheets within the secondary structure of protein

37. _____ Several complicated "knots" in a tertiary protein structure

38. _____ An example of a functional protein

39. _____ Shape of protein

40. _____ When these bonds are broken during catabolic reactions, the energy released is used to form new compounds.

41. _____ Steroid found in the plasma membrane surrounding every body cell

42. _____ Abnormally high concentration of triglycerides in the blood

CHAPTER 5
Cell Structure

Cells are the smallest structural units of living things. Because we are living, we are made up of a mass of cells. Human cells, which vary in shape and size, can only be seen under a microscope. The three main parts of a cell are the cytoplasmic membrane, the cytoplasm, and the nucleus. As you review this chapter, you will be amazed at the resemblance of a cell to the body as a whole. You will identify a miniature circulatory system, reproductive system, digestive system, lymphatic system, skeletal system, and many other structures that will aid in your understanding of these and other body systems in future chapters.

I—FUNCTIONAL ANATOMY OF CELLS

Multiple Choice—select the best answer.

1. Which of the following is *not* a main cellular structure?
   a. plasma membrane
   b. interstitial fluid
   c. cytoplasm (including organelles)
   d. nucleus

2. All of the following are examples of the plasma membrane function *except:*
   a. boundary of cell.
   b. self-identification.
   c. receptor sites.
   d. "power plants" of cell.

3. Which of the following is a functional characteristic of ribosomes?
   a. provision of ATP
   b. protein synthesis
   c. DNA replication
   d. binding site for steroid hormones

4. Production of ATP occurs within which organelle?
   a. smooth endoplasmic reticulum
   b. Golgi apparatus
   c. lysosomes
   d. mitochondria

5. Preparation of protein molecules for cellular exportation is the function of which of the following organelles?
   a. Golgi apparatus
   b. microvilli
   c. peroxisomes
   d. mitochondria

6. In nondividing cells DNA appears as threads that are referred to as:
   a. chromatin.
   b. nucleoplasm.
   c. nucleolus.
   d. none of the above.

7. The nucleolus is composed chiefly of:
   a. DNA.
   b. rRNA.
   c. tRNA.
   d. none of the above.

True or False

8. _____ The plasma membrane can be described as a triple layer of phospholipid molecules.

9. _____ The process by which cells translate the signal received by a membrane receptor into a specific chemical change in the cell is called *signal transportation.*

10. _____ Each and every cell always has one nucleus.

11. _____ Generally, the more active a cell is, the more mitochondria it will contain.

12. _____ Membranous bags that temporarily contain molecules for transport or later use are known as *peroxisomes.*

Matching—identify each cell structure with its corresponding function.

a. nucleolus
b. lysosome
c. cytoplasm
d. plasma membrane
e. endoplasmic reticulum
f. ribosome
g. mitochondria
h. nucleus

13. _____ forms ribosomes

14. _____ separates the cell from its environment

15. _____ acts as the cell's "digestive system"

16. _____ acts as a "protein factory"

17. _____ contains organelles

18. _____ contains DNA

19. _____ act as "power plants" of the cell

20. _____ classified as both smooth and rough

Labeling—from memory, label the parts of the typical cell on the diagram below.

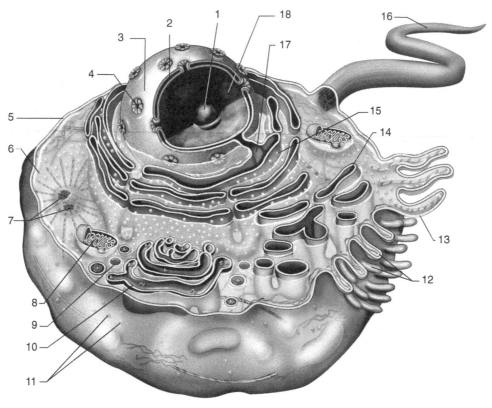

Animal cell.

1.

2.

3.

4.

5.

6.

7.

8.

9.

10.

11.

12.

13.

14.

15.

16.

17.

18.

➡ *If you had difficulty with this section, review pages 78-87.*

II—CYTOSKELETON

Fill in the blanks.

21. _____ is the cell's internal supporting framework.

22. _____ are the smallest cell fibers.

23. The thickest of the cell fibers are tiny, hollow tubes called _____.

24. The _____ is an area of the cytoplasm near the nucleus that coordinates the building and breaking of microtubules in the cell.

25. _____, _____, and _____ are cell extensions that appear on certain types of cells.

26. When membrane channels of adjacent plasma membranes connect to others, the formation is known as _____ _____.

27. _____ hold skin together.

➔ *If you had difficulty with this section, review pages 88-92.*

CROSSWORD PUZZLE

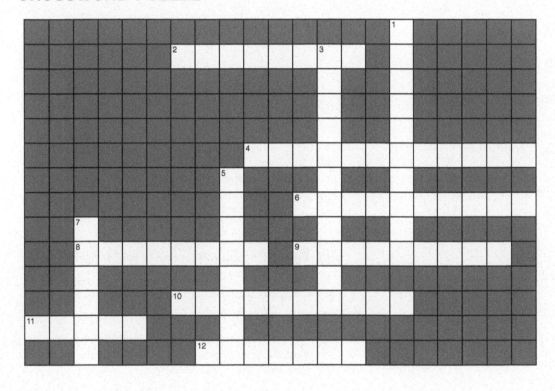

ACROSS
2. RNA; body
4. Thread; granule
6. Small; see; activity
8. Receive; agent
9. Whip
10. Protein; body
11. Star
12. Blister; little

DOWN
1. Center; body
3. Small; shaggy hair
5. Dissolution; body
7. Crest or fold

 APPLYING WHAT YOU KNOW

28. Brian is a sedentary, overweight cigarette smoker who has chest pain whenever he exerts himself. Upon examination, his cardiologist determines that Brian is suffering from heart disease. Which receptors in the cells that line the blood vessels of his heart are responsible? What type of cholesterol is responsible?

What other diseases may he be at risk for?

29. After several weeks of exercising in the weight room, Valerie notices that she has not only become stronger, but quite muscular as well. Which organelle has increased its density in the cytoplasm of the cells of her muscles in response to a greater demand for ATP production?

DID YOU KNOW?

- The largest single cell in the human body is the female sex cell, the ovum. The smallest single cell in the human body is the male sex cell, the sperm.
- There are more bacterial cells in the body than human cells. Scientists have estimated that about 95% of all the cells in the body are bacteria. The vast majority of these microbes can be found within the digestive tract.

 ONE LAST QUICK CHECK

Multiple Choice—select the best answer.

30. Which of the following cellular extensions are required when absorption is important?
    a. cilia
    b. microvilli
    c. flagella
    d. none of the above

31. Movement of the ovum within the female reproductive tract is largely as a result of:
    a. the flagella extending from the ovum.
    b. the cilia extending from the ovum.
    c. the cilia lining the uterine tubes.
    d. none of the above.

32. Skin cells are held tightly together by:
    a. gap junctions.
    b. desmosomes.
    c. tight junctions.
    d. adhesions.

33. Ribosomes are attached to:
    a. lysosomes.
    b. rough endoplasmic reticulum.
    c. peroxisomes.
    d. cilia.

34. The phospholipid area of the plasma membrane of a cell is:
    a. single layered.
    b. bilayered.
    c. trilayered.
    d. multilayered.

Matching—identify each term with its corresponding definition.

a. release hormones
b. transport oxygen
c. destroy bacteria
d. contract for movement
e. detect changes in the environment

35. _____nerve cells

36. _____muscle cells

37. _____red blood cells

38. _____gland cells

39. _____immune cells

Fill in the blanks.

40. A typical, or _____, cell exhibits the most important characteristics of cell types.

41. _____ is the term meaning "water-loving."

42. _____ is the process that allows a message to be carried across a membrane.

43. _____ detoxify harmful substances that enter cells.

44. The _____ is one of the largest cell structures and occupies the central portion of the cell.

45. Embedded within the phospholipid bilayer of the cell membrane are a variety of _____ _____ _____.

True or False

46. _____ Peroxisomes are small membranous sacs containing enzymes that detoxify harmful substances that enter the cells.

47. _____ Dynein, myosin, and kinesin are examples of proteasomes.

48. _____ Microfilaments serve as "cellular muscles."

49. _____ All cells contain thousands of ribosomes.

CHAPTER 6
Cell Function

Cells, just like humans, require water, food, gases, elimination of wastes, and numerous other substances and processes in order to survive. Cells must transport the substances within the cytoplasm and across cell membranes. The movement of these substances in and out of the cell is accomplished by two primary methods: passive transport and active transport. In passive transport, no cellular energy is required to effect movement through the cell membrane. However, in active transport, cellular energy is necessary to provide movement through the cell membrane.

Once nutrients enter the cells, a series of chemical reactions is necessary to prepare the materials to be utilized by the body. The chemical reaction that breaks down larger, more complex substances into simpler substances and releases energy from the food molecules is known as *catabolism*. Energy is essential because it provides the body with the power (ATP) to perform its tasks and to maintain body temperature.

Cellular respiration is the process by which cells break down glucose, or a nutrient that has been converted to glucose or one of its simpler products, into carbon dioxide and water. As the molecule breaks down, energy is released. Three main pathways are available to the cell to accomplish cellular respiration. These pathways are glycolysis, the citric acid cycle, and the electron transport system. The anatomy and physiology of the cells allow us to adapt successfully to our environment and maintain health. By working together harmoniously, the various structures and functions of cells ensure survival.

I—MOVEMENT OF SUBSTANCES THROUGH CELL MEMBRANES

Multiple Choice—select the best answer.

1. Which of the following is *not* a passive transport process?
   a. dialysis
   b. osmosis
   c. filtration
   d. pinocytosis

2. Diffusion of water through a selectively permeable membrane in the presence of at least one impermeant solute is referred to as:
   a. diffusion.
   b. osmosis.
   c. phagocytosis.
   d. dialysis.

3. The trapping of bacteria by specialized white blood cells is an example of:
   a. pinocytosis.
   b. exocytosis.
   c. phagocytosis.
   d. none of the above.

4. A hypertonic solution is one that contains:
   a. a greater concentration of solute than the cell.
   b. the same concentration of solute as the cell.
   c. a lesser concentration of solute as the cell.
   d. none of the above.

5. The force of a fluid pushing against a surface could be described as:
   a. facilitated diffusion.
   b. hydrostatic pressure.
   c. hypostatic pressure.
   d. none of the above.

True or False

6. _____ Facilitated diffusion is a metabolically expensive process.

7. _____ The sodium-potassium pump is an example of an active transport process.

8. _____ Cellular secretion can be achieved by exocytosis.

9. _____ Solutes are particles dissolved in a solvent.

10. _____ Osmosis is a form of filtration that results in the separation of small and large solute particles.

Matching—identify each item with its corresponding description.

a. isotonic
b. hypertonic
c. hypotonic
d. diffusion
e. endocytosis

11. _____ solution that draws water from a cell

12. _____ two fluids that have the same potential osmotic pressure

13. _____ solution that causes cells to swell

14. _____ passive transport

15. _____ active transport

→ *If you had difficulty with this section, review pages 99-108 and 117-118.*

Labeling—match each term with its corresponding number in the following diagram of cellular respiration.

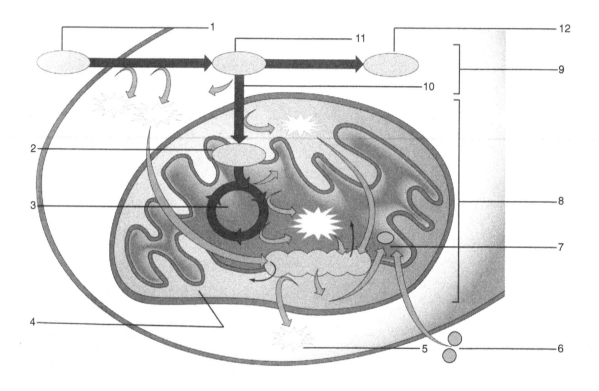

_____ aerobic
_____ glucose
_____ mitochondrion
_____ anaerobic
_____ pyruvic acid
_____ citric acid cycle

_____ lactic acid
_____ O_2
_____ ATP
_____ transition
_____ H_2O
_____ acetyl CoA

II—CELL METABOLISM

Multiple Choice—select the best answer.

16. Enzymes that cause essential chemical reactions to occur are called:
    a. metabolic agents.
    b. catalysts.
    c. substrates.
    d. initiators.

17. Molecules that are acted upon by enzymes are known as:
    a. diploid.
    b. hypertonic.
    c. introns.
    d. substrates.

18. In naming enzymes, the root name of the substance whose chemical reaction is catalyzed is followed by the suffix:
    a. -ase.
    b. -cin.
    c. -ose.
    d. -ous.

19. Most enzymes:
    a. are specific in their action.
    b. can alter their function by changing the shape of the molecule.
    c. are synthesized as inactive proenzymes.
    d. all of the above.

20. Which of the following activates enzymes by means of an allosteric effect?
    a. end-product inhibition
    b. kinases
    c. substrate
    d. pepsin

21. Enzymes are:
    a. fats.
    b. proteins.
    c. carbohydrates.
    d. minerals.

True or False

22. _____ The three processes that compose cellular respiration are glycolysis, the citric acid cycle, and the electron transport system.

23. _____ The portion of an enzyme molecule that chemically "fits" the substrate molecule(s) is referred to as the *active site*.

24. _____ The "lock and key" model is used to describe how DNA base pairs align.

25. _____ Protein anabolism is a major cellular activity.

26. _____ The citric acid cycle is also known as the *Krebs cycle*.

27. _____ Glycolysis is aerobic.

Multiple Choice—select the best answer.

28. Which of the following statements is *not* true of glycolysis?
    a. It occurs in the cytoplasm of the cell.
    b. It is also known as the *Krebs cycle*.
    c. It is anaerobic.
    d. Glycolysis splits one molecule of glucose into two molecules of pyruvic acid.

29. The Krebs cycle takes place in the:
    a. ribosome.
    b. cytoplasm.
    c. mitochondria.
    d. Golgi apparatus.

30. The third step in cellular respiration is:
    a. the electron transport system.
    b. transcription.
    c. the Krebs cycle.
    d. glycolysis.

➜ *If you had difficulty with this section, review pages 109-119.*

CROSSWORD PUZZLE

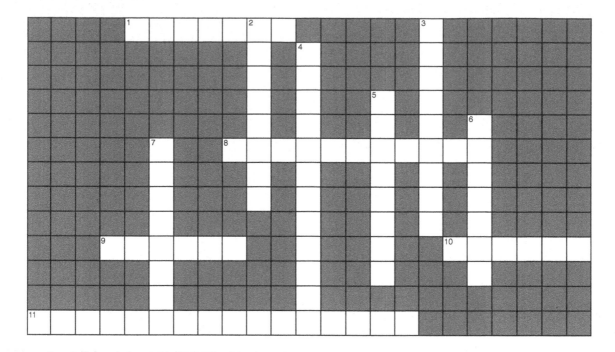

ACROSS
1. Air; life; relating to
8. Inward or within; cell; condition
9. In; ferment
10. Motion; enzyme
11. Against; across; carry (two words)

DOWN
2. Equal; tension; relating to
3. Spread out; process
4. Eat; cell; condition
5. Lower; loosen; actor
6. Push; condition
7. Together; in; ferment

 APPLYING WHAT YOU KNOW

31. Nurse Bricker was instructed to dissolve a pill in a small amount of liquid medication. As she dropped the capsule into the liquid, she was interrupted by the telephone. On her return to the medication cart, she found the medication completely dissolved and apparently scattered evenly throughout the liquid. This phenomenon did not surprise her because she was aware from her knowledge of cell transport that _____ had created this distribution.

32. Bobbi ran in the Boston marathon. During the race, she lost a lot of fluids through perspiration and became dehydrated. Would you expect her cells to shrink, swell, or remain the same?

? DID YOU KNOW?

- A human can detect one drop of perfume diffused throughout a three-room apartment.
- The longest living cells in the body are brain cells, which can live an entire lifetime.

✓ ONE LAST QUICK CHECK

Multiple Choice—select the best answer.

33. The energy required for active transport processes is obtained from:
   a. ATP.
   b. DNA.
   c. diffusion.
   d. osmosis.

34. Movement of substances from a region of high concentration to a region of low concentration is:
   a. active transport.
   b. passive transport.
   c. cellular energy.
   d. concentration gradient.

35. Osmosis is the _____ of water across a selectively permeable membrane.
   a. filtration
   b. equilibrium
   c. active transport
   d. diffusion

36. A molecule or other agent that alters enzyme function by changing its shape is called:
   a. an allosteric effector.
   b. a kinase.
   c. an anabolic agent.
   d. a proenzyme.

37. Glycolysis is a catabolic pathway that begins with glucose and ends with:
   a. oxygen.
   b. filtration.
   c. pyruvic acid.
   d. sodium.

38. Which movement always occurs down a hydrostatic pressure gradient?
   a. osmosis
   b. filtration
   c. dialysis
   d. facilitated diffusion

39. The "uphill" movement of a substance through a living cell membrane is:
   a. osmosis.
   b. diffusion.
   c. active transport.
   d. passive transport.

40. Membrane pumps are an example of which type of movement?
   a. gravity
   b. hydrostatic pressure
   c. active transport
   d. passive transport

41. An example of a cell that performs phagocytosis is the:
   a. white blood cell.
   b. red blood cell.
   c. muscle cell.
   d. bone cell.

42. A saline solution that contains a higher concentration of salt than living red blood cells would be:
   a. hypotonic.
   b. hypertonic.
   c. isotonic.
   d. homeostatic.

43. A red blood cell becomes engorged with water and will eventually lyse, releasing hemoglobin into the solution. This solution is _____ to the red blood cell.
   a. hypotonic
   b. hypertonic
   c. isotonic
   d. homeostatic

Matching—match the statement with the proper selection. (Only one answer is correct.)

   a. molecule able to diffuse across a particular membrane
   b. protein "tunnels"
   c. enzyme
   d. facilitated diffusion
   e. "cell drinking"
   f. phagocytosis
   g. type of membrane channel
   h. enzymes that add or remove carbon dioxide
   i. glycolysis

44. _____ membrane channels

45. _____ endocytosis

46. _____ pepsin

47. _____ carboxylases

48. _____ pinocytosis

49. _____ aquaporins

50. _____ carrier-mediated passive transport

51. _____ first stage of cellular respiration

52. _____ permeant

CHAPTER 7

Cell Growth and Development

Cell reproduction completes the study of cells. A basic explanation of DNA, the "hereditary molecule," gives us a proper respect for the capability of the cell to transmit physical and mental traits from generation to generation. Cell reproduction is essential for an organism to maintain itself or grow. When a cell divides, it must be able to replicate the DNA in its genome so that the two daughter cells have the same genetic information as the parent cell. Reproduction of the cell—mitosis—is a complex process requiring several stages. These stages are outlined and diagrammed in the text to facilitate learning. Understanding cell growth, reproduction, and physiology will help you comprehend the physiology of the body as a whole.

I—PROTEIN SYNTHESIS AND CELL GROWTH

Multiple Choice—select the best answer.

1. Protein synthesis:
   a. is required for cell growth.
   b. begins with reading of the genetic "master code" in the cell's DNA.
   c. influences all cell structures and functions.
   d. all of the above.

2. In the DNA molecule, a sequence of three base pairs forms a(n):
   a. codon.
   b. anticodon.
   c. polymerase.
   d. none of the above.

3. Transcription can best be described as the:
   a. synthesis of DNA.
   b. synthesis of any RNA molecule.
   c. reading of any mRNA codons by tRNA.
   d. entire set of DNA.

4. Which of the following statements is true?
   a. Complex polypeptide chains form tRNA.
   b. The site of transcription is within the nucleus, whereas the site of translation is in the cytoplasm.
   c. Uracil is present in DNA in the place of thymine.
   d. None of the above is true.

5. A DNA molecule is characterized by all of the following *except:*
   a. double-helix shape.
   b. obligatory base pairing.
   c. ribose sugar.
   d. phosphate groups.

6. Which of the following is *not* a characteristic of RNA?
   a. It is single-stranded.
   b. It contains uracil, not thymine.
   c. The obligatory base pairs are adenine-uracil and guanine-cytosine.
   d. Its molecules are larger than those of DNA.

7. Nucleic acids are synthesized directly on the DNA molecule with the help of:
   a. enzymes.
   b. prophase.
   c. neoplasms.
   d. lipids.

Matching—identify the term related to protein synthesis with its corresponding definition.

   a. mRNA
   b. ribosome
   c. tRNA
   d. translation
   e. transcription
   f. complementary base pair

8. _____ Process that occurs when the double strands of a DNA segment separate and RNA nucleotides pair with DNA nucleotides

9. _____ The type of RNA that carries information in groups of three nucleotides called *codons,* each of which codes for a specific amino acid

10. _____ The type of RNA that has an anticodon and binds to a base pair–specific amino acid

11. _____ The process involving the movement of mRNA with respect to the ribosome

12. _____ Uracil-adenine

13. _____ The site of translation

Labeling—label the following illustration of a DNA molecule.

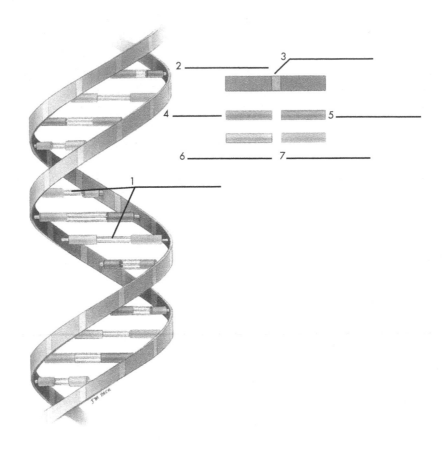

➡ *If you had difficulty with this section, review pages 121-128.*

II—CELL REPRODUCTION

Circle the word or phrase that does not belong.

14. mitosis	meiosis	M phase	enzyme
15. anaphase	end phase	apart	2 chromosomes
16. meiosis	sex cells	telophase	oogonia
17. zygote	mitosis	diploid	46 chromosomes
18. metaphase	prophase	telophase	interphase

Multiple Choice—select the best answer.

19. The correct order of mitosis is:
    a. prophase, metaphase, anaphase, telophase.
    b. anaphase, telophase, metaphase, prophase.
    c. prophase, anaphase, metaphase, telophase.
    d. none of the above.

20. The total of 46 chromosomes per cell is referred to as:
    a. haploid.
    b. diploid.
    c. myoid.
    d. none of the above.

21. A type of cell division that occurs only in primitive sex cells during the process of becoming mature sex cells is:
    a. mitosis.
    b. meiosis.
    c. gamete.
    d. differentiation.

22. Splitting of the plasma membrane and cytoplasm into two during cell reproduction is called:
    a. mitosis.
    b. meiosis.
    c. anaphase.
    d. cytokinesis.

23. Cell reproduction is sometimes referred to as the:
    a. A phase.
    b. R phase.
    c. M phase.
    d. X phase.

Fill in the blanks.

24. The phase of mitosis known as the *completion phase* is _____.

25. The phase of mitosis known as the *apart phase* is _____.

26. The *position-changing phase* of mitosis is _____.

27. When a cell is not experiencing mitosis and is "between phases," it is said to be in _____.

28. When a cell begins to divide, it is said to be in the *before phase*, or _____.

Labeling—on the following diagram, label the phases of mitosis. Remember that interphase and DNA replication occur before mitosis begins!

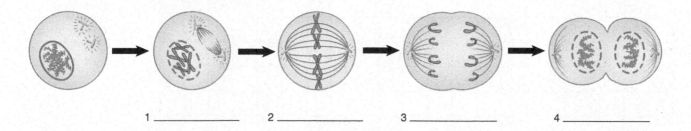

1 _____ 2 _____ 3 _____ 4 _____

➜ *If you had difficulty with this section, review pages 128-131.*

III—MECHANISMS OF DISEASE

True or False

29. _____ *Atrophy* refers to a decrease in cell size.

30. _____ Genetic disorders are mutations in a cell's genetic code.

31. _____ Cell death due to injury or a pathologic condition is known as *necrosis*.

32. _____ Viruses do not contain DNA or RNA.

33. _____ A blood disease caused by the production of abnormal hemoglobin is known as *sickle cell anemia*.

➡ *If you had difficulty with this section, review pages 132-133.*

❓ DID YOU KNOW?

- Our entire DNA sequence would fill two hundred 1000-page New York City telephone directories.
- A complete 3 billion base genome would take 3 gigabytes of storage space.

✏ APPLYING WHAT YOU KNOW

34. Mrs. McWilliam's home pregnancy test indicated that she was pregnant. She made an appointment with her doctor to confirm the results. While she was there, she inquired about ordering genetic testing while she was pregnant. What information might these tests reveal?

35. Dan broke his arm playing high school football and had to wear a cast for 6 weeks. When the doctor finally removed his cast, he was shocked to see that his arm had shrunk remarkably. His shock and disappointment were visible to the doctor. What should the doctor tell him about his arm?

CROSSWORD PUZZLE

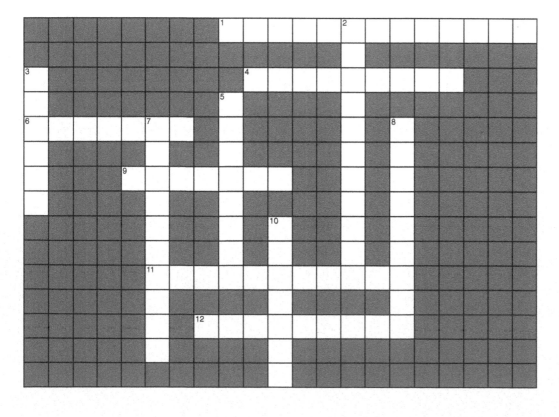

ACROSS
1. Across; write; process
4. Away; falling
6. Becoming smaller
9. Without; nourishment; state
11. Excessive; shape
12. End; stage

DOWN
2. Cell; normal
3. Sexual union
5. First; stage
7. Between; stage
8. Change; stage
10. Double; form

ONE LAST QUICK CHECK

Multiple Choice—select the best answer.

36. The genetic code for a particular protein is passed from DNA to mRNA by a process known as:
    a. transcription.
    b. translation.
    c. interphase.
    d. genome.

37. If a strand of DNA has a base sequence of AGGC, the complementary pair for that strand will be:
    a. TCCG.
    b. CCTG.
    c. TTCG.
    d. TUUG.

38. The spindle fibers attach to each chromatid during which stage of mitosis?
    a. prophase
    b. anaphase
    c. telophase
    d. metaphase

39. Which of the following is *not* true of RNA?
    a. It is a single strand.
    b. It contains uracil rather than thymine.
    c. The base pairs are adenine and uracil and guanine and cytosine.
    d. It contains deoxyribose sugar.

40. During which stage of mitosis does the cleavage furrow begin to develop?
    a. prophase
    b. metaphase
    c. anaphase
    d. telophase

41. All of the DNA in each cell of the body is called the:
    a. tissue typing.
    b. genome.
    c. gene.
    d. genetic code.

42. If the sequence of bases in a nucleic acid were AUCGA, which of the following statements would be true?
    a. The nucleic acid would contain deoxyribose.
    b. It is a strand of DNA.
    c. It is a strand of RNA.
    d. It will remain in the nucleus of the cell.

43. In which stage of mitosis do chromosomes move to opposite ends of the cells along the spindle fibers?
    a. anaphase
    b. metaphase
    c. prophase
    d. telophase

44. The synthesis of proteins by ribosomes using information coded in the mRNA molecule is called:
    a. translation.
    b. transcription.
    c. replication.
    d. crenation.

45. Translation can be inhibited or prevented by a process called:
    a. cytokinesis.
    b. cell division.
    c. RNA interference.
    d. meiosis.

Circle the word or phrase that does not belong.

46. DNA   adenine   uracil   thymine

47. RNA   ribose   thymine   uracil

48. translation   protein synthesis mRNA   interphase

49. cleavage furrow   anaphase   prophase   2 daughter cells

50. metaphase   prophase   telophase   gene

Fill in the blanks.

51. The DNA molecular structure allows only two combinations of bases to occur. This is known as _____ _____ _____.

52. The complete set of proteins synthesized by a cell is called the _____ of the cell.

53. The shape of a DNA molecule is referred to as a _____ _____.

54. _____ is the type of cell division that occurs only in primitive sex cells during the process of becoming mature sex cells.

55. Mature sex cells are called _____.

CHAPTER 8

Introduction to Tissues

After successfully completing the study of the cell, you are ready to progress to the next level of anatomical structure: tissues. Four principal types of tissues—epithelial, connective, muscle, and nervous—perform multiple functions to ensure that homeostasis is maintained. Among these functions are protection, absorption, excretion, support, insulation, conduction of impulses, movement of bones, and destruction of bacteria. This variety of functions gives us a real appreciation for the complexity of this level.

Our study continues with a review of body membranes and their function in the body. Membranes are thin layers of epithelial and/or connective tissue that cover and protect the body surfaces, line body cavities, and cover the internal surfaces of hollow organs. These major membranes—cutaneous, serous, mucous, and synovial—are also critical to homeostasis and body survival. An understanding of tissues and membranes is necessary to successfully bridge your knowledge between the cell and the study of body organs.

I—INTRODUCTION TO TISSUES AND EXTRACELLULAR MATRIX

Multiple Choice—select the best answer.

1. A tissue is:
   a. a membrane that lines body cavities.
   b. a group of similar cells that perform a common function.
   c. a thin sheet of cells embedded in a matrix.
   d. the most complex organizational unit of the body.

2. The four principal types of tissues include all of the following *except:*
   a. nervous.
   b. muscle.
   c. cartilage.
   d. connective.

3. The most complex tissue in the body is:
   a. muscle.
   b. blood.
   c. connective.
   d. nervous.

4. In tissues, the material between cells that is made up of water and a variety of proteins is referred to as:
   a. intercellular material.
   b. extracellular matrix.
   c. lacunae.
   d. none of the above.

5. Which of the following is *not* a primary germ layer?
   a. endoderm
   b. periderm
   c. mesoderm
   d. ectoderm

6. Which tissue lines body cavities and protects body surfaces?
   a. epithelial
   b. connective
   c. muscular
   d. nervous

True or False

7. _____ The biology of tissues is referred to as *histology.*

8. _____ Proteins in the extracellular matrix include various types of structural protein fibers such as collagen and elastin.

9. _____ Sweat and sebaceous glands are formed by connective tissue.

10. _____ During embryonic development, new kinds of cells can be formed from a special kind of undifferentiated cell called a *stem cell.*

➔ *If you had difficulty with this section, review pages 138-144.*

II—TISSUE REPAIR

Fill in the blanks.

11. _____ is the growth of new tissue (as opposed to scarring).

12. A _____ is an unusually thick scar.

13. Tissues usually repair themselves by allowing _____ cells to remove dead or injured cells.

14. Epithelial and _____ tissues have the greatest capacity to regenerate.

15. Like muscle tissue, _____ tissue has a very limited capacity to regenerate.

➡ *If you had difficulty with this section, review pages 144-145.*

III—BODY MEMBRANES

Multiple Choice—select the best answer.

16. Which of the following is *not* an example of epithelial membrane?
    a. synovial membrane
    b. cutaneous membrane
    c. serous membrane
    d. mucous membrane

17. Pleurisy is a condition that affects which membrane?
    a. cutaneous membrane
    b. serous membrane
    c. mucous membrane
    d. none of the above

True or False

18. _____ Parietal membranes cover the surface of organs.

19. _____ Synovial membrane is an example of connective tissue membrane.

➡ *If you had difficulty with this section, review pages 145-148.*

IV—TUMORS AND CANCER

Circle the correct answer.

20. Benign tumors usually grow (slowly or quickly).

21. Malignant tumors (are or are not) encapsulated.

22. An example of a benign tumor that arises from epithelial tissue is (papilloma or lipoma).

23. Malignant tumors that arise from connective tissues are generally called (melanoma or sarcoma).

24. A cancer specialist is an (osteologist or oncologist).

25. Chemotherapy uses (cytotoxic or cachexic) compounds to destroy malignant cells.

➡ *If you had difficulty with this section, review pages 149-151.*

CROSSWORD PUZZLE

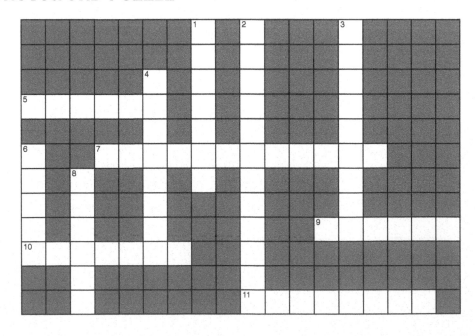

ACROSS
5. Kind
7. Protein; polysaccharide
9. Crab
10. Flesh; tumor
11. Together; egg; relating to

DOWN
1. Change; produce
2. Tissue; origin
3. Without; shape
4. Inward or within; skin
6. Slime
8. Womb

APPLYING WHAT YOU KNOW

26. Bruce is a sedentary, cigarette smoking, middle-aged man who is complaining of chest pain. Ultimately, he is diagnosed with lung cancer. What tests may have been utilized to determine his diagnosis? Which type of treatment might be involved?

27. Joe had experienced a recent respiratory infection but felt he was responding well to over-the-counter medications. He still had a low-grade fever, however. He was awakened during the night with pain in the thoracic region. Fearful that the symptoms might indicate a heart attack, he called 911 and was transported to the emergency department. On the way to the hospital, the paramedic advised Joe that his EKG was normal. After all tests for cardiac illness and pathology returned negative, Joe was sent home on antibiotics, pain medication, and with recommended bed rest. From your study of tissues and membranes, what might be the reason for this treatment?

 DID YOU KNOW?

- Muscle tissue is three times more efficient at burning calories than fat.
- As many as 500,000 Americans die from cancer each year. That's more than all the lives lost in the past 100 years by the U.S. military forces. Half of all cancers are diagnosed in people under the age of 67.
- Embryonic stem cells are derived from eggs fertilized in the laboratory, not in a woman's body.

 ONE LAST QUICK CHECK

Matching—select the best answer.

a. Cutaneous
b. Serous
c. Mucous
d. Synovial

28. ____ Directly exposed to outside environment

29. ____ Lubricates cavities not open to outside environment

30. ____ Dense fibrous connective tissue

31. ____ Lubricates cavities open to the outside environment

32. ____ Skin

33. ____ Lines joint cavities

34. ____ Thermoregulation

35. ____ Peritoneum

36. ____ Digestive tract

37. ____ Respiratory tract

Fill in the blanks.

The three primary germ layers are (38) _____,
(39) _____, and (40) _____.

41. The biology of tissues is _____.

42. Tissue cells are surrounded by or embedded in extracellular material called _____.

43. An atypical thick scar that may develop in the lower layer of skin is a _____.

44. _____ tissue is often replaced, when damaged, with fibrous connective tissue instead of the original tissue.

45. _____ is the growth of functional new tissue.

46. _____ is a glandular benign tumor.

47. _____ is the name for "cancer genes."

Matching—match the clue with the proper selection. (Only one answer is correct.)

   a. tumor markers
   b. computed tomography
   c. staging
   d. immunotherapy
   e. chemotherapy
   f. cachexia
   g. radiotherapy
   h. monoclonal antibodies
   i. biopsy
   j. laser

48. _____ Involves classifying a tumor based on the size and extent of the spread

49. _____ X-ray scanning

50. _____ Substances produced by cancer cells

51. _____ Removal and examination of living tissue

52. _____ Cytotoxic compound used to destroy malignant cells

53. _____ Gamma radiation used to destroy cancer cells

54. _____ Intense beam of light to destroy a tumor

55. _____ Bolsters the body's own defenses against cancer cells

56. _____ Herceptin and Erbitux

57. _____ Loss of appetite

CHAPTER 9

Tissue Types

As we progress in our review of histology, we begin to have an appreciation for the variety of tissues within the body. As mentioned in the prior chapter, four major tissues provide multiple functions for the body such as protection, secretion, absorption, excretion, sensory functions, support, transportation, regulation, and the integration of body activities. To provide these functions, tissues must come in various sizes and textures and have numerous capabilities. This chapter reviews the major tissues of the body; their location, structure, and functions; and their importance in the homeostasis and survival of the human body.

I—EPITHELIAL TISSUE

Multiple Choice—select the best answer.

1. Which of the following is *not* a function of membranous epithelium?
   a. secretion
   b. protection
   c. absorption
   d. all are functions of the membranous epithelium

2. Which of the following is *not* a structural example of epithelium?
   a. stratified squamous
   b. simple transitional
   c. stratified columnar
   d. pseudostratified columnar

3. The simple columnar epithelium lining the intestines contains plasma membranes that extend into thousands of microscopic extensions called:
   a. villi.
   b. microvilli.
   c. cilia.
   d. flagella.

4. Epithelial cells can be classified according to shape. Which of the following is *not* a characteristic shape of epithelium?
   a. cuboidal
   b. rectangular
   c. squamous
   d. columnar

5. Keratinized stratified squamous epithelium is found in the:
   a. mouth.
   b. vagina.
   c. skin.
   d. all of the above.

6. Endocrine glands discharge their products into:
   a. body cavities.
   b. blood.
   c. organ surfaces.
   d. none of the above.

7. Which of the following is *not* a functional classification of exocrine glands?
   a. alveolar
   b. apocrine
   c. holocrine
   d. merocrine

8. The functional classification of salivary glands is:
   a. endocrine.
   b. apocrine.
   c. holocrine.
   d. merocrine.

9. This epithelial tissue readily allows diffusion, as in the linings of blood and lymphatic vessels.
   a. simple squamous
   b. stratified squamous
   c. simple columnar
   d. pseudostratified columnar

True or False

10. _____ Epithelial tissue is attached to an underlying layer of connective tissue called the *basement membrane.*

11. _____ Epithelium is rich with blood supply.

12. _____ Exocrine glands discharge their products directly into the blood.

Matching—identify the arrangement of epithelial cells with its corresponding description.

a. simple squamous
b. simple cuboidal
c. simple columnar
d. pseudostratified columnar
e. stratified squamous
f. stratified cuboidal
g. stratified columnar
h. transitional

13. _____ single layer of cube-shaped cells

14. _____ multiple layers of cells with flat cells at the outer surface

15. _____ single layer of cells in which some are tall and thin and able to reach the free surface and others are not

16. _____ layers of cells that appear cubelike when an organ is relaxed and flat or distended by fluid, such as the walls of the urinary bladder. This tissue is typically found in body areas subjected to stress and tension changes.

17. _____ single layer of flat, scalelike cells

18. _____ single layer of tall, thin cells that compose the surface of mucous membranes

Labeling—label the following images and identify the principal tissue type of each. Be as specific as possible. Consult your textbook if you need assistance.

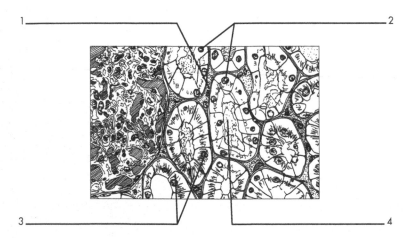

1 _____   2 _____
3 _____   4 _____

Tissue type: _____

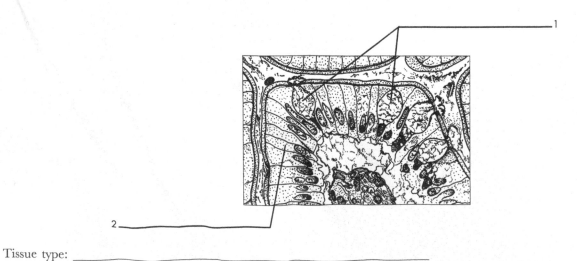

1 _____
2 _____

Tissue type: _____

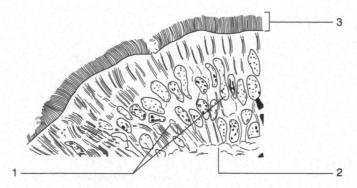

Tissue type: _____

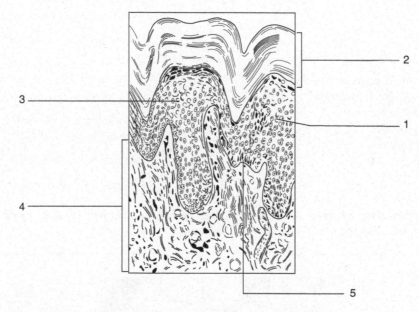

Tissue type: _____

 If you had difficulty with this section, review pages 156-162.

II—CONNECTIVE TISSUE

Multiple Choice—select the best answer.

19. Which of the following is *not* an example of connective tissue?
    a. transitional
    b. reticular
    c. blood
    d. bone

20. Which of the following fibers is *not* found in connective tissue matrix?
    a. collagenous
    b. elastic
    c. fibroblastic
    d. reticular

21. Fibroblasts are usually present in the greatest numbers in which type of connective tissue?
    a. adipose
    b. loose fibrous
    c. reticular
    d. dense

22. Adipose tissue performs which of the following functions?
    a. insulation
    b. protection
    c. support
    d. all of the above

23. Which of the following connective tissue types forms the framework of the spleen, lymph nodes, and bone marrow?
    a. loose
    b. adipose
    c. reticular
    d. areolar

24. The mature cells of bone are called:
    a. fibroblasts.
    b. osteoclasts.
    c. osteoblasts.
    d. osteocytes.

25. The basic structural unit of bone is the microscopic:
    a. osteon.
    b. lacunae.
    c. lamellae.
    d. canaliculi.

26. Mature bone grows and is reshaped by the simultaneous activity of which two cells?
    a. osteoblasts and osteocytes
    b. osteoblasts and osteoclasts
    c. osteocytes and osteoclasts
    d. none of the above

27. The most prevalent type of cartilage is:
    a. hyaline cartilage.
    b. fibrous cartilage.
    c. elastic cartilage.
    d. none of the above.

28. When mast cells encounter an allergen, they release the chemical:
    a. benedryl.
    b. allergra.
    c. zyflo.
    d. histamine.

True or False

29. _____ The most prevalent types of cells in areolar connective tissue are fibroblasts and macrophages.

30. _____ The terms *osteon* and *Haversian system* are synonymous.

31. _____ The long bones of the body are formed through the process of intramembranous ossification.

32. _____ Cartilage is perhaps the most vascular tissue in the human body.

33. _____ Ligaments attach bone to bone.

34. _____ Bone-forming cells are osteoclasts.

Labeling—label the following images and identify the principal tissue type of each. Be as specific as possible. Consult your textbook if you need assistance.

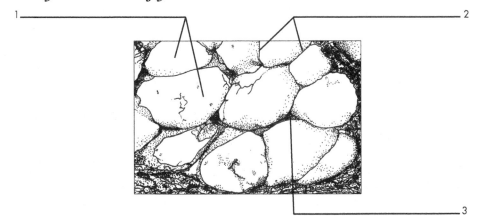

Tissue type: _____

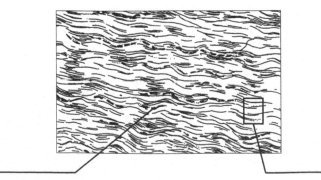

Tissue type: _____

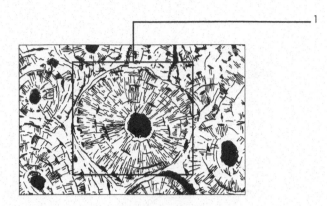

Tissue type: _____

➜ *If you had difficulty with this section, review pages 159 and 162-170.*

III—MUSCLE TISSUE

Matching—identify the type of muscle tissue with its corresponding definition.

   a. cardiac muscle
   b. skeletal muscle
   c. smooth muscle

35. _____ cylindrical, striated, voluntary cells

36. _____ nonstriated, involuntary, narrow fibers with only one nucleus per fiber

37. _____ striated, branching, involuntary cells with intercalated disks

38. _____ responsible for willed body movements

39. _____ also called *visceral muscle*

40. _____ found in the walls of hollow internal organs

Labeling—label the following images and identify the principal tissue type of each. Be as specific as possible. Consult your textbook if you need assistance.

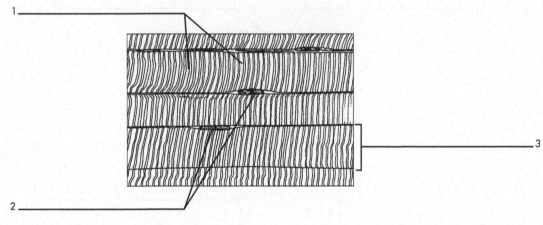

Tissue type: _____

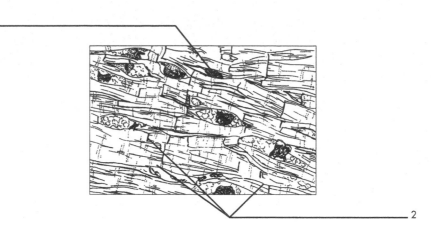

Tissue type: _____

 If you had difficulty with this section, review pages 170-172.

IV—NERVOUS TISSUE

Matching—match each term with its corresponding description.

  a. neuron
  b. neuroglia
  c. axon
  d. soma
  e. dendrite

41. _____ the cell body of the neuron

42. _____ supportive cells

43. _____ cell process that transmits nerve impulses away from the cell body

44. _____ the conducting cells of the nervous system

45. _____ cell process that carries nerve impulses toward the cell body

Labeling—label the following image and identify the principal tissue type. Be as specific as possible. Consult your textbook if you need assistance.

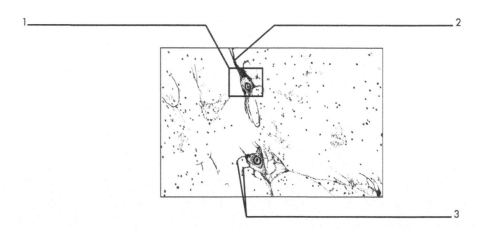

Tissue type: _____

 If you had difficulty with this section, review page 172.

CROSSWORD PUZZLE

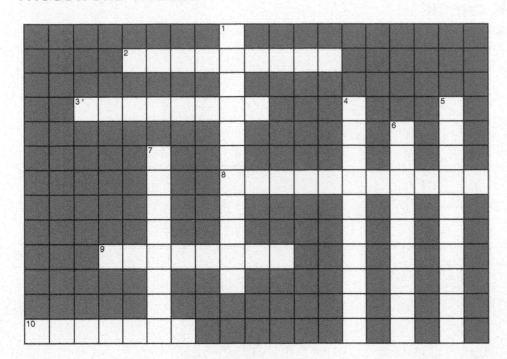

ACROSS
2. Tissue; ammonia compound
3. Cube-like; relating to
8. Cartilage; cell
9. Put together
10. Fat; full of

DOWN
1. Channel; little
4. Fiber; bud
5. On or upon; nipple; thing
6. Separate; process
7. Scale; characterized by

 APPLYING WHAT YOU KNOW

46. Holly is a bodybuilder who is obsessed with her physique. She exercises daily and eats a very low-fat diet. A personal fitness trainer has assessed her body fat at 12%. Determine whether she is too lean or too fat. Explain the relationship between her body fat percentage and lifestyle.

47. Billy is a teenager who has had asthma since he was 7 years old. His doctor recently suggested adding Singulair to his medication regimen. What is the reason for Singulair, and what action does it serve in the body?

? DID YOU KNOW?

- Approximately 32,000 pints of blood are used each day in the United States.
- Based on current information, a woman must have a minimum percent body fat of 13%–17% for regular menstruation. If a woman's percent body fat is too low, her periods may stop and she may experience infertility.

ONE LAST QUICK CHECK

Labeling—label the following images and identify the principal tissue type of each. Be as specific as possible. Consult your textbook if you need assistance.

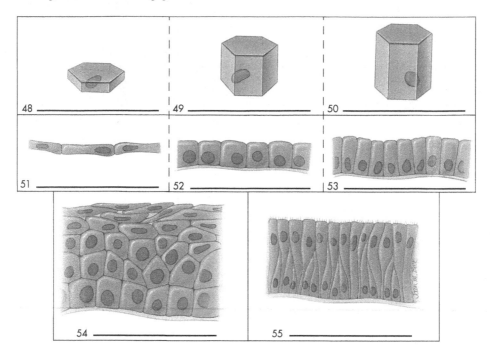

Multiple Choice—select the best answer.

56. Which of the following is *not* an example of connective tissue?
    a. glands
    b. blood
    c. fat
    d. bone

57. Stratified squamous (nonkeratinized) epithelium can be found in all of the following *except*:
    a. vagina.
    b. mouth.
    c. esophagus.
    d. skin.

58. The most abundant and widespread tissue is:
    a. epithelial.
    b. connective.
    c. muscle.
    d. nervous.

59. Loose connective tissue is also known as:
    a. voluntary.
    b. hyaline.
    c. areolar.
    d. visceral.

60. Tissue that insulates to conserve body heat is:
    a. reticular.
    b. fibrous.
    c. adipose.
    d. osseous.

61. What statement regarding blood is true?
    a. Erythrocytes are white blood cells.
    b. Thrombocytes are also known as *platelets*.
    c. Leukocytes are red blood cells.
    d. Formed elements are known as *plasma*.

Matching—match the term with the corresponding description.

    a. sebaceous
    b. matrix
    c. squamous
    d. membranous
    e. erythrocytes
    f. adipocytes

62. _____ extracellular substance of tissue cells

63. _____ type of epithelial tissue

64. _____ cell shape

65. _____ type of holocrine gland

66. _____ fat cell

67. _____ red blood cell

CHAPTER 10

Skin

More of our time, attention, and money are spent on this system than any other. Every time we look into a mirror we become aware of the integumentary system, as we observe our skin, hair, nails, and the appendages that give luster and comfort to this system. The discussion of the skin begins with the structure and function of the two primary layers called the *epidermis* and *dermis*. It continues with an examination of the appendages of the skin, which include the hair, receptors, nails, sebaceous glands, and sudoriferous glands.

Your study of the skin concludes with a review of one of the most serious and frequent threats to the skin—burns. An understanding of the integumentary system provides you with an appreciation of the danger that severe burns or trauma can pose to this system.

I—STRUCTURE OF THE SKIN

Multiple Choice—select the best answer.

1. Beneath the dermis lies a loose layer of skin rich in fat and areolar tissue called the:
   a. dermo-epidermal junction.
   b. hypodermis.
   c. epidermis.
   d. none of the above.

2. The most important cells in the epidermis are the:
   a. keratinocytes.
   b. melanocytes.
   c. Langerhans cells.
   d. dermal papillae.

3. The order of the cells of the epidermis, from superficial to deep, are:
   a. stratum corneum, stratum lucidum, stratum spinosum, stratum granulosum, stratum basale.
   b. stratum corneum, stratum spinosum, stratum lucidum, stratum granulosum, stratum basale.
   c. stratum basale, stratum corneum, stratum lucidum, stratum spinosum, stratum granulosum.
   d. stratum corneum, stratum lucidum, stratum granulosum, stratum spinosum, stratum basale.

4. In which area of the body would you expect to find an especially thick stratum?
   a. back of the hand
   b. thigh
   c. abdomen
   d. sole of the foot

5. In which layer of the skin do cells divide by mitosis to replace cells lost from the outermost surface of the body?
   a. stratum basale
   b. stratum corneum
   c. stratum lucidum
   d. stratum spinosum

6. Smooth muscles that produce "goose bumps" when they contract are:
   a. papillary muscles.
   b. hair muscles.
   c. follicular muscles.
   d. arrector pili muscles.

7. Keratin is found in which layer of the skin?
   a. dermis
   b. epidermis
   c. subcutaneous
   d. serous

8. Meissner's corpuscles are specialized nerve endings that make it possible for skin to detect:
   a. heat.
   b. cold.
   c. light touch.
   d. deep pressure.

9. The basic determinant of skin color is the quantity of:
   a. keratin.
   b. melanin.
   c. albinin.
   d. none of the above.

10. Which of the following is *not* a contributing factor to skin color?
    a. exposure to sunlight
    b. genetics
    c. place of birth
    d. volume of blood in skin capillaries

True or False

11. _____ Most of the body is covered by thick skin.

12. _____ A surgeon would most likely prefer to make an incision parallel to Langer cleavage lines.

13. _____ If the enzyme tyrosinase is absent from birth because of a congenital defect, a condition called *albinism* results.

14. _____ The epidermis is the "true skin" and is composed of two layers.

15. _____ *Subcutaneous layer* and *hypodermis* are synonymous terms.

Labeling—match each term with its corresponding number on the following diagram of a cross section of skin. Terms may be used more than once.

_____ dermal papillae
_____ shaft of hair
_____ root of hair
_____ friction ridge
_____ sulcus
_____ ridges of dermal papillae
_____ subcutaneous adipose tissue
_____ blood vessels

_____ dermis
_____ dermo-epidermal junction
_____ sweat duct
_____ opening of sweat duct
_____ epidermis
_____ reticular layer of dermis
_____ papillary layer of dermis
_____ hypodermis

_____ sweat gland
_____ lamellar (Pacini) corpuscle
_____ arrector pili muscle
_____ hair follicle
_____ sebaceous gland
_____ nerve fibers

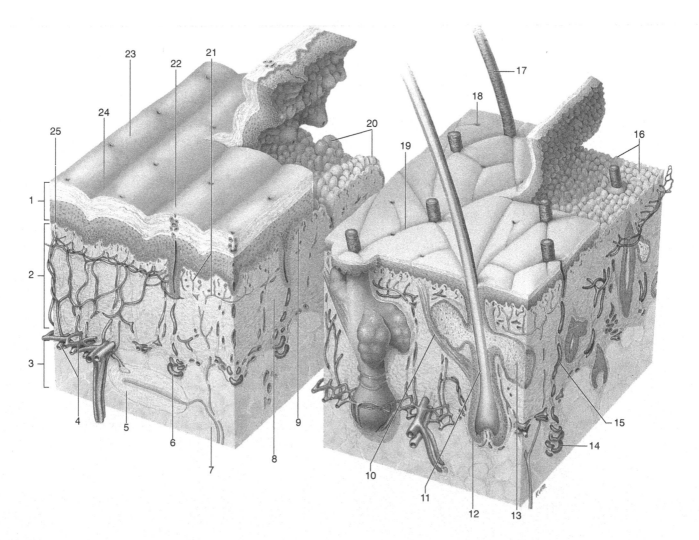

➜ *If you had difficulty with this section, review pages 181-190.*

II—FUNCTIONS OF THE SKIN

Multiple Choice—select the best answer.

16. Which of the following is not a function of the skin?
    a. sensation
    b. excretion
    c. immunity
    d. all of the above are skin functions

17. Which of the following vitamins is synthesized by the skin?
    a. vitamin A
    b. vitamin B
    c. vitamin C
    d. vitamin D

18. Which of the following is *not* a mechanism of heat loss by the skin?
    a. evaporation
    b. radiation
    c. vasoconstriction
    d. convection

19. Vitamin D fulfills the requirements necessary for a substance to be classified as a(n):
    a. hormone
    b. mineral
    c. nucleic acid
    d. enzyme

20. Which structure compares actual body temperature with set point temperature and then sends out appropriate correction signals to effectors?
    a. pituitary
    b. hypothalamus
    c. thalamus
    d. none of the above

True or false

21. _____ Skin is a minor factor in the body's thermoregulatory mechanism.

22. _____ In most circumstances, skin plays a major role in the overall excretion of body wastes.

23. _____ To help dissipate heat during exercise, sweat production can reach as much as 3 liters per hour.

➜ *If you had difficulty with this section, review pages 190-194.*

III—APPENDAGES OF THE SKIN

Multiple Choice—select the best answer.

24. The developing fetus is covered by an extremely fine, soft hair coat called:
    a. vellus.
    b. lanugo.
    c. fatalis follicle.
    d. none of the above.

25. Which of the following is associated with hair?
    a. sebaceous glands
    b. ceruminous glands
    c. eccrine glands
    d. none of the above

26. Ceruminous glands are found in the:
    a. axillae.
    b. soles of feet.
    c. ear canal.
    d. none of the above.

27. The most numerous, important, and widespread sweat glands in the body are:
    a. apocrine.
    b. eccrine.
    c. ceruminous.
    d. sebaceous.

28. Hair growth is stimulated by:
    a. cutting it frequently.
    b. shaving.
    c. increasing melanin production.
    d. none of the above.

True or False

29. _____ The visible portion of a hair is the shaft.

30. _____ The inner core of the hair is called the *cortex.*

31. _____ Sweat, or sudoriferous, glands are the most numerous of the skin glands.

32. _____ One of the factors associated with male pattern baldness is androgens.

33. _____ Growth of nails is due to mitosis in the stratum basale.

➜ *If you had difficulty with this section, review pages 194-199.*

IV—MECHANISMS OF DISEASE

Matching—identify the term with the corresponding description.

    a. papillomavirus
    b. furuncle
    c. ringworm
    d. hard skin
    e. symptom of underlying condition
    f. staph or strep infection
    g. bedsores
    h. hives

34. _____ impetigo

35. _____ tinea

36. _____ warts

37. _____ boils

38. _____ decubitus ulcers

39. _____ urticaria

40. _____ scleroderma

41. _____ eczema

Fill in the blanks.

42. _____ is the term associated with an unusually high body temperature.

43. _____ _____ occurs when the body loses a large amount of fluid resulting from heat loss mechanisms.

44. _____ _____ is also known as *sunstroke.*

45. Local damage caused by extremely low temperatures is referred to as _____.

➔ *If you had difficulty with this section, review pages 199-202.*

V—BURNS

Multiple Choice—select the best answer.

46. The "rule of palms" assumes that the palm size of a burn victim equals about ____ of total body surface area.
    a. 1%
    b. 2%
    c. 5%
    d. none of the above

47. Blisters, severe pain, and generalized swelling are characteristic of which type of burn?
    a. first-degree burns
    b. second-degree burns
    c. third-degree burns
    d. none of the above

True or False

48. _____ According to the "rule of nines," the body is divided into nine areas of 9%.

49. _____ Immediately after injury, third-degree burns hurt less than second-degree burns.

Matching—identify each term with its corresponding description.

    a. first-degree burn
    b. second-degree burn
    c. third-degree burn
    d. partial-thickness burn
    e. full-thickness burn

50. _____ destroys both epidermis and dermis and may involve underlying tissue

51. _____ involves only the epidermis

52. _____ another name for first- and second-degree burns

53. _____ damage to epidermis and upper layers of dermis with blisters

54. _____ another name for third-degree burn

Labeling—using the "rule of nines" method, label the following diagram to estimate the amount of skin surface for each area.

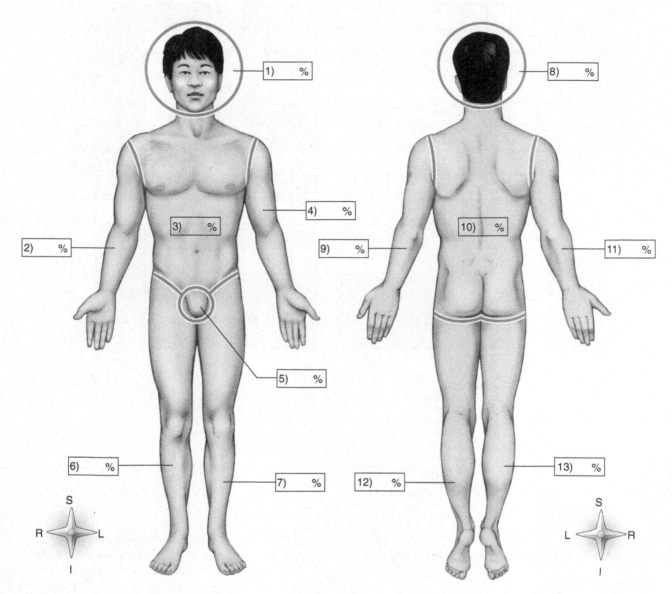

➜ *If you had difficulty with this section, review pages 202-203.*

CROSSWORD PUZZLE

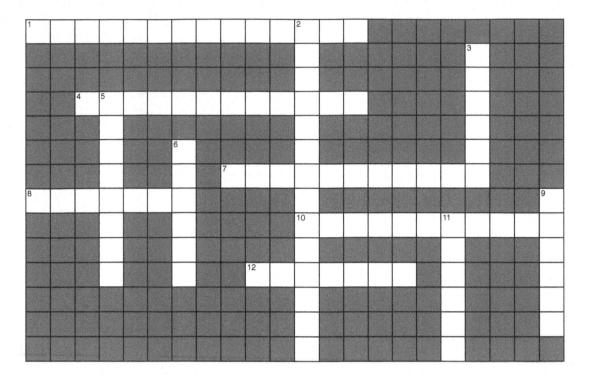

ACROSS
1. Excessive; horn; condition
4. Out; secrete; acorn (two words)
7. Under or below; heat; abnormal condition
8. Heat; produce
10. Hard; skin
12. Black; substance

DOWN
2. Tallow (hard animal fat); relating to; acorn (2 words)
3. To boil over
5. Blue; condition
6. Moon; small
9. Down
11. Skin

 APPLYING WHAT YOU KNOW

55. Mr. Ziven was admitted to the hospital with second- and third-degree burns. Both arms, the anterior trunk, right anterior leg, and genital region were affected by the burns. The doctor quickly estimated that _____% of Mr. Ziven's body had been burned.

56. After investigating the scene of the crime, Officer Gorski announced that dermal papillae were found that would help solve the case. What did he mean?

57. Bernie is 65 and was recently diagnosed with melanoma. He finds this diagnosis difficult to believe because has lived in Alaska for the past 20 years and gets very little exposure to sun. Can you suggest a possible explanation for his diagnosis?

 DID YOU KNOW?

- Because the dead cells of the epidermis are constantly being worn and washed away, we get a new outer skin layer every 27 days.
- The average person sheds 40 pounds of skin in a lifetime.

ONE LAST QUICK CHECK

Multiple Choice—select the best answer.

58. Which of the following statements about hair follicles is true?
    a. Arrector pili muscles are associated with them.
    b. Sudoriferous glands empty into them.
    c. They arise directly from the epidermal layer of skin.
    d. All of the above are true.

59. Which of the following statements about apocrine glands is true?
    a. They can be classified as sudoriferous.
    b. They can be found primarily in the armpit area, the areolae of the breasts, and around the anus.
    c. They enlarge and begin to function at puberty.
    d. All of the above are true.

60. Which of the following is found in the epidermal layer of the skin?
    a. nerves
    b. melanin
    c. blood vessels
    d. all of the above are found in the dermis

61. What characterizes second-degree burns?
    a. blisters
    b. swelling
    c. severe pain
    d. all of the above

62. Blackheads can result from the blockage of which of the following glands?
    a. lacrimal
    b. sebaceous
    c. ceruminous
    d. sudoriferous

63. A common type of skin cancer is:
    a. malignant melanoma.
    b. vitiligo.
    c. basal cell carcinoma.
    d. Kaposi sarcoma.

64. What is the fold of skin that hides the root of a nail called?
    a. lunula
    b. body
    c. cuticle
    d. papillae

65. Which of the following is *not* an important function of the skin?
    a. sense organ activity
    b. absorption
    c. protection
    d. temperature

66. Another name for the dermis is:
    a. corium.
    b. strata.
    c. subcutaneous.
    d. lunula.

67. The shedding of epithelial elements from the skin surface is called:
    a. desquamation.
    b. convection.
    c. cleavage lines.
    d. turnover.

Matching—identify the correct answer for each item.

    a. fingerprint
    b. pressure
    c. brown pigment
    d. perspiration
    e. oil
    f. follicle
    g. little moon
    h. axilla sweat glands
    i. fungal infection
    j. genetic inflammatory skin disorder

68. _____ melanin

69. _____ Pacini corpuscle

70. _____ sebaceous

71. _____ hair

72. _____ lunula

73. _____ dermal papillae

74. _____ sudoriferous

75. _____ apocrine

76. _____ tinea

77. _____ psoriasis

CHAPTER 11
Skeletal Tissues

How strange we would look without our skeleton! It is the skeleton that provides the rigid, supportive framework that gives shape to our bodies. But this is just the beginning, because the skeleton also protects the organs beneath it, maintains homeostasis of blood calcium, produces blood cells, and helps the muscular system provide movement for us.

After reviewing the microscopic structure of bone and cartilage, you will understand how skeletal tissues are formed, their differences, and their importance in the human body. Your microscopic investigation will make the study of this system easier as you logically progress from this view to macroscopic bone formation and growth and visualize the structure of long bones.

Bones are classified structurally by their shape: long bones, short bones, flat bones, irregular bones, and sesamoid bones. They are also classified by the types of cells that form the bone: compact bone and cancellous, or spongy, bone. Throughout life, bone formation (ossification) and bone destruction (resorption) occur concurrently to ensure a firm and comfortable framework for our bodies.

I—TYPES OF BONES

Matching—identify each structure with its corresponding description.

a. epiphysis
b. medullary cavity
c. carpal
d. articular cartilage
e. femur
f. endosteum
g. vertebra
h. diaphysis
i. patella
j. periosteum
k. sternum

1. _____ the thin membrane that lines the medullary cavity

2. _____ an example of a flat bone

3. _____ the shaft of the long bone

4. _____ an example of a long bone

5. _____ the thin layer that cushions jolts and blows

6. _____ an example of a sesamoid bone

7. _____ an attachment for muscle fibers

8. _____ an example of a short bone

9. _____ the end of a long bone

10. _____ the tubelike, hollow space in the diaphysis of long bones

11. _____ an example of an irregular bone

➡ *If you had difficulty with this section, review pages 210-212.*

II—BONE TISSUE STRUCTURE, BONE MARROW, AND REGULATION OF BLOOD CALCIUM LEVELS

Multiple Choice—select the best answer.

12. Which of the following is *not* a component of bone matrix?
    a. inorganic salts
    b. organic matrix
    c. collagenous fibers
    d. all of the above are components of bone matrix

13. Small spaces in which bone cells lie are called:
    a. lamellae.
    b. lacunae.
    c. canaliculi.
    d. interstitial lamellae.

14. The basic structural unit of compact bone is:
    a. trabeculae.
    b. cancellous bone.
    c. osteon.
    d. none of the above.

15. The cells that produce the organic matrix in bone are:
    a. chondrocytes.
    b. osteoblasts.
    c. osteocytes.
    d. osteoclasts.

16. The bones in an adult that contain red marrow include all of the following *except*:
    a. ribs.
    b. tarsals.
    c. pelvis.
    d. femur.

17. Low blood calcium evokes a response from:
    a. calcitonin.
    b. the thyroid.
    c. parathyroid hormone.
    d. none of the above.

True or False

18. _____ Haversian canals run lengthwise, whereas Volkmann's canals run transverse to the bone.

19. _____ Giant, multinucleate cells that are responsible for bone resorption are called *osteocytes*.

20. _____ Bone marrow is found not only in the medullary cavities of certain long bones but also in the spaces of cancellous bone.

21. _____ Calcitonin functions to stimulate osteoblasts and inhibit osteoclasts.

22. _____ *Hematopoiesis* is a term referring to the formation of new Haversian systems.

23. _____ Yellow marrow is found in almost all of the bones of an infant's body.

➡ *If you had difficulty with this section, review pages 210 and 212-218.*

III—BONE DEVELOPMENT, REMODELING, AND REPAIR
Multiple Choice—select the best answer.

24. The primary ossification center is located at the:
    a. epiphysis.
    b. diaphysis.
    c. articular cartilage.
    d. none of the above.

25. The primary purpose of the epiphyseal plate is:
    a. mending fractures.
    b. enlarging the epiphysis.
    c. providing bone strength.
    d. lengthening long bones.

26. The epiphyseal plate is composed mostly of:
    a. chondrocytes.
    b. osteocytes.
    c. osteoclasts.
    d. none of the above.

27. Bone loss normally begins to exceed bone gain between the ages of:
    a. 30 and 35 years.
    b. 35 and 40 years.
    c. 55 and 60 years.
    d. 65 and 70 years.

28. The first step to healing a bone fracture is:
    a. callus formation.
    b. fracture hematoma formation.
    c. alignment of the fracture.
    d. collar formation.

True or False

29. _____ The addition of bone to its outer surface resulting in growth in diameter is called *appositional growth*.

30. _____ Most bones of the body are formed by intramembranous ossification.

31. _____ Once an individual reaches skeletal maturity, the bones undergo years of metabolic rest.

32. _____ Lack of exercise tends to weaken bones through decreased collagen formation and excessive calcium withdrawal.

33. _____ When bones reach their full length, the epiphyseal plate disappears.

➡ *If you had difficulty with this section, review pages 217-224.*

IV—CARTILAGE
Multiple Choice—select the best answer.

34. The fibrous covering of cartilage is:
    a. periosteum.
    b. perichondrium.
    c. chondroclast.
    d. none of the above.

35. The external ear, epiglottis, and the auditory tube are composed of:
    a. hyaline cartilage.
    b. fibrocartilage.
    c. elastic cartilage.
    d. none of the above.

36. Vitamin D deficiency can result in:
    a. scurvy.
    b. rickets.
    c. osteochondroma.
    d. none of the above.

True or False

37. _____ Both bone and cartilage are well vascularized.

38. _____ The intervertebral discs are composed of fibrocartilage.

39. _____ The growth of cartilage occurs by both appositional and interstitial growth.

Labeling—label the following diagrams.

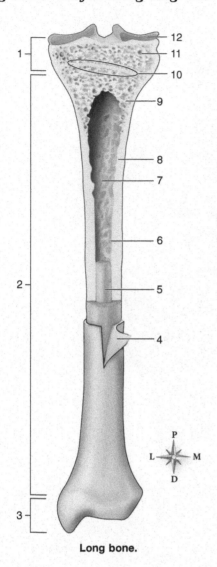

Long bone.

1. _____
2. _____
3. _____
4. _____
5. _____
6. _____
7. _____
8. _____
9. _____
10. _____
11. _____
12. _____

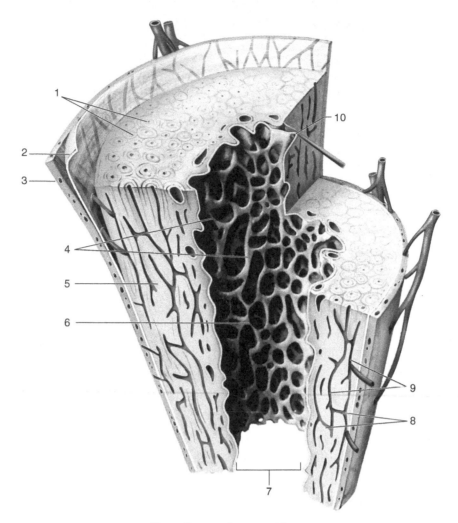

Cancellous and compact bone.

1. _____

2. _____

3. _____

4. _____

5. _____

6. _____

7. _____

8. _____

9. _____

10. _____

➔ *If you had difficulty with this section, review pages 225-228.*

V—MECHANISMS OF DISEASE

Fill in the blanks.

40. _____ is a malignant tumor of hyaline cartilage that arises from chondroblasts.

41. _____ is the most common primary malignant tumor of skeletal tissue.

42. _____ is a common bone disease often occurring in postmenopausal women and manifesting symptoms of porous, brittle, and fragile bones.

43. _____ is also known as *osteitis deformans.*

44. _____ is a bacterial infection of the bone and marrow tissue.

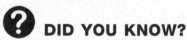 *If you had difficulty with this section, review pages 227-228.*

CROSSWORD PUZZLE

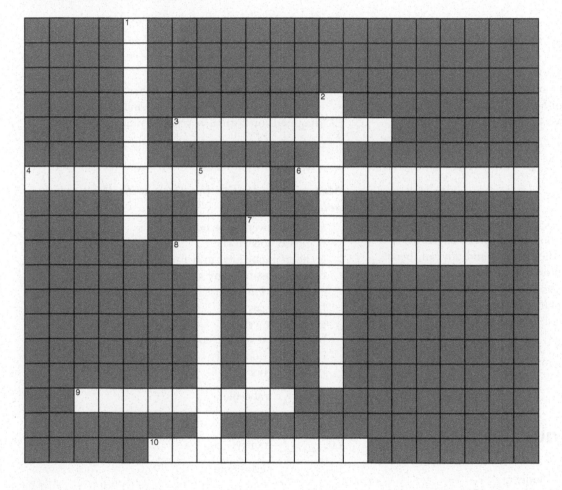

ACROSS
3. On; growth
4. Lattice; characterized by
6. Around; bone
8. Around; cartilage; thing
9. Bone; cell
10. Beam; little

DOWN
1. Within; bone
2. Bone; pore; condition
5. Bone; softening
7. Bind; result of action

❓ DID YOU KNOW?

• Approximately 25 million Americans have osteoporosis. Four out of five are women.

• Every second, our bone marrow produces 2 million red blood cells.

APPLYING WHAT YOU KNOW

45. Mrs. Harris is a 60-year-old white woman. She has noticed in recent years that her height has slightly decreased. Recently, she fractured her wrist in a slight fall. Which skeletal system disorder might she be suffering from? What techniques could be used to diagnose her condition? What treatments are available?

46. Mrs. Wiedeke had advanced cancer of the bone. As the disease progressed, Mrs. Wiedeke required several blood transfusions throughout her therapy. She asked the doctor one day to explain the necessity for the transfusions. What explanation might the doctor give to Mrs. Wiedeke?

47. Dr. Kennedy, an orthopedic surgeon, called the admissions office of the hospital and advised them that he would be admitting a patient in the next hour with an epiphyseal fracture. Without any other information, the patient is assigned to the pediatric ward. What prompted this assignment?

ONE LAST QUICK CHECK

Fill in the blanks.

48. Functions of bones include:
    _____,
    _____,
    _____,
    _____, and
    _____.

49. The _____ _____ is the hollow area inside the diaphysis of a bone.

50. A thin layer of cartilage covering each epiphysis is the _____ _____.

51. The _____ lines the medullary cavity of long bones.

52. _____ is used to describe the process of blood cell formation.

53. Blood cell formation is a vital process carried on in _____ _____ _____.

54. The _____ is a strong fibrous membrane that covers a long bone except at joint surfaces.

55. Bones may be classified by shape. Those shapes include _____, _____, _____, _____, and _____.

56. Bones serve as the major reservoir for _____, a vital substance required for normal nerve and muscle function.

57. _____ is the most abundant type of cartilage.

Matching—identify the term with the proper selection.

a. outer covering of bone
b. dense bone tissue
c. fibers embedded in a firm gel
d. criss-crossing bony branches of spongy bone
e. ends of long bones
f. connect lacunae
g. cartilage cells
h. structural unit of compact bone
i. mature bone cells
j. ring of bone

58. _____ trabeculae

59. _____ compact

60. _____ spongy

61. _____ periosteum

62. _____ cartilage

63. _____ osteocytes

64. _____ canaliculi

65. _____ lamellae

66. _____ chondrocytes

67. _____ Haversian system

CHAPTER 12
Axial Skeleton

The skeletal system may be compared to a large, 206-piece puzzle. Each bone, as with each puzzle piece, is unique in size and shape. And again, just like with a puzzle, pieces or bones are not interchangeable. They have a lock-and-key concept that allows them to fit in only one area of the skeletal frame and perform functions necessary for that location.

The skeleton is divided into two main areas: the axial skeleton and the appendicular skeleton. All of the 206 bones of the human body may be classified into one of these two areas. We begin with the axial skeleton. Eighty bones make up this division of the skeleton. The word *axial* is taken from the word *axis* and is so named because the bones are close to or along the central axis of the body. Included in the axial skeleton are the bones of the skull, vertebral column, middle ear (ossicles), ribcage, sternum, and the hyoid bone.

Bones are unique, with markings to identify them in relationship to others. Of special uniqueness to the axial skeleton is the hyoid bone, which is the only bone in the body that does not articulate directly with any other bone. It serves as a movable base for the tongue and certain muscles of the floor of the mouth. When you have a thorough understanding and retention of the bones of the axial skeleton, you will be prepared to continue your study of the remaining bones, known as the *appendicular skeleton*.

I—DIVISIONS OF THE SKELETON

Matching—identify each term with its associated division of the skeleton.

a. axial skeleton
b. appendicular skeleton

1. _____ coccyx

2. _____ 80 bones

3. _____ 126 bones

4. _____ vertebral column

5. _____ carpals

6. _____ scapula

7. _____ auditory ossicles (ear bones)

8. _____ shoulder girdle

9. _____ skull

10. _____ clavicles

➔ *If you had difficulty with this section, review pages 233-236.*

II—THE SKULL

Multiple Choice—select the best answer.

11. The squamous suture connects which two bones?
    a. frontal and parietal
    b. parietal and temporal
    c. temporal and sphenoid
    d. sphenoid and frontal

12. The mastoid sinuses are found in which bone?
    a. frontal
    b. sphenoid
    c. parietal
    d. temporal

13. The skull bone that articulates with the first cervical vertebrae is the:
    a. occipital.
    b. sphenoid.
    c. ethmoid.
    d. none of the above.

14. A *meatus* can be described as a:
    a. large bony prominence.
    b. shallow groove.
    c. tubelike opening or channel.
    d. raised, rough area.

15. Separation of the nasal and cranial cavities is achieved by the:
    a. cribriform plate of the ethmoid bone.
    b. sella turcica of the sphenoid bone.
    c. foramen magnum of the occipital bone.
    d. palatine process of the maxilla.

16. Which of the following is *not* a bone of the orbit?
    a. ethmoid
    b. nasal
    c. lacrimal
    d. frontal

True or False

17. _____ The sphenoid is a bone of the face.

18. _____ A specialized adaptation of the infant skull is called a *fontanel*.

19. _____ The cheek is shaped by the zygomatic, or malar, bone.

20. _____ The hyoid is one of several bones that do not articulate with any other bones.

21. _____ The external acoustic meatus is located within the temporal bone.

Multiple Choice—select the best answer.

22. Which of the following is *not* a marking on facial bones?
    a. mental foramen
    b. sinus
    c. coronoid process
    d. suture

23. The palatine process:
    a. forms the cheekbones.
    b. forms part of the hard palate.
    c. forms the upper part of the bridge of the nose.
    d. forms the posterior portion of the nasal septum.

24. The foundation or keystone in the architecture of the face is the:
    a. mandible.
    b. maxillae.
    c. zygomatic.
    d. lacrimal bone.

25. The shape of the nose is formed by the nasal bones and the:
    a. costal cartilage.
    b. sella turcica.
    c. septal cartilage.
    d. cribriform plate.

26. Which marking does *not* appear on the mandible?
    a. ramus
    b. condylar process
    c. alveolar process
    d. horizontal plate

Labeling—using the terms provided, label the following diagrams.

optic foramen of sphenoid bone
sphenoid bone
perpendicular plate of ethmoid bone
vomer
frontal bone
nasal bone

glabella
maxilla
mental foramen of mandible
ethmoid bone
parietal bone
mandible

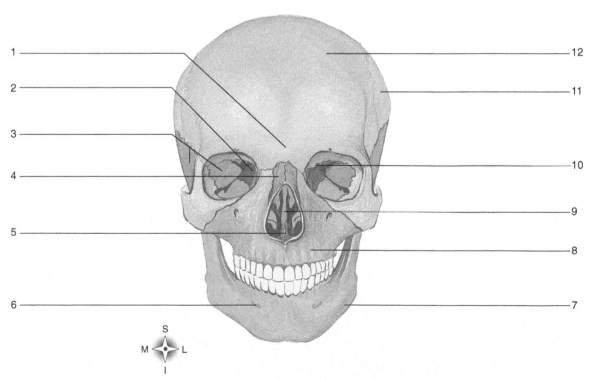

Anterior view of the skull.

foramen spinosum
jugular foramen
occipital bone
superior orbital fissure
foramen magnum
greater wing
foramen lacerum
petrous part of temporal bone
crista galli of ethmoid bone
optic foramen

sella turcica
sphenoid bone
foramen ovale
internal acoustic meatus
parietal bone
temporal bone
lesser wing
ethmoid bone
cribriform plate
frontal bone

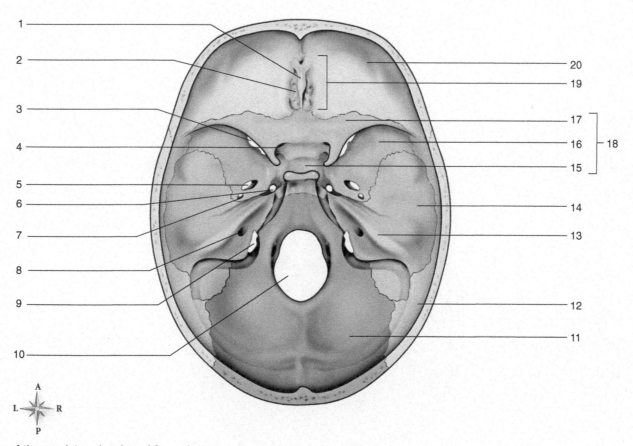

Floor of the cranial cavity viewed from above.

mastoid process
foramen lacerum
incisive foramen of maxilla
temporal bone
medial pterygoid plate of sphenoid
zygomatic arch
foramen magnum
occipital condyle
zygomatic process of temporal bone
horizontal plate of palatine bone
parietal bone
occipital bone

stylomastoid foramen
hard palate
styloid process
mastoid foramen
jugular foramen
vomer
palatine process of maxilla
foramen ovale
zygomatic process of maxilla
lateral pterygoid plate of sphenoid
temporal process of zygomatic bone
carotid canal

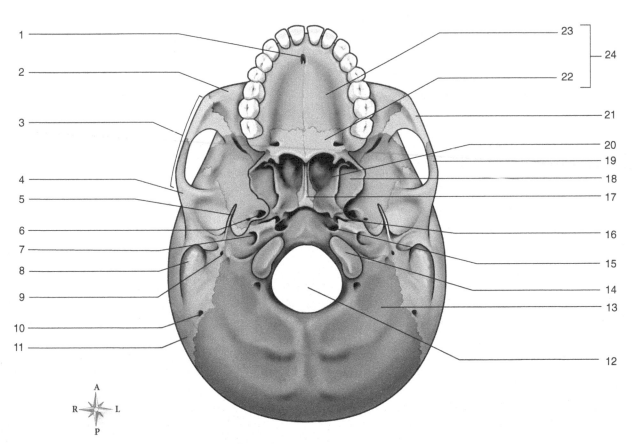

Skull viewed from below.

occipital bone
parietal bone
maxilla
sphenoid bone
lambdoid suture
external acoustic meatus of temporal bone
mental foramen of mandible
mastoid process of temporal bone
lacrimal bone
zygomatic bone
condyloid process of mandible

squamous suture
coronal suture
ethmoid bone
coronoid process of mandible
pterygoid process of sphenoid bone
mandible
nasal bone
frontal bone
temporal bone
styloid process

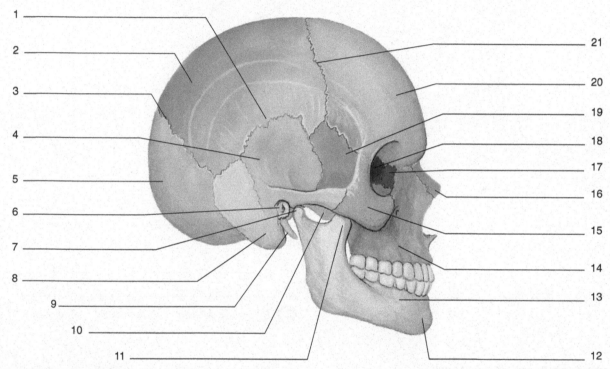

Skull viewed from the right side.

Labeling—label the following diagram.

Bones of left orbit.

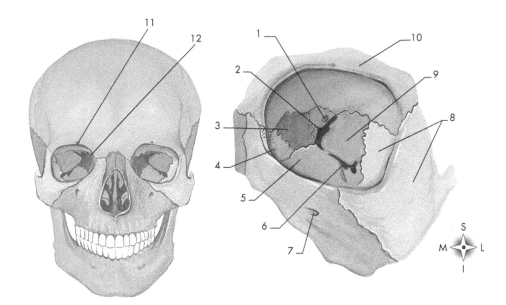

1. _____
2. _____
3. _____
4. _____
5. _____
6. _____

7. _____
8. _____
9. _____
10. _____
11. _____
12. _____

➔ *If you had difficulty with this section, review pages 236-254.*

III—VERTEBRAL COLUMN

Multiple Choice—select the best answer.

27. Lamina is a posterior portion of the:
    a. hyoid.
    b. maxilla.
    c. vertebra.
    d. zygomatic.

28. Which of the following is *not* a part of the vertebral column?
    a. cervical curvature
    b. thoracic curvature
    c. lumbar curvature
    d. coccyx curvature

29. The dens projects from the body of the:
    a. first vertebra.
    b. second vertebra.
    c. coccyx.
    d. first thoracic vertebra.

30. The vertebral column is curved:
    a. to increase the carrying strength of the column.
    b. to protect certain structures that are beneath.
    c. to accommodate the shape of the body.
    d. to accommodate head, neck, and hip movements.

31. The first cervical vertebra is known as the:
    a. axis.
    b. primary vertebra.
    c. atlas.
    d. pedicle.

Labeling—label the following diagrams of the vertebral column. Be sure to identify the spinal regions, spinal curves, and quantity of vertebrae for each region.

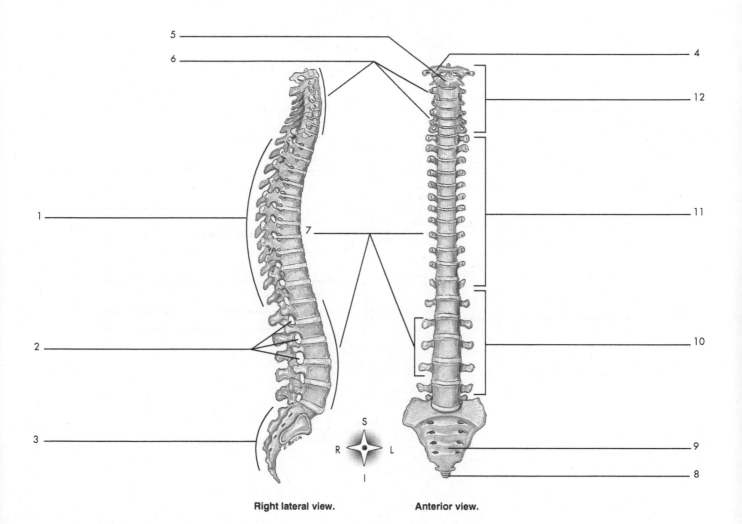

Right lateral view.

Anterior view.

Labeling—label the following images of vertebrae.

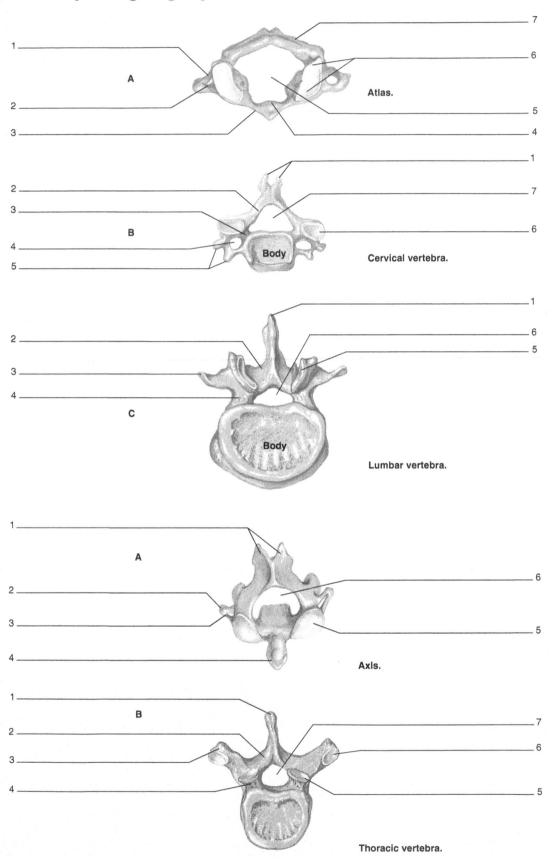

Atlas.

Cervical vertebra.

Lumbar vertebra.

Axis.

Thoracic vertebra.

➡ *If you had difficulty with this section, review pages 250-258.*

IV—STERNUM AND RIBS

Matching—identify each term with its corresponding description.

a. body
b. false ribs
c. floating ribs
d. manubrium
e. true ribs
f. xiphoid process
g. costal cartilage

32. _____ first seven pairs of ribs that attach directly to the sternum

33. _____ eleventh and twelfth ribs, which have no attachment to the sternum

34. _____ middle part of the sternum

35. _____ most superior part of the sternum

36. _____ the blunt, cartilaginous, lower tip of the sternum

37. _____ the five pairs of ribs that do not attach directly to the sternum

38. _____ tissue that attaches ribs directly or indirectly to the sternum

Labeling—label the following diagram.

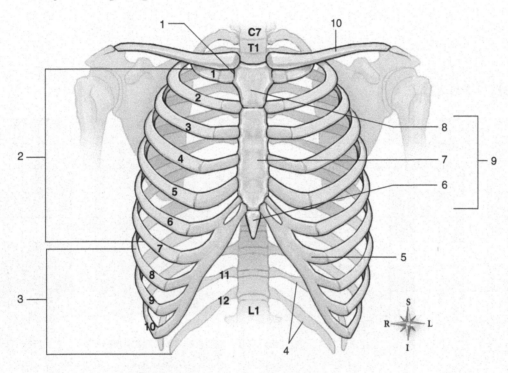

Thoracic cage.

1. _____
2. _____
3. _____
4. _____
5. _____

6. _____
7. _____
8. _____
9. _____
10. _____

→ *If you had difficulty with this section, review pages 254-260.*

V—MECHANISMS OF DISEASE

Multiple Choice—select the best answer.

39. Another name for "hunchback" is:
    a. scoliosis.
    b. kyphosis.
    c. lordosis.
    d. Osgood-Schlatter disease.

40. Which of the following abnormal curvatures can interfere with breathing, posture, and other vital functions?
    a. scoliosis
    b. lordosis
    c. kyphosis
    d. all of the above

41. Mastoiditis involves the:
    a. occipital bone.
    b. temporal bone.
    c. parietal bone.
    d. frontal bone.

42. Otitis media is usually treated with:
    a. surgery.
    b. steroids.
    c. antibiotics.
    d. laser treatments.

True or False

43. _____ *Swayback* and *kyphosis* are synonymous terms.

44. _____ Normal curvature of the spine is convex posteriorly through the thoracic region and concave posteriorly through the cervical and lumbar regions.

➔ *If you had difficulty with this section, review pages 260-261.*

CROSSWORD PUZZLE

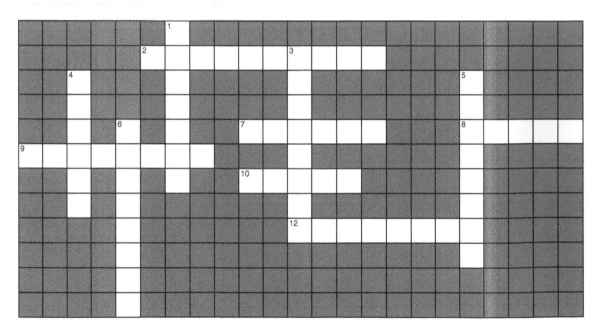

ACROSS
2. Sieve; shape
7. Seam
8. Nose; relating to
9. Wall; relating to
10. Hollow
12. Tear; relating to

DOWN
1. Forehead; relating
3. Fountain; little
4. Chest
5. To chew
6. That which turns

APPLYING WHAT YOU KNOW

45. Spring was in full bloom and Joe's sinuses were bothering him. He was able to control the drainage with medication, but his head felt heavy and the sinus areas were very painful. What is the explanation for this?

46. Leroy is a football player, and during his game he broke his nose. He said he felt fine and was ready to return to the team, but the coach and doctor wanted him to have additional tests to determine the extent of trauma to his nose. If Leroy feels ready to play, what is the concern of the doctor regarding his nose?

 DID YOU KNOW?

- Humans and giraffes have the same number of bones in their neck.
- The bones of the middle ear are mature at birth.
- The skeleton of an average 160-pound body weighs about 29 pounds.

 ONE LAST QUICK CHECK

*Circle the one that does **not** belong.*

47. cervical	thoracic	coxal	coccyx
48. frontal	occipital	maxilla	sphenoid
49. malleus	vomer	incus	stapes
50. ulna	ilium	ischium	pubis
51. ethmoid	parietal	occipital	nasal
52. anvil	atlas	axis	cervical

Matching—identify the bone with its marking. There may be more than one correct answer.

a. mastoid
b. pterygoid process
c. foramen magnum
d. sella turcica
e. mental foramen
f. conchae
g. xiphoid process
h. frontal sinuses
i. coronoid process

53. _____ occipital

54. _____ sternum

55. _____ temporal

56. _____ sphenoid

57. _____ ethmoid

58. _____ frontal

59. _____ mandible

Fill in the blanks.

60. All vertebra have a central opening called the _____ _____.

61. The upper part of the sternum is called the _____.

62. The skull bone that articulates with the atlas is the _____.

63. Part of the lateral wall of the cranium and part of the floor of each orbit are formed by the _____ bone.

True or False

64. _____ The skull consists of two major divisions: the cranium and the face.

65. _____ There are four pairs of paranasal sinuses: frontal, sphenoid, ethmoid, and parietal.

66. _____ The middle ear bones are referred to as *auditory ossicles.*

CHAPTER 13
Appendicular Skeleton

As mentioned in the prior chapter, the skeleton is divided into two main areas. You reviewed the first area, the axial skeleton, in the previous chapter. The remaining 126 bones of the 206 total bones in the human body are known as the *appendicular skeleton*. *Appendicular* is the adjective of the word *appendage*, which means "joined to something larger." The "appendicular" skeleton (appendages) is attached to the body frame, or "axial" (trunk) skeleton. It is made up of the bones of the arms and legs, the pectoral girdle, and the pelvis. The bones of the appendicular skeleton are involved primarily in motion and the manipulation of objects.

Although we can neatly divide the skeleton into these two main areas—axial and appendicular—there are subtle differences that exist between a man's and a woman's skeleton that provide us with insight into the functional differences between the sexes. An understanding of the skeletal system gives us an appreciation of the complex and interdependent functions that make this system essential for maintaining homeostasis and sustaining life.

I—THE APPENDICULAR SKELETON/ UPPER EXTREMITY

Multiple Choice—select the best answer.

1. Which of the following is *not* part of the shoulder girdle?
   a. clavicle
   b. sternum
   c. scapula
   d. none of the above

2. The coronoid fossa is a:
   a. depression on the thumb.
   b. projection of the ulna.
   c. region on the spine.
   d. depression on the humerus.

3. The arm socket is the:
   a. coronoid fossa.
   b. olecranon fossa.
   c. coracoid process.
   d. glenoid cavity.

4. The bone on the thumb side of the forearm is the:
   a. radius.
   b. ulna.
   c. carpal.
   d. metacarpal.

5. Of the five metacarpal bones, which forms the most freely movable joint with the carpal bones?
   a. index finger
   b. small finger
   c. ring finger
   d. thumb

6. Which two bones compose the shoulder girdle?
   a. clavicle and sternum
   b. clavicle and scapula
   c. clavicle and 3rd vertebra
   d. clavicle and humerus

True or False

7. _____ The two bones that form the framework of the forearm are the radius and ulna.

8. _____ The wrist is composed of small bones called *metacarpals*.

9. _____ The medial forearm bone in the anatomical position is the ulna.

10. _____ The most evident carpal bone is the triquetrum.

Labeling—label the following diagrams.

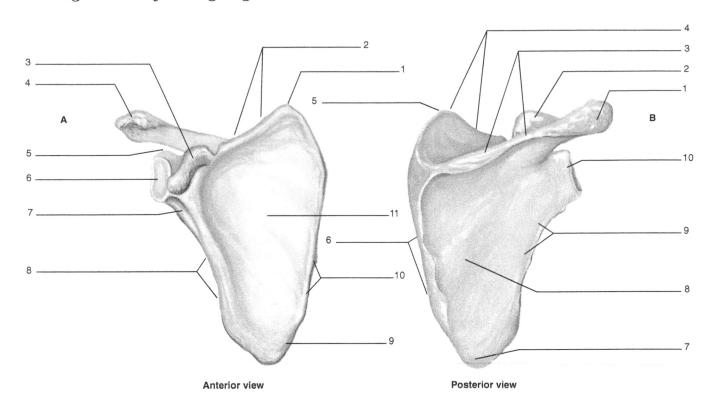

Anterior view

Posterior view

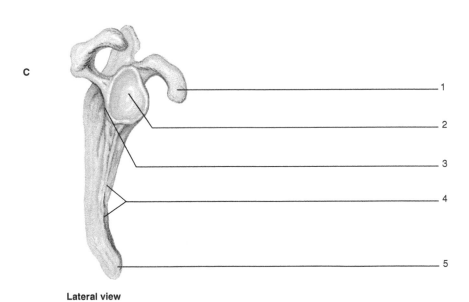

Lateral view

Scapula.

Labeling—match each term with its corresponding number on the following diagrams.

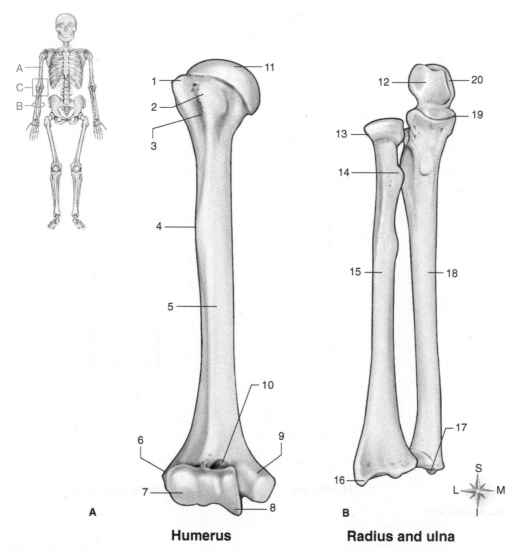

A

Humerus

B

Radius and ulna

Bones of the arm (anterior view).

_____ deltoid tuberosity
_____ capitulum
_____ coronoid fossa
_____ radial tuberosity
_____ coronoid process
_____ intertubercular groove
_____ humerus
_____ radius
_____ head of radius
_____ lesser tubercle

_____ lateral epicondyle
_____ greater tubercle
_____ medial epicondyle
_____ styloid process of ulna
_____ trochlea
_____ head
_____ olecranon process
_____ trochlear notch
_____ styloid process of radius
_____ ulna

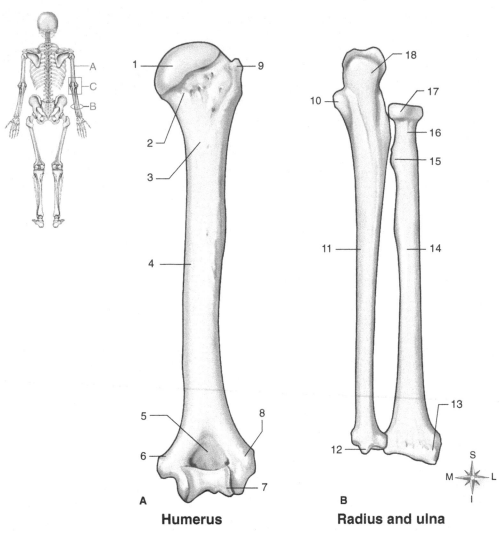

A

Humerus

B

Radius and ulna

Bones of the arm (posterior view).

_____ greater tubercle	_____ lateral epicondyle
_____ head of radius	_____ coronoid process
_____ anatomical neck	_____ ulna
_____ styloid process of ulna	_____ head
_____ medial epicondyle	_____ olecranon fossa
_____ trochlea	_____ olecranon process
_____ surgical neck	_____ radius
_____ humerus	_____ neck
_____ radial tuberosity	_____ styloid process of radius

Labeling—match each term with its corresponding number on the following diagrams. Some terms may be used more than once.

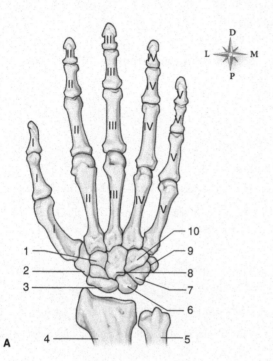

_____ ulna
_____ hamate
_____ proximal phalanx
_____ trapezium
_____ scaphoid
_____ distal phalanx
_____ metacarpal bone
_____ capitate
_____ triquetrum
_____ radius
_____ trapezoid
_____ lunate
_____ pisiform
_____ middle phalanx

➡ *If you had difficulty with this section, review pages 264-269.*

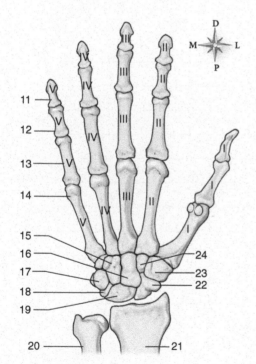

Bones of the hand and wrist.

II—THE APPENDICULAR SKELETON/ LOWER EXTREMITY

Multiple Choice—select the best answer.

11. Which of the following is *not* one of the bones of the pelvic girdle?
    a. ilium
    b. acetabulum
    c. ischium
    d. pubis

12. The greater trochanter is a bony landmark of the:
    a. femur.
    b. tibia.
    c. pubis.
    d. ramus.

13. During childbirth the infant passes through an imaginary plane called the:
    a. pelvic outlet.
    b. symphysis pubis.
    c. pelvic brim.
    d. ilium.

14. Which of the following is *not* a tarsal bone?
    a. talus
    b. cuneiform
    c. scaphoid
    d. navicular

15. The strongest and lowermost portion of the coxal bones is the:
    a. ilium.
    b. ischium.
    c. pubis.
    d. pubic symphysis.

True or False

16. _____ The largest coxal bone is the ischium.

17. _____ The most distal portion of the fibula is composed of a bony landmark called the *medial malleolus.*

18. _____ The *longitudinal arch* refers to a structure within the pelvic inlet.

19. _____ Each toe contains three phalanges.

20. _____ The fibula is also known as the *shin bone.*

Labeling—label the following diagrams.

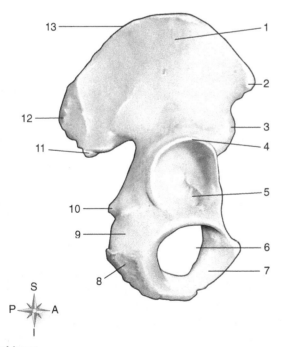

Coxal bone.

1. _____
2. _____
3. _____
4. _____
5. _____
6. _____
7. _____
8. _____
9. _____
10. _____
11. _____
12. _____
13. _____

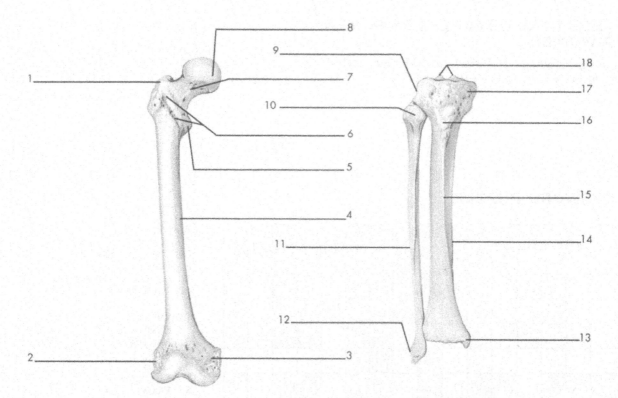

Femur

Fibula and tibia

Bones of the thigh and leg.

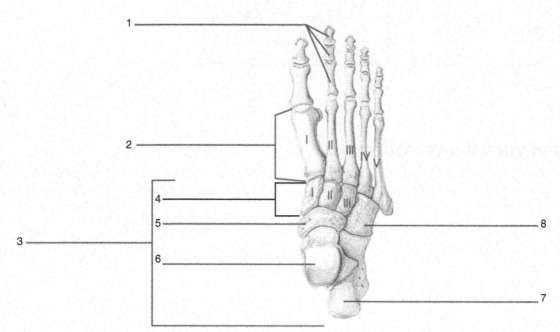

Bones of the foot.

➜ *If you had difficulty with this section, review pages 270-276.*

III—SKELETAL DIFFERENCES IN MEN AND WOMEN

Matching—identify the skeletal characteristics with the appropriate gender.

a. male skeleton
b. female skeleton

21. _____ elongated forehead

22. _____ small pelvic inlet

23. _____ subpubic angle less than 90 degrees

24. _____ more massive muscle attachment sites

25. _____ more movable coccyx

➡ *If you had difficulty with this section, review pages 277-278.*

CROSSWORD PUZZLE

ACROSS
2. Thigh
6. Shoulder blade
8. Flank
11. Beyond; wrist; relating to
12. Wrist; relating to

DOWN
1. Basin
3. Key; little
4. Arm
5. Clasp
7. Dish; small
9. Elbow
10. Shin bone

✏ APPLYING WHAT YOU KNOW

26. While playing football, Bill was involved in a tackle that caused a forced hyperextension of his elbow joint. Which skeletal structures could he have injured?

27. Amanda loves to wear extremely high-heeled shoes. How does this affect the weight distribution on the bones of her feet? Which skeletal structures are at risk of being damaged?

DID YOU KNOW?

- The bones of the hands and feet make up more than half of the total 206 bones of the body.

- The femur (thigh bone) is the longest bone in the body and makes up one quarter of the body's total height.

✓ ONE LAST QUICK CHECK

*Circle the one that does **not** belong.*

28. pelvic girdle	ankle	wrist	axial
29. scapula	pectoral girdle	ribs	clavicle
30. carpal	phalanges	metacarpal	ethmoid
31. humerus	radius	talus	carpal
32. condyles	head	acetabulum	greater trochanter

Matching—identify the bone with its marking. There may be more than one correct answer, and not all letters may be used.

a. ischium
b. scapula
c. olecranon process
d. symphysis pubis
e. greater trochanter
f. calcaneus
g. glenoid cavity
h. ilium
i. medial malleolus
j. acetabulum

33. _____ coxal

34. _____ femur

35. _____ ulna

36. _____ tarsals

37. _____ scapula

38. _____ tibia

Fill in the blanks.

39. Eight _____ bones form the wrist.

40. The heel bone is the _____.

41. The tarsal bone that articulates with the tibia and fibula is the _____.

42. The largest sesamoid bone in the body is the _____.

43. The larger and stronger of the two lower leg bones is the _____.

True or False

44. _____ A nondisplaced, or closed, fracture is also known as a *simple fracture.*

45. _____ One type of incomplete fracture common in children is the impacted fracture.

46. _____ *Pectoral girdle* and *shoulder girdle* are synonymous.

47. _____ The structure above the pelvic inlet is the *true pelvis.*

48. _____ A stress fracture is clearly visible on x-ray.

CHAPTER 14
Articulations

We conclude our study of bones with a chapter on joints, or articulations. A joint, or articulation, is a point of contact between bones. Sitting, walking, and running are just a few examples of movements that would not be possible without the successful functioning of articulations. Joints also permit us to lift heavy objects and perform fine motor skills such as needlepoint. The unusual and unique shape and size of articulations are responsible for the variety and degree of motion that we expect from our body.

Joints may be classified according to structure (fibrous and cartilaginous) or according to function (synarthrosis—immovable; amphiarthrosis—slightly movable; diarthrosis—freely movable). Proper functioning of articulations is necessary for us to adapt to our environment with controlled, smooth, and pain-free movements.

I—CLASSIFICATION OF JOINTS

Multiple Choice—select the best answer.

1. The articulation between the root of a tooth and the alveolar process of the mandible or maxilla is called the:
   a. suture.
   b. gomphosis.
   c. synchondrosis.
   d. symphysis.

2. Immovable joints are called:
   a. synarthroses.
   b. amphiarthroses.
   c. diarthroses.
   d. none of the above.

3. The radioulnar articulation is classified as which type of articulation?
   a. syndesmosis
   b. synchondrosis
   c. symphysis
   d. diarthrosis

4. The most movable joints in the body are:
   a. symphyses.
   b. sutures.
   c. synovial joints.
   d. synchondroses.

5. An example of a symphysis is:
   a. the articulation between the pubic bones.
   b. the articulation between the bodies of adjacent vertebrae.
   c. both a and b.
   d. none of the above.

6. The inner surface of the joint capsule is lined with:
   a. bursae.
   b. a joint cavity.
   c. periosteum.
   d. synovial membrane.

7. The joint that allows for the widest range of movement is a _____ joint.
   a. gliding
   b. saddle
   c. ball-and-socket
   d. hinge

8. An example of a pivot joint is the:
   a. first metacarpal articulating with the trapezium.
   b. humerus articulating with the trapezium.
   c. interphalangeal joints.
   d. head of the radius articulating with the ulna.

True or False

9. _____ *Diarthrosis* and *synovial joint* refer to basically the same structure.

10. _____ The elbow joint is a ball-and-socket joint.

11. _____ The ability to oppose the fingers and thumb is achieved by a saddle joint.

12. _____ *Articulation* and *joint* are synonymous terms.

13. _____ Diarthrotic joints are the least common type of joint in the body.

14. _____ There are several examples of suture articulations throughout the entire body.

15. _____ Menisci are composed of hyaline cartilage.

16. _____ The shoulder joint is a ball-and-socket joint.

Matching—identify each joint or description with its corresponding classification.

   a. amphiarthroses
   b. diarthroses
   c. synarthroses

17. _____ joint between bodies of vertebrae

18. _____ symphysis pubis

19. _____ hip joint

20. _____ fibrous joint

21. _____ immovable joint

22. _____ cartilaginous joint

23. _____ thumb

24. _____ joints between skull bones

25. _____ freely movable joint

26. _____ synovial joint

27. _____ slightly movable joint

28. _____ the most prevalent type of joint in the body

Matching—identify each joint with its corresponding functional classification.

   a. ball and socket
   b. condyloid
   c. gliding
   d. hinge
   e. pivot
   f. saddle

29. _____ elbow

30. _____ joints between facets of adjacent vertebrae

31. _____ ellipsoidal

32. _____ dens of axis/atlas joint

33. _____ knee joint

34. _____ least movable group of the synovial joints

35. _____ hip joint

36. _____ shoulder joint

37. _____ joint between first metacarpal and trapezium

Labeling—label the structures of the synovial joint on the following diagram.

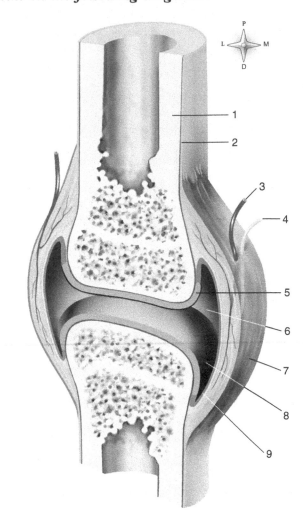

1. _____

2. _____

3. _____

4. _____

5. _____

6. _____

7. _____

8. _____

9. _____

➡ *If you had difficulty with this section, review pages 284-289.*

II—REPRESENTATIVE SYNOVIAL JOINTS

Multiple Choice—select the best answer.

38. The glenoid labrum is associated with which joint?
    a. hip
    b. knee
    c. shoulder
    d. vertebral

39. Perhaps the strongest ligament in the body is the:
    a. rotator cuff.
    b. iliofemoral.
    c. pubofemoral.
    d. intertrochanteric.

40. The largest and most complex joint of the body is the:
    a. shoulder.
    b. knee.
    c. hip.
    d. ankle.

41. The anterior cruciate ligament of the knee connects the:
    a. anterior tibia with the posterior femur.
    b. posterior tibia with the anterior femur.
    c. anterior fibula with the posterior femur.
    d. anterior fibula with the anterior femur.

42. Vertebral bodies are connected by:
    a. the anterior longitudinal ligament.
    b. the posterior longitudinal ligament.
    c. the ligamentum flavum.
    d. both a and b.

43. Protrusion of the nucleus pulposus through the annulus fibrosus results in:
    a. bursitis.
    b. housemaid's knee.
    c. herniated disk.
    d. none of the above.

44. The medial and lateral menisci are:
    a. ligaments.
    b. cartilage.
    c. bursae.
    d. none of the above.

45. "Joint mice" are structurally:
    a. impinged bursae.
    b. loose pieces of synovial membrane.
    c. loose pieces of articular cartilage.
    d. cracks in the articular cartilage.

Labeling—label the following diagrams of synovial joints.

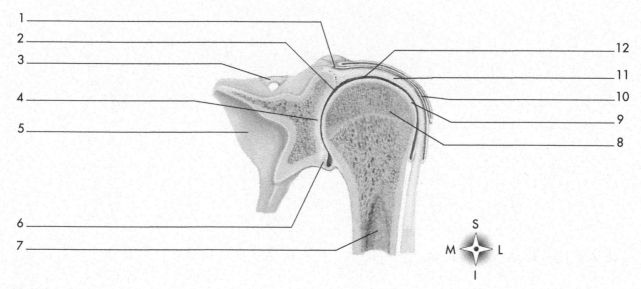

Shoulder joint.

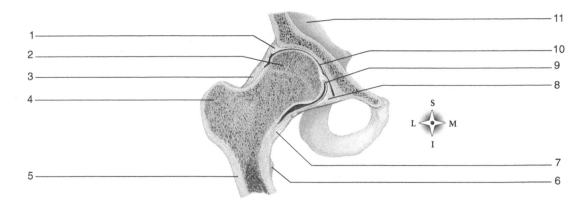

Hip joint.

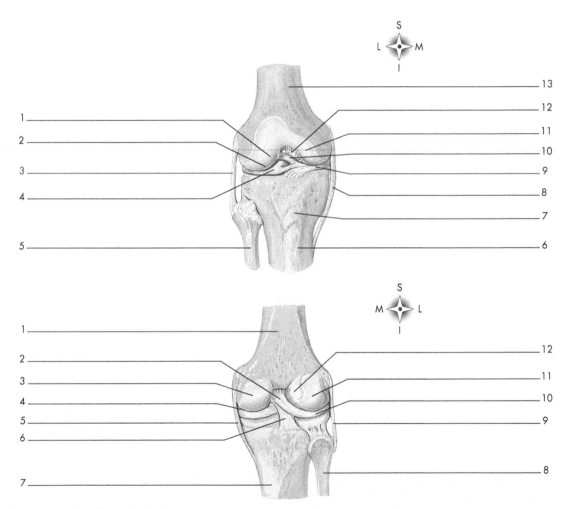

Knee joint. A, anterior view. B, posterior view.

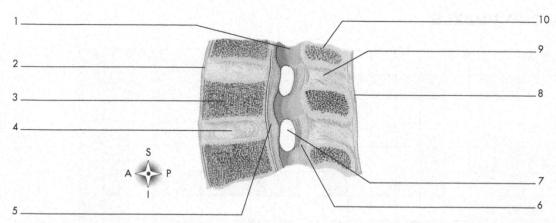

1 _____

2 _____

3 _____

4 _____

5 _____

S
A ◆ P
I

10 _____

9 _____

8 _____

7 _____

6 _____

Vertebrae and their ligaments.

 If you had difficulty with this section, review pages 289-298 and 306.

III—MOVEMENT AT SYNOVIAL JOINTS

Matching—identify each term with its corresponding definition or description.

a. plantar flexion
b. extension
c. abduction
d. hyperextension
e. goniometer
f. rotation
g. flexion
h. inversion
i. depression
j. adduction

46. _____ instrument that measures range of motion

47. _____ lifting the arms away from the midline

48. _____ turning the head as to say "no"

49. _____ elbow movement, as when lifting weights during a "bicep curl"

50. _____ increasing joint angle

51. _____ moving beyond extension

52. _____ causes extension of the leg as a whole

53. _____ turning sole of foot inward

54. _____ opening your mouth

55. _____ bringing fingers together

 If you had difficulty with this section, review pages 298-306.

IV—MECHANISMS OF DISEASE

Fill in the blanks.

56. _____ is an imaging technique that allows a physician to examine the internal structure of a joint without the use of extensive surgery.

57. The most common noninflammatory joint disease is _____, or _____ _____ _____.

58. A general name for many different inflammatory joint diseases is _____.

59. A metabolic type of inflammatory arthritis is _____ _____.

60. An acute musculoskeletal injury to the ligamentous structure surrounding a joint and disrupting the continuity of the synovial membrane is a _____.

 If you had difficulty with this section, review pages 306-308.

CROSSWORD PUZZLE

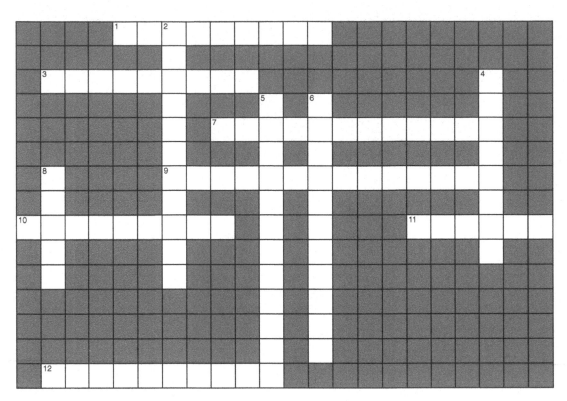

ACROSS
1. Away; lead; process
3. Stretch; process
7. Back; bend; process
9. Both sides; joint; condition
10. Bend forward; process
11. Seam
12. Lying on the back; process

DOWN
2. Apart; to place; process
4. Crescent
5. Joint; little; state
6. Between; joint; condition
8. Purse

 APPLYING WHAT YOU KNOW

61. Lowell is afflicted with severely inflamed joints because of arthritis. If he is suffering from the chronic systemic version of this disease, what symptoms would he be experiencing? Which joints are most likely involved and what is the most likely cause?

62. Sam is suffering from a type of arthritis associated with excess blood levels of uric acid. What type of arthritis is this? What symptoms might he experience, which joints would be affected, and how is this form of arthritis treated?

? DID YOU KNOW?

- The average person uses the leg joints to walk an average of 115,000 miles during his or her lifetime.
- Finger joints have wrinkles and creases only if the joint moves. If a finger joint stops moving, the creases eventually flatten out.

✓ ONE LAST QUICK CHECK

Circle the correct answer.

63. Freely movable joints are (amphiarthroses or diarthroses).

64. The sutures in the skull are (synarthrotic or amphiarthrotic).

65. All (diarthrotic or amphiarthrotic) joints have a joint capsule, a joint cavity, and a layer of cartilage over the ends of the two adjoining bones.

66. (Ligaments or tendons) grow out of periosteum and attach two bones together.

67. The (articular cartilage or epiphyseal cartilage) cushions surfaces of bones.

68. Gliding joints are the (least movable or most movable) of the diarthrotic joints.

69. The knee is the (largest or smallest) joint.

70. Hinge joints allow motion in (two or four) directions.

71. The saddle joint at the base of each of our thumbs allows for greater (strength or mobility).

72. When you rotate your head, you are using a (gliding or pivot) joint.

True or False

73. _____ A uniaxial joint is a synovial joint.

74. _____ Joints identified as *synchondroses* are synovial joints.

75. _____ Inflammation of the bursa is referred to as *pleurisy*.

76. _____ The main bursa of the shoulder joint is the subdeltoid bursa.

77. _____ Angular movements change the size of the angle between articulating bones.

78. _____ Pronation is a circular movement.

79. _____ Gliding movements are the most complex of movements.

80. _____ Protraction is an angular movement.

81. _____ Juvenile rheumatoid arthritis is more common in boys.

82. _____ The knee joint has a "baker's dozen," or 13, bursae, which serve as protective pads around it.

CHAPTER 15
Axial Muscles

Over 600 skeletal muscles make up what is commonly referred to as the "power system." They are attached snugly over the skeletal frame to shape and mold the contours of our body. Like the skeleton, muscles may be divided into two major divisions: the axial muscles and the appendicular muscles. The axial muscles have both their origin and insertions on parts of the axial skeleton.

Skeletal muscles constitute 40% to 50% of our body weight. And although memorizing the names and locations of skeletal muscles appears to be an overwhelming task, it is comforting to learn that muscles are named and categorized quite simply. Classification and identification are focused upon location, function, shape, direction of fibers, number of heads or divisions, or points of attachment. This chapter helps you understand the structure of skeletal muscles and the logical approach to muscle recognition.

I—SKELETAL MUSCLE STRUCTURE

Multiple Choice—select the best answer.

1. An entire skeletal muscle is covered by a coarse sheath called:
   a. endomysium.
   b. perimysium.
   c. epimysium.
   d. aponeurosis.

2. Muscles that are arranged like the feathers in a plume are described as:
   a. parallel.
   b. convergent.
   c. sphincter.
   d. pennate.

3. An aponeurosis is:
   a. broad and flat.
   b. tube shaped.
   c. featherlike.
   d. none of the above.

4. Antagonists are muscles that:
   a. oppose prime movers.
   b. facilitate prime movers.
   c. stabilize muscles.
   d. directly perform movements.

5. A fixed point about which a rod moves is called a:
   a. lever.
   b. bone.
   c. belly.
   d. fulcrum.

6. In first-class levers, the:
   a. fulcrum is between the pull and the load.
   b. load is between the fulcrum and the force.
   c. force is between the fulcrum and the load.
   d. load and force are equal.

True or False

7. _____ The origin of a muscle is the point of attachment that moves when the muscle contracts.

8. _____ Skeletal muscles usually act in groups rather than individually.

9. _____ *Prime mover* and *agonist* are synonymous.

10. _____ The optimum angle of pull of a muscle is generally parallel to the long axis of the bone.

11. _____ Tipping the head back, as in looking up at the sky, is an example of the function of a first-class lever.

→ *If you had difficulty with this section, review pages 314-320.*

II—HOW MUSCLES ARE NAMED

Matching—identify each muscle with the appropriate characteristic.

    a. location
    b. function
    c. shape
    d. direction of fibers
    e. number of heads
    f. points of attachment
    g. size of muscle

12. _____ deltoid

13. _____ brachialis

14. _____ sternocleidomastoid

15. _____ quadriceps

16. _____ gluteus maximus

17. _____ adductor

18. _____ rectus

 If you had difficulty with this section, review pages 321-323.

III—IMPORTANT SKELETAL MUSCLES: MUSCLES OF THE HEAD AND NECK

Matching—identify each muscle with its appropriate body movement.

    a. buccinator
    b. corrugator supercilii
    c. epicranius
    d. orbicularis oculi
    e. pterygoids
    f. sternocleidomastoid

19. _____ wrinkling the forehead vertically

20. _____ grating the teeth during mastication

21. _____ kissing

22. _____ raising the eyebrows

23. _____ flexing the head

24. _____ closing the eyes

Labeling—label the following diagram.

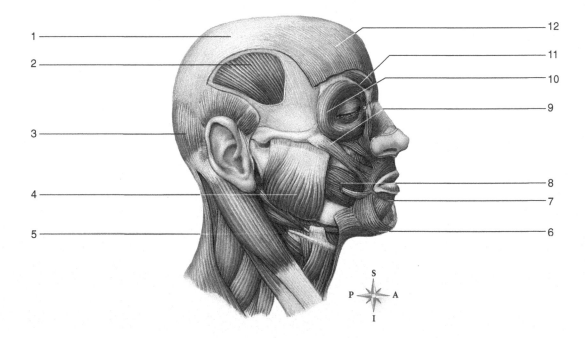

Facial muscles: lateral view.

 If you had difficulty with this section, review pages 324-326.

IV—TRUNK MUSCLES

True or False

25. _____ The external oblique compresses the abdomen.

26. _____ The rectus abdominis flexes the trunk.

27. _____ The levator ani closes the anal canal.

28. _____ The external intercostals elevate the ribs.

29. _____ The coccygeus muscles and levator ani form most of the pelvic floor.

30. _____ The muscles of the anterior and lateral abdominal wall are arranged in three layers.

Labeling—label the following diagrams.

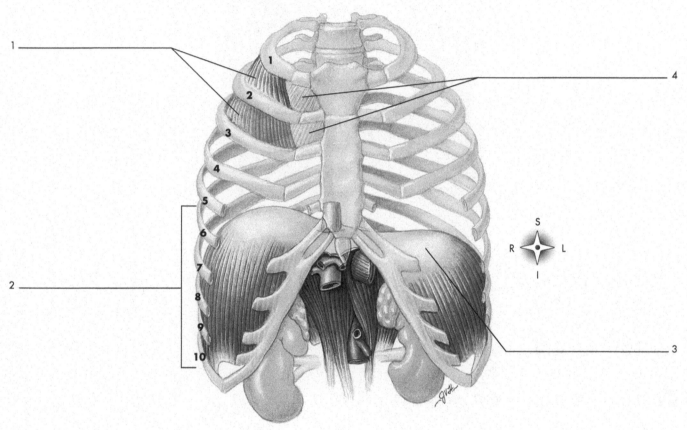

Muscles of the thorax.

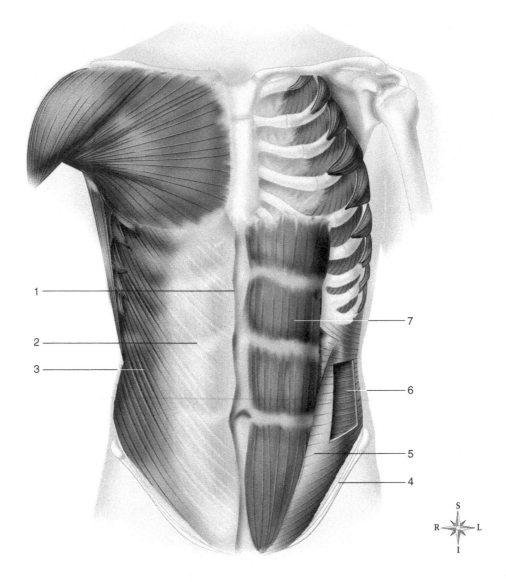

Muscles of the trunk and abdominal wall.

 If you had difficulty with this section, review pages 327-333.

CROSSWORD PUZZLE

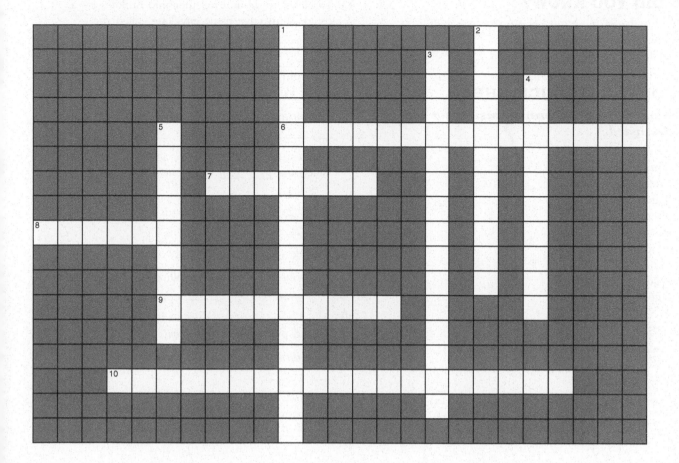

ACROSS
6. Breast; relating to; lesser
7. Buttocks; relating to
8. Band or bundle
9. Trumpeter
10. Breastbone; key; breast; like

DOWN
1. Back of head; forehead; relating to
2. Chew; process
3. Lifter; of the shoulder blade (2 words)
4. Temple of head; relating to
5. Line; white (2 words)

 APPLYING WHAT YOU KNOW

31. Jack played football and was tackled so severely that he had "the wind knocked out of him," according to his coach. What muscles of respiration might have been temporarily affected by this tackle?

32. Alex broke his humerus while playing lacrosse. The break was healing well, but there was also significant damage to the brachialis muscle that concerned his doctor. Alex was referred to physical therapy for rehabilitation. What is the principle used to assess muscle action in a lever system? To assess brachialis muscle strength correctly, the forearm should be in what position?

DID YOU KNOW?

- The muscles of the hand begin to grow rapidly between 6 and 7 years of age.
- A cat has 32 muscles in each ear.

 ONE LAST QUICK CHECK

Matching—choose the proper answer for the muscles listed.

   a. sternocleidomastoid
   b. semispinalis capitis
   c. external intercostals
   d. diaphragm
   e. internal oblique
   f. erector spinal group
   g. quadratus lumborum
   h. levator ani
   i. zygomaticus major
   j. rectus abdominis

33. _____ bends head and neck laterally

34. _____ elevates ribs

35. _____ enlarges thorax

36. _____ "prayer" muscle

37. _____ provides important postural function

38. _____ flexes trunk

39. _____ depresses last rib

40. _____ extends vertebral column

41. _____ helps form the floor of the pelvic cavity

42. _____ assists in laughing

Fill in the blanks.

43. Fascicles are bound together into bundles by a tough connective tissue envelope called the _____.

44. _____ muscles have fascicles that radiate out from a small to a wider point of attachment, much like the blades in a fan.

45. The prime mover is also known as the _____.

46. When a muscle shortens, the central body portion called the _____ contracts.

47. Lever systems have four component parts: (1) a lever, (2) a fulcrum, (3) a load, and (4) a _____.

48. During _____ the diaphragm flattens.

49. The muscular pelvic floor filling the diamond-shaped outlet is called the _____.

50. A _____ is any rigid bar free to turn about a fixed point called its *fulcrum*.

51. The *deltoid* is so-named because of its descriptive _____.

52. The powerful muscles that either elevate or retract the mandible are the _____ and the _____.

CHAPTER 16

Appendicular Muscles

After mastering a basic knowledge of the axial muscles, you should now progress to the study of the appendicular muscles. The appendicular muscles control the movements of the upper and lower limbs, the pectoral girdle, and the pelvic girdle.

As mentioned in the last chapter, the muscular system is often referred to as the "power system," and rightfully so, because it is this system that provides the force necessary to move the body and perform organic functions. Just as an automobile relies on the engine to provide motion, the body depends on the muscular system to perform both voluntary and involuntary types of movements. The power of this system is impressive indeed, for if we were able to direct all of our muscles in one direction, it is estimated that we would have the power to move 25 tons.

After reviewing and mastering the appendicular muscles, you will progress to the next chapter to learn how muscles contract and how they contribute to our survival.

I—UPPER LIMB MUSCLES

Multiple Choice—select the best answer.

1. All of the following are rotator cuff muscles *except:*
   a. deltoid.
   b. infraspinatus.
   c. supraspinatus.
   d. teres minor.

2. The muscle that shrugs the shoulders is the:
   a. sternocleidomastoid.
   b. deltoid.
   c. trapezius.
   d. pectoralis minor.

3. The posterior arm muscle that extends the forearm is the:
   a. triceps brachii.
   b. triceps surae.
   c. brachialis.
   d. biceps brachii.

4. The olecranon of the ulna is a site of insertion for the:
   a. biceps brachii.
   b. brachialis.
   c. brachioradialis.
   d. triceps brachii.

True or False

5. _____ Intrinsic muscles of the hand originate on the forearm and insert on the metacarpals.

6. _____ Carpal tunnel syndrome affects the median nerve.

7. _____ The deltoid is a good example of a multifunctional muscle.

8. _____ The pectoralis major flexes the upper arm.

9. _____ The biceps brachii is an extensor muscle.

Labeling—using the terms provided, label the following illustrations. Some terms may be used more than once.

levator scapulae
serratus anterior
rhomboid major
teres minor
seventh cervical vertebra
teres major (cut)
latissimus dorsi (cut)

rhomboid minor
trapezius
pectoralis minor (cut)
pectoralis minor
subscapularis
latissimus dorsi

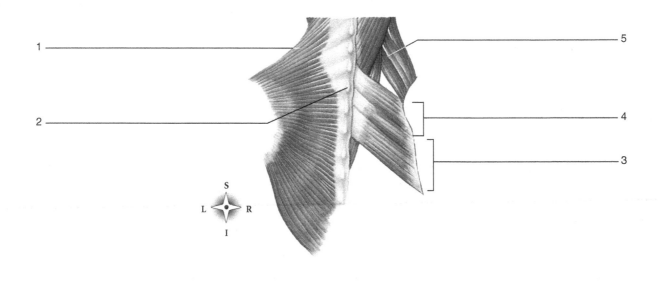

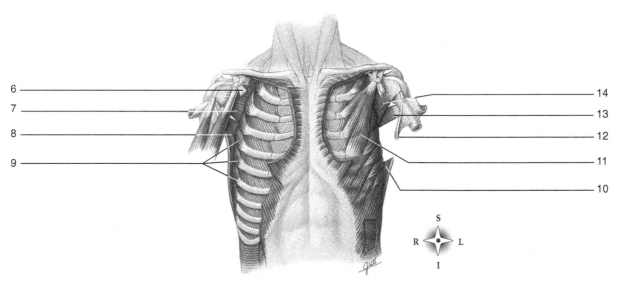

Muscles acting on the shoulder girdle.

Labeling—using the terms provided, label the following illustration.

subscapularis
acromion process
coracoid process
greater tubercle
intertubercular (bicipital) groove
teres minor

humerus
supraspinatus
lesser tubercle
infraspinatus
clavicle

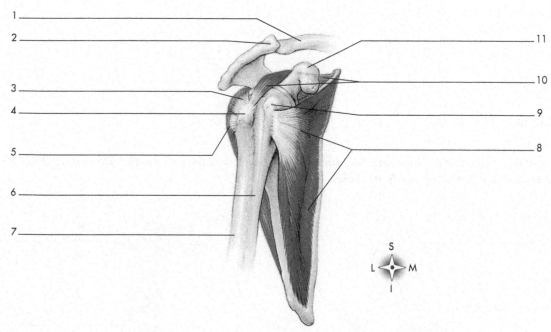

Rotator cuff muscles.

Labeling—label the following illustrations.

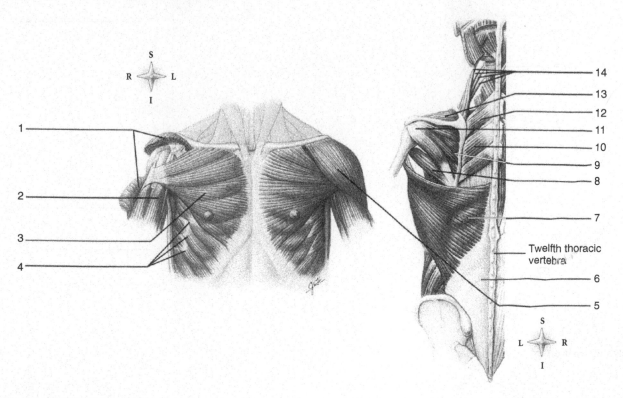

Twelfth thoracic vertebra

Muscles that move the upper arm.

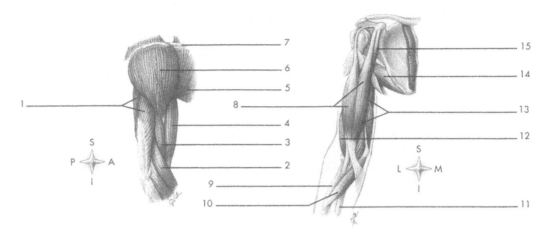

Muscles of the upper arm.

Labeling—on the following illustrations, label the muscles that act on the forearm. Also label the origin and insertion point of each muscle.

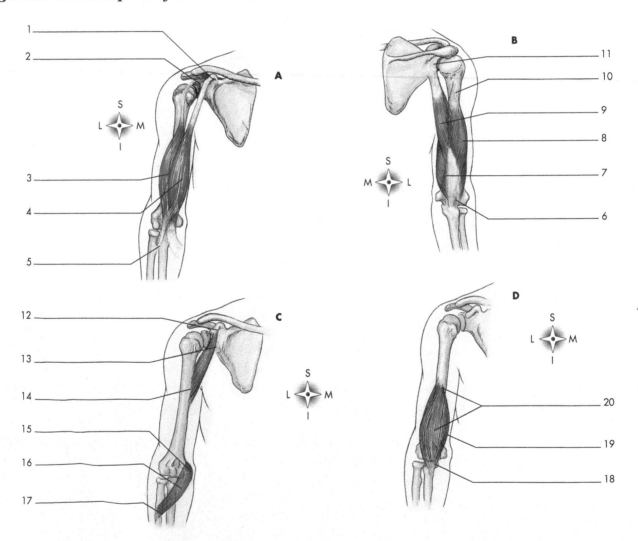

Muscles that act on the forearm.

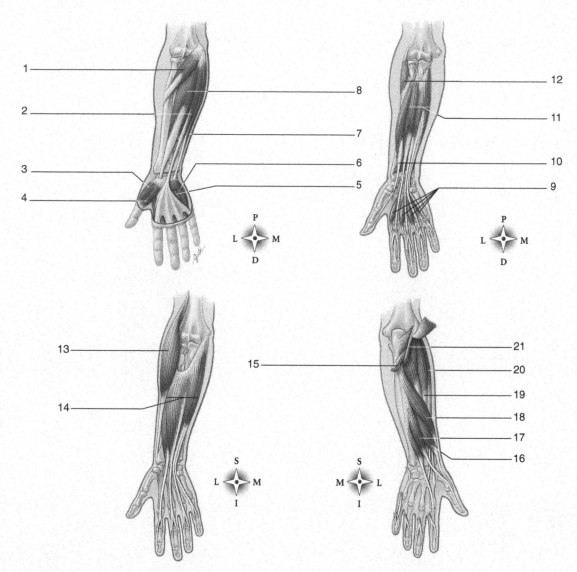

Muscles of the forearm.

 If you had difficulty with this section, review pages 337-348.

II—LOWER LIMB MUSCLES

Multiple Choice—select the best answer.

10. The muscles of the quadriceps femoris include all of the following *except:*
    a. vastus intermedius.
    b. vastus medialis.
    c. vastus lateralis.
    d. vastus femoris.

11. The anterior superior iliac spine is the site of origin for the:
    a. sartorius.
    b. rectus femoris.
    c. gracilis.
    d. iliacus.

12. A common site for intramuscular injections is the:
    a. gluteus maximus.
    b. gluteus minimus.
    c. gluteus medius.
    d. tensor fasciae latae.

13. Plantar flexion of the foot is achieved by the:
    a. tibialis anterior.
    b. tibialis posterior.
    c. peroneus brevis.
    d. soleus.

14. The muscles of the hamstrings include all of the following *except* the:
    a. iliopsoas.
    b. semitendinosus.
    c. semimembranosus.
    d. biceps femoris.

True or False

15. _____ The Achilles tendon is common to both the gastrocnemius and soleus.

16. _____ The iliopsoas is composed solely of the psoas major and the iliacus.

17. _____ The vastus intermedius originates on the posterior surface of the femur.

Labeling—label the following illustrations.

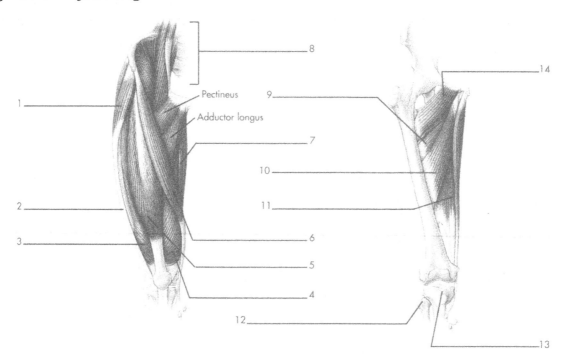

Pectineus

Adductor longus

Muscles of the thigh.

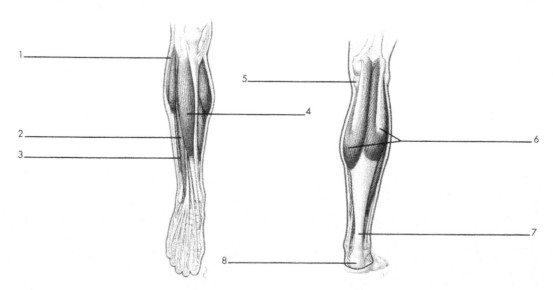

Muscles of the lower leg.

 If you had difficulty with this section, review pages 349-360.

CROSSWORD PUZZLE

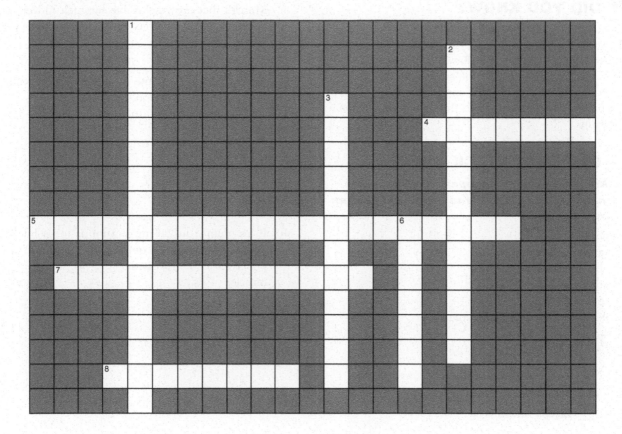

ACROSS
4. Position
5. Wrist; relating to; together; running or (race) course (3 words)
7. Belly; leg
8. Stretch or tension; relating to; state

DOWN
1. Shinbone; relating to; front; more; quality (2 words)
2. Pulled tight; together; egg white; inflammation
3. Sole of foot; mouse; little (2 words)
6. Triangle; like

 APPLYING WHAT YOU KNOW

18. Mr. Lynch spends hours typing on his computer. As of late, he is experiencing weakness, pain, and tingling in the palm and radial aspect of the hand. What condition may he be experiencing? Which anatomical structures are most likely involved? Which options for treatment are available?

19. The nurse was preparing an injection for Mrs. Tatakis. The amount to be given was 2 mL. What area of the body will the nurse most likely select for the injection?

20. Al is analyzing the musculature involved in the athletes he coaches. Today he is observing a basketball player executing a jump shot. Which muscles are involved at the hips, knees, and ankles as the athlete jumps? Which muscles are involved at the shoulders, elbows, and wrists as the athlete shoots the basketball?

DID YOU KNOW?

- Muscles cannot push, they can only pull. The reason the arm can push is because of muscles in the back of the arm pulling on the elbow!
- The smallest muscles, like the smallest bones, are found in the middle ear. Examples of these are the tensor tympani (connected to the eardrum) and the stapedius.

 ONE LAST QUICK CHECK

Matching—choose the proper function(s) for the muscles listed. Each may have more than one answer.

a. flexor
b. extensor
c. abductor
d. adductor
e. rotator
f. dorsiflexor or plantar flexor

21. _____ Trapezius

22. _____ Rhomboid major

23. _____ Gastrocnemius

24. _____ Biceps brachii

25. _____ Gluteus medius

26. _____ Soleus

27. _____ Iliopsoas

28. _____ Pectoralis major

29. _____ Gluteus maximus

30. _____ Triceps brachii

31. _____ Deltoid

32. _____ Fibularis longus

33. _____ Gracilis

Fill in the blanks.

34. Muscles that are responsible for such movements as dorsiflexion, plantar flexion, inversion, and eversion of the foot are the _____ _____ _____.

35. Another common name for the calcaneal tendon is the _____ tendon.

The rotator cuff muscles are:

36. _____

37. _____

38. _____ _____

39. _____

40. If less than 2 mL of medication is to be injected into the muscle, the common muscle that is preferred as the site is the_____ muscle.

CHAPTER 17

Muscle Contraction

Although the muscular system has several functions, the primary purpose is to provide movement or power. Muscles produce power by contracting. The ability of a large muscle or muscle group to contract depends on the ability of microscopic muscle fibers to contract within the larger muscle. To accomplish the mechanism of contraction, muscle fibers progress through a series of events during excitation of the sarcolemma, contraction and relaxation.

Three types of muscles provide us with a variety of motions. When skeletal or voluntary muscles contract, they provide movement of bones, heat production, and posture. Smooth muscles are found throughout the viscera of our body and assist with involuntary functions such as peristalsis. Cardiac muscle is the third and final type. It makes up the wall of the heart and provides the pumping action necessary for life. Our muscles must be used to keep the body healthy and in good condition. Scientific evidence keeps pointing to the fact that the proper use and exercise of muscles may prolong life. An understanding of the structure and function of the muscular system may, therefore, add quality and quantity to our lives.

I—FUNCTION OF SKELETAL MUSCLE TISSUE

Multiple Choice—select the best answer.

1. Which of the following is *not* a general function of muscle tissue?
   a. movement
   b. protection
   c. heat production
   d. posture

2. The skeletal muscle fiber characteristic of *excitability* directly results in these cells being capable of:
   a. responding to nerve signals.
   b. shortening.
   c. returning to resting length after contracting.
   d. producing heat.

3. The correct order of arrangement of skeletal muscle cells, from largest to smallest, is:
   a. fiber, myofibril, myofilament.
   b. myofibril, myofilament, fiber.
   c. myofilament, myofibril, fiber.
   d. fiber, myofilament, myofibril.

4. Sarcoplasmic reticulum is:
   a. a system of transverse tubules that extend at a right angle to the long axis of the cell.
   b. a segment of the myofibril between two successive Z lines.
   c. a unique name for the plasma membrane of a muscle fiber.
   d. none of the above.

5. Which of the following are myofilament proteins?
   a. troponin
   b. tropomyosin
   c. a and b
   d. none of the above

6. The contractile unit of a myofibril is the:
   a. sarcomere.
   b. triad.
   c. sarcolemma.
   d. cross-bridge.

7. The chief function of the T tubule is to:
   a. provide nutrients to the muscle fiber.
   b. allow the fiber to contract.
   c. allow the electrical signal to move deep into the cell.
   d. allow the generation of new muscle fibers.

8. Myosin heads are also called:
   a. cross-bridges.
   b. motor endplates.
   c. synapses.
   d. motor neurons.

9. During muscle contraction, Ca^{++} is released from the:
   a. synaptic cleft.
   b. mitochondria.
   c. sarcoplasmic reticulum.
   d. sarcoplasm.

10. The region of a muscle fiber where a motor neuron connects to the muscle fiber is called the:
    a. synaptic vesicle.
    b. motor endplate.
    c. H band.
    d. none of the above.

True or False

11. _____ The thick myofilament is made up of myosin.

12. _____ Skeletal muscle has a poor ability to stretch.

13. _____ A T tubule sandwiched between sacs of sarcoplasmic reticulum is called a *codon*.

14. _____ Actin, troponin, and tropomyosin are present on the thin myofilament.

15. _____ The I band resides within a single sarcomere.

16. _____ Rigor mortis is caused by a lack of ATP to "turn off" muscle contraction.

17. _____ The cell membrane of a muscle fiber is called the *sarcoplasmic reticulum*.

18. _____ Anaerobic respiration is the first choice of the muscle cell for the production of ATP.

19. _____ During rest, excess oxygen molecules in the sarcoplasm are attracted to a large protein molecule called *myoglobin*.

20. _____ Anaerobic respiration results in the formation of an incompletely catabolized molecule called *lactic acid*.

Labeling—match each term with its corresponding number on the following diagram of the structure of skeletal muscle. The answer blanks are on page 109.

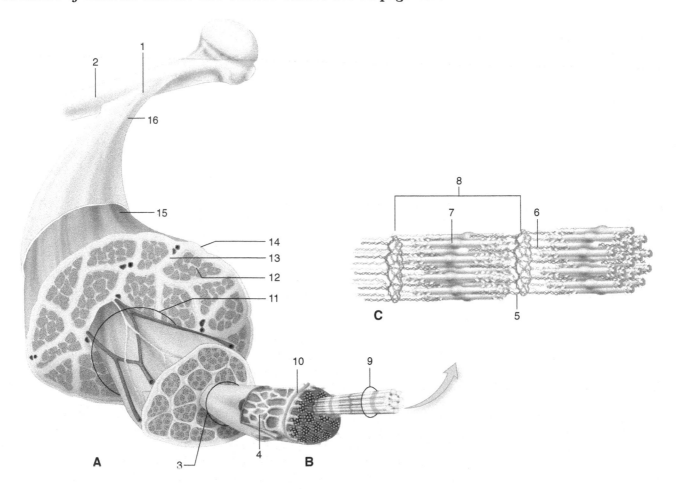

_____ sarcomere
_____ sarcoplasmic reticulum
_____ myofibril
_____ thin filament
_____ bone
_____ T tubule
_____ fascicle
_____ fascia

_____ muscle fiber (muscle cell)
_____ perimysium
_____ epimysium
_____ Z disk
_____ thick filament
_____ tendon
_____ endomysium
_____ muscle

Labeling—using the terms provided, label the following diagrams.

sarcoplasm
synaptic vesicles (continuing Ach)
sarcoplasmic reticulum
motor neuron fiber
Ach receptor sites
Schwann cell
motor endplate

sarcomere
sarcolemma
myelin sheath
synaptic cleft
myofibril
mitochondria
T tubule

1 _____
2 _____
3 _____
4 _____
5 _____
6 _____
8 _____
7 _____

Neuromuscular junction.

9 _____
15 _____
10 _____
11 _____
12 _____
14 _____
13 _____

Skeletal muscle cell.

 If you had difficulty with this section, review pages 362-373.

II—FUNCTION OF SKELETAL MUSCLE ORGANS

Multiple Choice—select the best answer.

21. The principal component(s) of a motor unit is/are:
    a. one somatic motor neuron.
    b. the muscle fibers supplied by a somatic motor neuron.
    c. none of the above.
    d. both a and b.

22. The staircase phenomenon is also known as:
    a. tetanus.
    b. electromyography.
    c. wave summation.
    d. treppe.

23. Skeletal muscles are innervated by:
    a. somatic motor neurons.
    b. autonomic motor neurons.
    c. both a and b.
    d. internal stimulation.

24. Which of the following statements concerning isometric contractions is true?
    a. The length of the muscle changes.
    b. Muscle tension decreases.
    c. Joint movements are swift.
    d. Muscle length remains constant.

25. Physiologic muscle fatigue is caused by:
    a. relative lack of ATP.
    b. oxygen debt.
    c. lack of will.
    d. none of the above.

26. Increase in muscle size is called:
    a. hyperplasia.
    b. atrophy.
    c. hypertrophy.
    d. treppe.

27. Endurance training is also called:
    a. isometrics.
    b. hypertrophy.
    c. aerobic training.
    d. anaerobic training.

True or False

28. _____ A muscle contracts the instant it is stimulated.

29. _____ Isotonic contraction is one in which the tone or tension within a muscle remains the same, but the length of the muscle changes.

30. _____ One method of studying muscle contraction is called *myography*.

31. _____ Muscles with more tone than normal are described as *flaccid*.

Labeling—using the terms provided, label the following illustration of a motor unit.

myofibrils
neuromuscular junction
nucleus
motor neuron

myelin sheath
muscle fibers
Schwann cell

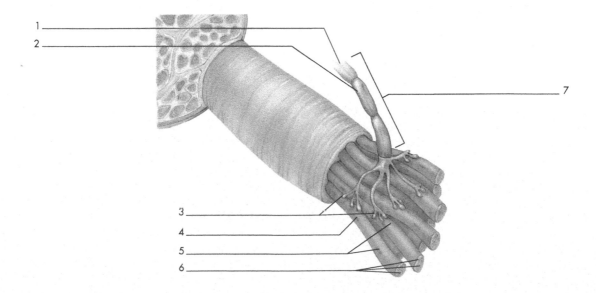

⊙ *If you had difficulty with this section, review pages 373-380.*

III—FUNCTION OF CARDIAC AND SMOOTH MUSCLE TISSUE

Matching—identify each muscle tissue with its corresponding characteristics.

a. cardiac muscle tissue
b. skeletal muscle tissue
c. smooth muscle tissue

32. _____ located in the walls of hollow organs

33. _____ contains many nuclei near the sarcolemma

34. _____ voluntary

35. _____ not striated

36. _____ striated; contains a single nucleus

37. _____ a principal function: peristalsis

38. _____ has larger-diameter T tubules that form diads with sarcoplasmic reticulum

39. _____ principal functions: movement of bones, heat production, and posture

40. _____ contains intercalated disks

41. _____ has loosely organized sarcoplasmic reticulum

Labeling—label the following diagram of a cardiac muscle fiber.

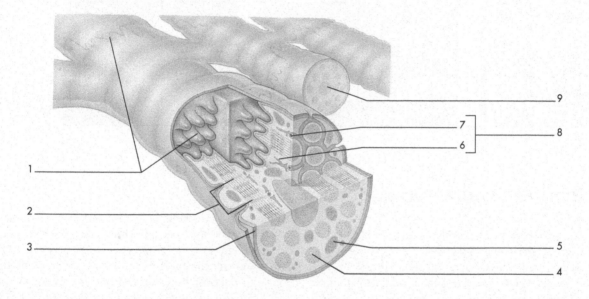

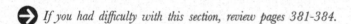

➤ *If you had difficulty with this section, review pages 381-384.*

IV—MECHANISMS OF DISEASE

Circle the correct answer.

42. Muscle strains are characterized by (myalgia or fibromyositis).

43. Crush injuries can cause (hemoglobin or myoglobin) to accumulate in the blood and result in kidney failure.

44. A viral infection of the nerves that control skeletal muscle movement is known as (poliomyelitis or muscular dystrophy).

45. (Muscular dystrophy or myasthenia gravis) is a group of genetic diseases characterized by atrophy of skeletal muscle tissues.

46. (Muscular dystrophy or myasthenia gravis) is an autoimmune disease in which the immune system attacks muscle cells at the neuromuscular junction.

➤ *If you had difficulty with this section, review pages 384-385.*

CROSSWORD PUZZLE

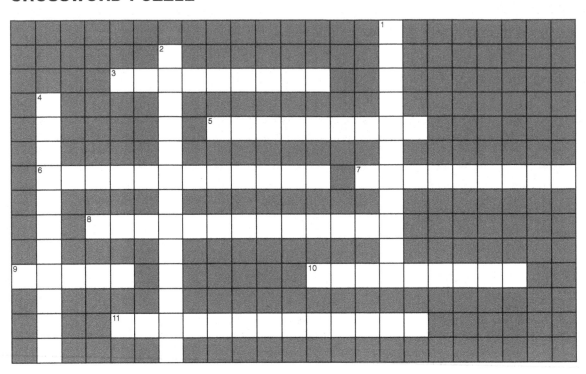

ACROSS
3. Muscle; ball; substance
5. Muscle; fiber; little
6. Arouse; capable; state
7. Flesh; part
8. Vinegar; bile; made of
9. To stretch; relating to
10. Bruise; result
11. Outward; stretch; capable; state

DOWN
1. Muscle; thread; thing
2. Together; drag or draw; of or like; quality of
4. Excessive; nourishment; state

 APPLYING WHAT YOU KNOW

47. Throughout Linda's life, she wanted to be a star in the 100-meter dash. However, no matter how hard she trained, she could never excel in this sport. On the other hand, she *did* achieve great success in much longer track events, especially the 10-kilometer race. Explain Linda's situation from the aspect of which skeletal muscle fiber type she may possess disproportionately by virtue of her genetics.

48. John is working in a hospital while he is studying to become a physician. One of his duties is to transport recently deceased patients to the morgue. While moving the patients onto the gurney, he is surprised to discover how stiff the bodies can be. Which physiologic phenomenon is responsible for this stiffness? Exactly why is it that these muscles can temporarily display stiffness?

? DID YOU KNOW?

- The simple act of walking requires the use of 200 muscles in the human body.
- People who are on bedrest or totally inactive lose approximately 1% of muscle strength per day.

✓ ONE LAST QUICK CHECK

Multiple Choice—select the best answer.

49. When a muscle does not shorten and no movement results, the contraction is:
    a. isometric.
    b. isotonic.
    c. twitch.
    d. tetanic.

50. Pushing against a wall is an example of which type of contraction?
    a. isotonic
    b. isometric
    c. twitch
    d. tetanic

51. Prolonged inactivity causes muscles to shrink in mass, a condition called:
    a. hypertrophy.
    b. disuse atrophy.
    c. paralysis.
    d. muscle fatigue.

52. Muscle fibers usually contract to about _____% of their starting length.
    a. 50
    b. 60
    c. 70
    d. 80

53. Which statement is true of smooth muscle?
    a. It lines the walls of many hollow organs.
    b. It is striated.
    c. It is voluntary.
    d. There are many T tubules throughout smooth muscle.

54. What is a quick, jerky response of a given muscle to a single stimulus called?
    a. isometric
    b. lockjaw
    c. tetanus
    d. twitch

True or False

55. _____ The energy required for muscular contraction is obtained by hydrolysis of amino acids.

56. _____ A motor neuron together with the cells it innervates is called a *motor unit.*

57. _____ If muscle cells are stimulated repeatedly without adequate periods of rest, the strength of the muscle contraction will decrease, resulting in fatigue.

58. _____ The minimum level of stimulation required to cause a fiber to contract is called the *threshold stimulus.*

59. _____ Weakness of abdominal muscles can lead to a hernia.

60. _____ There are two types of smooth muscle: visceral and multiunit.

61. _____ Cardiac muscle is also known as *striated involuntary.*

62. _____ The length/tension relationship states that the maximal strength a muscle can develop is related to the length of the fibers.

63. _____ Skeletal muscles have little effect on body temperature.

CHAPTER 18

Nervous System Cells

The nervous system organizes and coordinates the millions of stimuli received each day to make communication with and enjoyment of our environment possible. There are two main classes of cells that compose the nervous system: neurons and glia. Neurons process information, and glia provide neurons with mechanical and metabolic support.

Three types of neurons exist—sensory, motor, and interneurons—which are classified according to the direction in which they transmit impulses. Nerve impulses travel over routes made up of neurons and provide the rapid communication necessary for maintaining life.

The other main classification of cells in the nervous system is glia. Unlike neurons, glia cells do not conduct impulses but instead support the neurons in various ways. Glia means "glue," but glia do far more than provide the "glue" or support for the nervous system. They also supply nutrients and oxygen to neurons, insulate one neuron from another, destroy pathogens, and remove dead neurons. Five major types of glia are astrocytes, microglia, ependymal cells, oligo-dendrocytes, and Schwann cells. An understanding of the basic cells of the nervous system is necessary before you can study the complex and critical signaling and transmission of stimuli throughout the nervous system.

I—ORGANIZATION OF THE NERVOUS SYSTEM

Matching—identify each part of the nervous system with its definition.

- a. afferent division
- b. autonomic nervous system
- c. central nervous system
- d. efferent nervous system
- e. parasympathetic division
- f. peripheral nervous system
- g. somatic nervous system
- h. sympathetic division

1. _____ consists of the brain and spinal cord

2. _____ composed of nerves arising from the brain and spinal cord

3. _____ PNS subdivision that transmits incoming information from the sensory organs to the CNS

4. _____ produces the "fight or flight" response

5. _____ subdivision that carries information from the CNS to skeletal muscle

6. _____ subdivision of efferent division that transmits information to smooth muscle, cardiac muscle, and glands

7. _____ consists of all outgoing motor pathways

8. _____ coordinates the body's normal resting activities

➤ *If you had difficulty with this section, review pages 393-395.*

II—GLIA, NEURONS, AND REFLEX ARC

Matching—identify each type of cell with its characteristics. Answers may be used more than once.

- a. astrocyte
- b. microglia
- c. oligodendrocyte
- d. Schwann cell

9. _____ has the ability of phagocytosis

10. _____ helps to form the blood-brain barrier

11. _____ produces fatty myelin sheath in the PNS

12. _____ largest and most numerous of the neuroglial cells

13. _____ produces myelin sheath in the CNS

14. _____ type of neuroglia that forms the neurilemma

15. _____ "star cell"

16. _____ disorder of this cell associated with multiple sclerosis

Multiple Choice—select the best answer.

17. Which of the following is/are classified as nerve fibers?
    a. axon
    b. dendrites
    c. both a and b
    d. none of the above

18. Which of the following conduct impulses toward the cell body?
    a. axons
    b. dendrites
    c. Nissl bodies
    d. none of the above

19. A neuron with one axon and several dendrites is a:
    a. multipolar neuron.
    b. unipolar neuron.
    c. bipolar neuron.
    d. none of the above.

20. Which type of neuron lies entirely within the CNS?
    a. afferent
    b. efferent
    c. interneuron
    d. none of the above

21. Which sequence best represents the course of an impulse over a reflex arc?
    a. receptor, synapse, sensory neuron, motor neuron, effector
    b. effector, sensory neuron, synapse, motor neuron, receptor
    c. receptor, motor neuron, synapse, sensory neuron, effector
    d. receptor, sensory neuron, interneuron, motor neuron, effector

Labeling—label the following illustration showing the structure of a typical neuron.

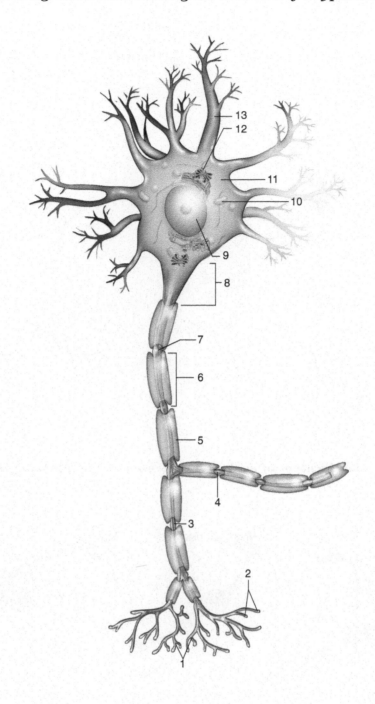

1. _____

2. _____

3. _____

4. _____

5. _____

6. _____

7. _____

8. _____

9. _____

10. _____

11. _____

12. _____

13. _____

Labeling—using the terms provided, label the following illustration of a myelinated axon.

neurilemma (sheath of Schwann cell)   myelin sheath
plasma membrane of axon   node of Ranvier
nucleus of Schwann cell   neurofibrils, microfilaments, and microtubules

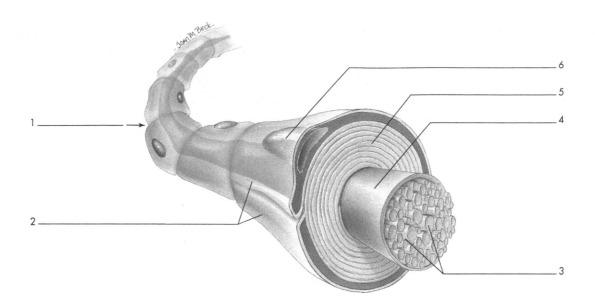

Labeling—identify the classification of each type of neuron in the following illustrations.

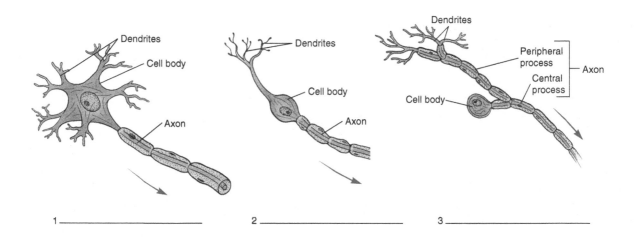

1 _____   2 _____   3 _____

Labeling—using the terms provided, label the following illustration of a reflex arc.

motor neuron axon
cell body
interneuron
dendrite
spinal nerve

sensory neuron axon
white matter
synapse
gray matter

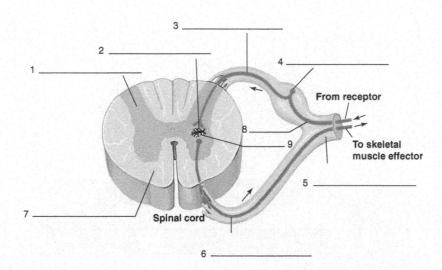

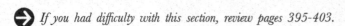

➔ *If you had difficulty with this section, review pages 395-403.*

III—NERVES AND TRACTS

Multiple Choice—select the best answer.

22. A complete nerve, consisting of numerous fascicles and their blood supply, is held together by a fibrous coat called the:
    a. endoneurium.
    b. perineurium.
    c. epineurium.
    d. fascicles.

23. Small, distinct regions of gray matter within the CNS are usually called:
    a. white matter.
    b. nuclei.
    c. ganglia.
    d. fascicles.

24. Nerves that contain mostly efferent fibers are called:
    a. sensory nerves.
    b. motor nerves.
    c. mixed nerves.
    d. Schwann nerves.

25. Gray matter in the CNS consists of:
    a. nerve fibers.
    b. neuroglia.
    c. axons.
    d. cell bodies.

26. Most nerves in the human nervous system are:
    a. sensory nerves.
    b. motor nerves.
    c. mixed nerves.
    d. reflex nerves.

➔ *If you had difficulty with this section, review page 404.*

IV—REPAIR OF NERVE FIBERS

True or False

27. _____ Evidence now indicates that neurons may be replaced.

28. _____ Regeneration of nerve fibers will occur if the cell body is intact and the fibers have a neurilemma.

29. _____ There are no differences between the CNS and PNS concerning the repair of damaged fibers.

➔ *If you had difficulty with this section, review pages 403-406.*

V—MECHANISMS OF DISEASE

Fill in the blanks.

30. _____ _____ is a disorder of the nervous system that involves the glia, rather than neurons.

31. _____ is a common type of brain tumor that is usually benign but may still be life-threatening.

32. A highly malignant form of astrocytic tumor is known as _____ _____.

33. An inherited glial disease characterized by numerous benign fibrous neuromas throughout the body is known as _____ _____.

34. Most disorders of the nervous system cells involve _____ rather than neurons.

→ *If you had difficulty with this section, review page 407.*

CROSSWORD PUZZLE

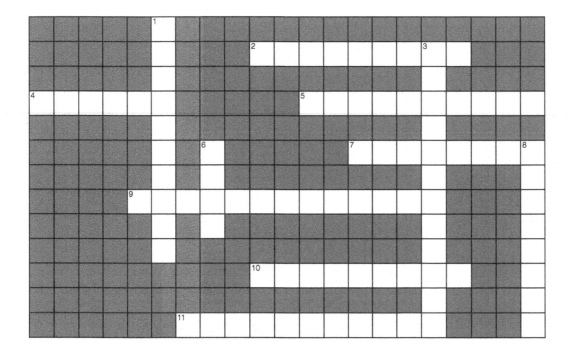

ACROSS
2. Star-shaped cell
4. Marrow; substance
5. Neuron; sheath
7. Tree; part (branch) of
9. Two; pole; relating to; nerve (2 words)
10. Small; glue
11. Between; nerve

DOWN
1. Upon; nerve; thing
3. End; part (branch) of
6. Axle
8. Away; carry; relating to

APPLYING WHAT YOU KNOW

35. Jim is experiencing muscular weakness, loss of coordination, visual impairment, and speech disturbances. Which disease of the CNS could he be experiencing? Which nervous tissue cells are most likely involved? What specifically occurs to both the neurons and neuroglia of the CNS? What are the possible treatments and what are the theories as to the cause of this disease?

36. Lee Roy is a professional football player who, as a result of a severe compression blow to the head, lost the ability to move his lower body. He was rushed to the hospital, where the doctors suspected crushing and bruising of the spinal cord. What are the chances of the damaged nervous tissue repairing itself?

 DID YOU KNOW?

- In the adult human body, there are 46 miles of nerves.
- The longest cells in the human body are the motor neurons. They can be up to 4.5 feet (1.37 meters) long and run from the lower spinal cord to the big toe.
- There are more nerve cells in the human brain than there are stars in the Milky Way.

 ONE LAST QUICK CHECK

Circle the correct answer.

37. The somatic motor division carries information to the (skeletal or smooth) muscles.

38. Incoming sensory pathways are (afferent or efferent).

39. The (sympathetic or parasympathetic) division coordinates the body's normal resting activities and is sometimes referred to as the "rest and repair" division.

40. The myelin sheath is produced by (ependymal or oligodendrocytes) in the CNS.

41. The (Schwann cells or microglia) are found only in peripheral neurons.

42. Myelin sheath gaps are often called (nodes of Ranvier or neurilemma).

43. Energy for the neuron is provided by (mitochondria or Golgi apparatus).

44. Myelinated fibers are (white or gray).

45. (Interneurons or efferent neurons) lie entirely within the central nervous system.

46. All electrical signals that start in receptors (do or do not) invariably travel over a complete reflex arc and terminate in effectors.

Matching—select the best choice for the following words and insert the correct letter in the blanks.

   a. neurons
   b. neuroglia

47. _____ axon

48. _____ supporting cells

49. _____ astrocytes

50. _____ sensory

51. _____ conduct impulses

52. _____ form the myelin sheath around central nerve fibers

53. _____ phagocytosis

54. _____ efferent

55. _____ multiple sclerosis

56. _____ multipolar

CHAPTER 19
Nerve Signaling

It is critical for nerves to be able to transfer information quickly and efficiently. Within about seven milliseconds an impulse travels through a neuron and is transmitted to the next neuron. A nerve impulse response is similar to a light switch. It is either on or off. If a stimulus is strong enough, it will trigger a programmed response, but increasing the strength of the stimulus beyond this point will not increase the intensity of the response. A weak stimulus will not trigger a response at all.

Conducting impulses is only one of the complex tasks assigned to neurons. Interneurons located within the central nervous system (brain and spinal cord) are capable of remembering or learning new responses, generating rational and creative thought, and implementing many other complex processes.

Your study of nerve signaling and transmission begins with the simplest concept of impulse conduction, known as the *reflex arc*, and progresses to the more complex pathways that often occur in the divergence/convergence of neural networks. The coordination of nerve cells, signaling, and transmission is critical to the communication and responses of impulses necessary for life.

I—ELECTRICAL NATURE OF NEURONS

Multiple Choice—select the best answer.

1. Compared with the inside of the cell, the outside of most cell membranes is:
   a. positive.
   b. negative.
   c. equal.
   d. none of the above.

2. The difference in electrical charge across a plasma membrane is called:
   a. depolarization.
   b. membrane potential.
   c. both a and b.
   d. none of the above.

3. A neuron's resting membrane potential is:
   a. 70 mV.
   b. −70 mV.
   c. 30 mV.
   d. −30 mV.

4. Which of the following statements is true concerning the sodium-potassium pump?
   a. Three sodium ions are pumped out of the neuron for every two potassium ions pumped into the neuron.
   b. Two sodium ions are pumped out of the neuron for every three potassium ions pumped into the neuron.
   c. Three sodium ions are pumped out of the neuron for every three chloride ions pumped into the neuron.
   d. Three sodium ions are pumped out of the neuron for every three potassium ions pumped into the neuron.

True or False

5. _____ A membrane that exhibits a membrane potential is said to be *polarized*.

6. _____ A slight shift away from the resting membrane potential in a specific region of the plasma membrane is often called a *stimulus-gated channel*.

7. _____ Chlorine ions (Cl^-) are the dominant extracellular cations.

→ *If you had difficulty with this section, review pages 413-414.*

II—ACTION POTENTIAL

Multiple Choice—select the best answer.

8. During a relative refractory period:
   a. an action potential is impossible.
   b. an action potential is possible only in response to a very strong stimuli.
   c. an action potential is occurring.
   d. none of the above.

9. Voltage-gated channels are:
   a. membrane channels that close during voltage fluctuations.
   b. ion channels that open in response to voltage fluctuations.
   c. membrane channels that are altered from an extremely high stimulus.
   d. none of the above.

10. When current leaps across an insulating myelin sheath from node of Ranvier to node of Ranvier, the type of impulse conduction is:
    a. repolarization.
    b. refraction.
    c. saltatory conduction.
    d. diffusion.

11. The larger the diameter of a nerve fiber:
    a. the slower the speed of conduction.
    b. the faster the speed of conduction.
    c. Fiber diameter does not influence speed of conduction.
    d. the more the speed fluctuates.

True or False

12. _____ Action potential and nerve impulse are synonymous.

13. _____ When repolarization has occurred, an impulse cannot be conducted.

14. _____ The action potential is an all-or-none response.

15. _____ Many anesthetics function by inhibiting the opening of sodium channels and thus blocking the initiation and conduction of nerve impulses.

➔ *If you had difficulty with this section, review pages 415-419.*

III—SYNAPTIC TRANSMISSION

Multiple Choice—select the best answer.

16. Which of the following structures is *not* a main component of a chemical synapse?
    a. synaptic knob
    b. synaptic cleft
    c. synaptic process
    d. plasma membrane of postsynaptic neuron

17. A synaptic knob is located on the:
    a. synaptic cleft.
    b. axon.
    c. dendrite.
    d. cell body.

18. Which of the following is true of spatial summation?
    a. Neurotransmitters released simultaneously from several presynaptic knobs converge on one postsynaptic neuron.
    b. Simultaneous stimulation of more than one postsynaptic neuron occurs.
    c. Impulses are fired in a rapid succession by the same neuron.
    d. Speed of impulse transmission is increased when several neurotransmitters are released.

True or False

19. _____ In an adult, the nervous system is replete with both electrical synapses and chemical synapses.

20. _____ Rapid-succession stimulation of a postsynaptic neuron by a synaptic knob can have a cumulative effect over time that can result in an action potential.

21. _____ Ca^{++} ions cause the release of neurotransmitters across the synaptic cleft.

Labeling—match each term with its corresponding number on the following illustration of a chemical synapse.

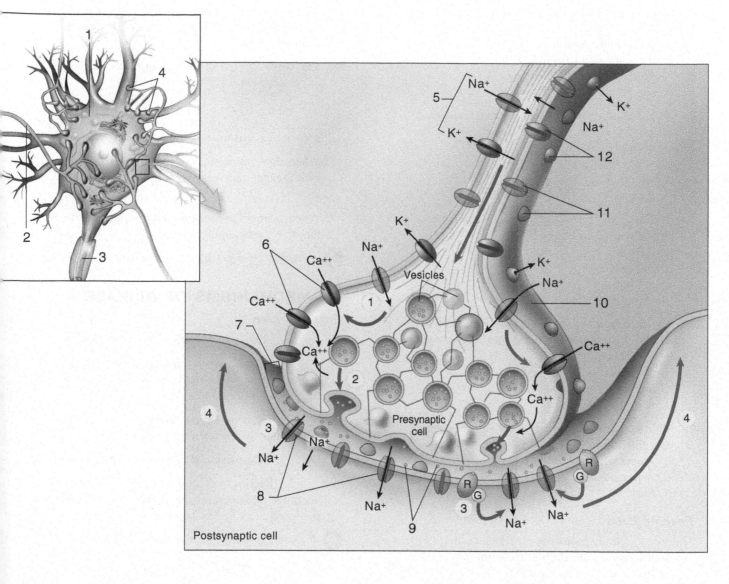

_____ axon of motor neuron

_____ synaptic knob

_____ stimulus-gated Na⁺ channels

_____ synaptic cleft

_____ action potential

_____ voltage-gated K⁺ channels

_____ axon of presynaptic neuron

_____ voltage-gated Ca⁺⁺ channels

_____ neurotransmitters

_____ voltage-gated Na⁺ channels

_____ motor neuron cell body

_____ synaptic knobs

➔ *If you had difficulty with this section, review pages 418-423.*

IV—NEUROTRANSMITTERS

Multiple Choice—select the best answer.

22. Neurotransmitters are released in a synapse and bind to:
    a. presynaptic terminals.
    b. the synaptic cleft.
    c. the base of the axon.
    d. receptors on the postsynaptic terminal.

23. The main chemical classes of neurotransmitters include all of the following *except:*
    a. acetylcholine.
    b. norepinephrine.
    c. amino acids.
    d. amines.

24. Which of the following is *not* an example of an amine neurotransmitter?
    a. serotonin
    b. histamine
    c. glycine
    d. dopamine

25. Severe depression can be caused by a deficit in which of the following neurotransmitters?
    a. acetylcholine
    b. amino acids
    c. amines
    d. neuropeptides

26. Which of the following is *not* a catecholamine?
    a. epinephrine
    b. norepinephrine
    c. dopamine
    d. serotonin

True or False

27. _____ Many biologists now believe that neuropeptides are the most common neurotransmitters in the CNS.

28. _____ Cocaine produces a temporary feeling of well-being by blocking the uptake of dopamine.

➡ *If you had difficulty with this section, review pages 424-428.*

V—NEURAL NETWORKS

Fill in the blanks

29. Neuroscience has advanced to a point at which the neuron doctrine has been expanded to include concepts of the _____ _____.

30. The concentration of neurotransmitters at synapses in certain neural pathways can affect _____.

31. _____ are nerve growth factors that are released by various cells of the body.

32. When more than one presynaptic axon synapses with a single postsynaptic neuron, _____ occurs.

33. When a single presynaptic axon synapses with many different postsynaptic neurons, _____occurs.

➡ *If you had difficulty with this section, review pages 429-430.*

VI—MECHANISMS OF DISEASE

True or False

34. _____ Multiple sclerosis is a myelin disorder.

35. _____ Physical injury, causing nerve damage, can cause local or widespread loss of sensation and/or motor control.

36. _____ Nerve conduction does not occur due to fluctuations in the concentration of ions.

37. _____ Myasthenia gravis is a bacterial disorder.

38. _____ Parkinson disease is a failure to release adequate dopamine at the synapse of certain motor pathways.

➡ *If you had difficulty with this section, review page 431.*

CROSSWORD PUZZLE

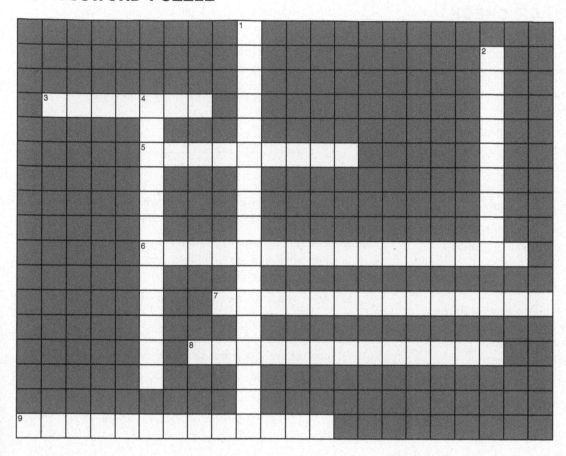

ACROSS
3. Together; join
5. Leap; relating to
6. Nerves; across; send; agent
7. Opposite; pole; relating to; process
8. Melt; alcohol; ammonia compound
9. Vinegar; bile; made of

DOWN
1. Thin skin; power; relating to (2 words)
2. Single; ammonia compound
4. After; together; join; relating to

 APPLYING WHAT YOU KNOW

39. Tracey was having a root canal procedure. Her dentist assured her that he would give her an anesthetic such as Marcaine that would keep her pain free the entire time. How does Marcaine prevent pain?

40. Susan was a cocaine abuser. Explain how the temporary feeling of well-being is achieved and the risk that abusing cocaine can be to the body.

 DID YOU KNOW?

- In the adult human body, there are 46 miles of nerves.
- The longest cells in the human body are the motor neurons. They can be up to 4.5 feet (1.37 meters) long and run from the lower spinal cord to the big toe.

ONE LAST QUICK CHECK

Circle the correct answer.

41. A synaptic knob is a tiny bulge at the end of the (presynaptic or postsynaptic) neuron's axon.

42. Acetylcholine is an example of a (neurotransmitter or protein molecule receptor).

43. Neurotransmitters are chemicals that allow neurons to (communicate or reproduce) with one another.

44. Neurotransmitters are distributed (randomly or specifically) into groups of neurons.

45. Endorphins and enkephalins are neurotransmitters that inhibit conduction of (fear or pain).

46. A synonym commonly used for action potential is (nerve impulse or depolarization).

47. In myelinated fibers, action potentials in the membrane occur only at the nodes of Ranvier. This type of impulse conduction is called (saltatory conduction or postsynaptic conduction).

48. A membrane that exhibits a membrane potential is said to be (polarized or myelinated)

Fill in the blanks.

49. A wave of electrical fluctuation that travels along the plasma membrane is called a _____ _____.

50. The membrane potential maintained by a nonconducting neuron's plasma membrane is called the _____ _____ _____ .

51. Movement of the membrane potential away from zero (thus below the usual RMP) is called _____.

Three structures make up a chemical synapse. They are: (52.) _____ _____, (53.) _____ _____, and the (54.) _____ _____.

55. Long-term memories (months or years) require _____ changes in the synapse, such as more vesicles or more vesicle release sites.

56. The unique neurotransmitter that combines acetate with choline is acetylcholine. It is deactivated by _____.

57. An example of a catecholamine is _____.

58. Two major function classifications of neurotransmitters are excitatory neurotransmitters and _____ _____.

True or False

59. _____ The function of a neurotransmitter is determined by the postsynaptic receptor.

60. _____ Neurotrophins stimulate neuron development but also can act as neurotransmitters or neuromodulators.

CHAPTER 20

Central Nervous System

Approximately one hundred billion neurons make up the brain. Everything we are and everything we hope to become are centered in this structure, which is about the size of a small bowling ball. Our personality, communication skills, memory, and sensations depend upon the successful functioning of the brain. We are still in the infancy of our knowledge of this unique organ, as it still holds many mysteries for scientists to uncover. We are fascinated by the fact that although all pain is felt and interpreted in the brain, the brain itself has no pain sensation—even when cut! This simple example illustrates the complexity of the brain and some of the challenges ahead in identifying and understanding its capabilities for our body.

The central nervous system (CNS) is made up of the spinal cord and brain. The spinal cord provides access to and from the brain by means of ascending and descending tracts. In addition, the spinal cord functions as the primary reflex center of the body. The brain consists of the brain stem, cerebellum, diencephalon, and cerebrum. These areas provide the extraordinary network necessary to receive, interpret, and respond to most stimuli. Your study of the CNS will give you an appreciation of the complex mechanisms necessary to perform your daily tasks.

I—COVERINGS OF THE BRAIN AND SPINAL CORD

Multiple Choice—select the best answer.

1. From superficial to deep, which is the correct order of location of the meninges?
   a. dura mater, arachnoid membrane, pia mater
   b. pia mater, arachnoid membrane, dura mater
   c. arachnoid membrane, pia mater, dura mater
   d. dura mater, pia mater, arachnoid membrane

2. The falx cerebri separates the:
   a. two hemispheres of the cerebellum.
   b. cerebellum from the cerebrum.
   c. two hemispheres of the cerebrum.
   d. dura mater from the arachnoid.

3. The cerebrospinal fluid resides in the:
   a. epidural space.
   b. subarachnoid space.
   c. subdural space.
   d. piarachnoid space.

4. The layer of the meninges that serves as the inner periosteum of the cranial bones is the:
   a. pia mater.
   b. arachnoid membrane.
   c. dura mater.

Labeling—label the coverings of the brain on the following diagram.

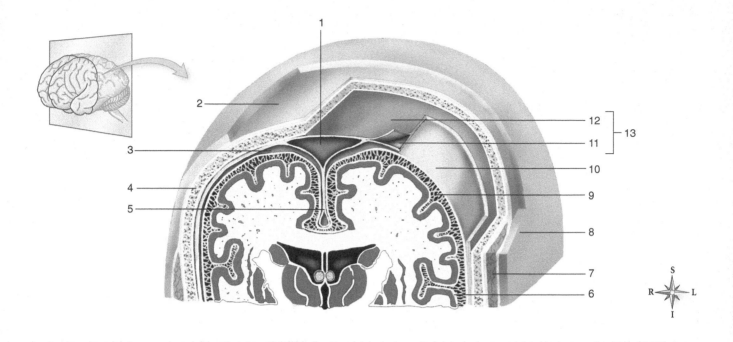

1. _____

2. _____

3. _____

4. _____

5. _____

6. _____

7. _____

8. _____

9. _____

10. _____

11. _____

12. _____

13. _____

➜ *If you had difficulty with this section, review pages 436-439.*

II—CEREBROSPINAL FLUID

Multiple Choice—select the best answer.

5. Formation of the cerebrospinal fluid (CSF) occurs mainly in the:
   a. cerebral aqueduct.
   b. superior sagittal sinus.
   c. choroid plexuses.
   d. median foramen.

6. The lateral ventricles are located within the:
   a. cerebrum.
   b. cerebellum.
   c. spinal cord.
   d. none of the above.

7. CSF is absorbed into the venous blood via the:
   a. cisterna magna.
   b. choroid plexus.
   c. falx cerebri.
   d. arachnoid villus.

8. CSF is *not* found in the:
   a. central canal.
   b. subarachnoid space.
   c. third ventricle.
   d. subdural space.

True or False

9. _____ The four large, fluid-filled spaces within the brain are called ventricles.

10. _____ Interference of CSF circulation, causing the fluid to accumulate in the subarachnoid space, is referred to as external hydrocephalus.

Labeling—label the following illustration of the fluid spaces of the brain.

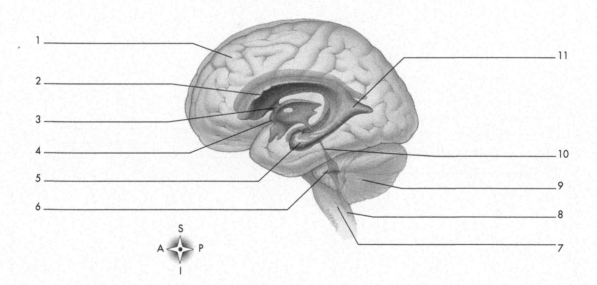

Labeling—using the terms provided, label the following illustrations depicting the flow of CSF and the layers of the brain.

cerebral aqueduct
cisterna magna
superior sagittal sinus (venous blood)
choroid plexus of third ventricle
subarachnoid space
falx cerebri (dura mater)
pia mater
choroid plexus of fourth ventricle
cerebral cortex

dura mater
arachnoid villus
choroid plexus of lateral ventricle
interventricular foramen
median foramen
central canal of spinal cord
lateral foramen
arachnoid layer

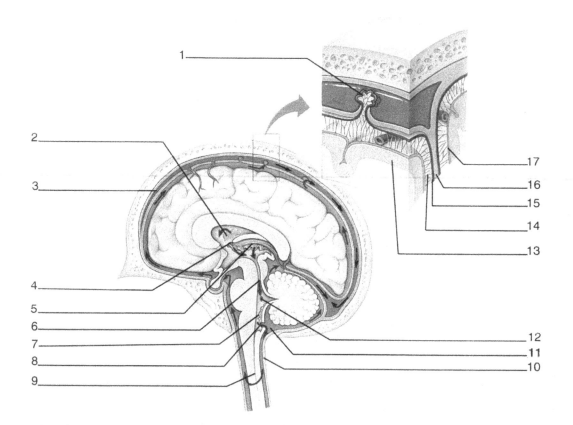

➡️ *If you had difficulty with this section, review pages 439-442.*

III—THE SPINAL CORD

Matching—identify each ascending, or sensory, tract with its corresponding function.

  a. lateral spinothalamic tract
  b. anterior spinothalamic tract
  c. fasciculi gracilis and cuneatus
  d. spinocerebellar tract

11. _____ transmits impulses of crude touch and pressure

12. _____ transmits impulses of subconscious kinesthesia

13. _____ transmits impulses of crude touch, pain, and temperature

14. _____ transmits impulses of discriminating touch and kinesthesia

Matching—identify each descending, or motor, tract with its corresponding function.

a. lateral corticospinal tract
b. anterior corticospinal tract
c. reticulospinal tract
d. tectospinal tract
e. rubrospinal tract

15. _____ transmits impulses that control voluntary movement of muscles on the same side of the body

16. _____ facilitates head and neck movement related to visual reflexes

17. _____ helps maintain posture during skeletal muscle movements

18. _____ transmits impulses that control voluntary movement of muscles on the opposite side of the body

19. _____ transmits impulses that coordinate body movements and maintenance of posture

Labeling—match each spinal cord term with its corresponding number in the following illustration.

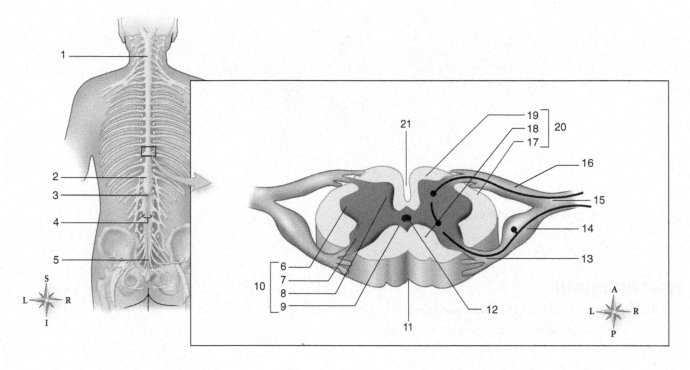

_____ white columns (funiculi)
_____ anterior median fissure
_____ cauda equina
_____ spinal nerve
_____ posterior column
_____ gray matter
_____ lumbar enlargement
_____ posterior median sulcus
_____ dorsal root ganglion
_____ lateral column
_____ posterior column

_____ cervical enlargement
_____ end of spinal cord
_____ anterior column
_____ central canal
_____ dorsal (posterior) nerve root
_____ filum terminale
_____ lateral column
_____ gray commissure
_____ ventral (anterior) nerve root
_____ anterior column

Labeling—using the terms provided, label the major tracts of the spinal cord on the following diagram.

fasciculus gracilis
anterior spinothalamic
lateral spinothalamic
lateral corticospinal
anterior corticospinal
rubrospinal
reticulospinal

fasciculus cuneatus
posterior spinocerebellar
anterior spinocerebellar
spinotectal
vestibulospinal
tectospinal

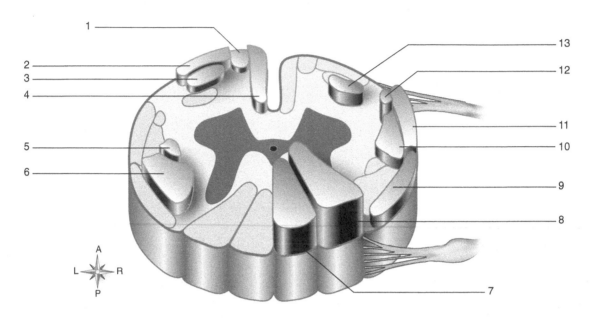

→ *If you had difficulty with this section, review pages 442-445.*

IV—THE BRAIN

Multiple Choice—select the best answer.

20. Which of the following is *not* a part of the brain stem?
    a. medulla oblongata
    b. hypothalamus
    c. pons
    d. midbrain

21. Which of the following is *not* a component of the midbrain?
    a. cerebral peduncles
    b. corpora quadrigemina
    c. superior colliculi
    d. all of the above are parts of the midbrain

22. The internal white matter of the cerebellum is the:
    a. arbor vitae.
    b. vermis.
    c. peduncle.
    d. none of the above.

23. The part of the brain that secretes releasing hormones is the:
    a. thalamus.
    b. hypothalamus.
    c. medulla.
    d. pons.

24. Regulation of the body's biological clock and production of melatonin is performed by the:
    a. pons.
    b. thalamus.
    c. cerebellum.
    d. pineal body.

25. The central sulcus divides the:
    a. temporal lobe and parietal lobe.
    b. cerebrum into two hemispheres.
    c. frontal lobe and parietal lobe.
    d. occipital lobe and parietal lobe.

26. The part of the cerebrum integral to consciousness is:
    a. Broca's area.
    b. the reticular activating system.
    c. the limbic system.
    d. the insula.

27. Commissural tracts compose the:
    a. corpus callosum.
    b. mammillary body.
    c. hippocampus.
    d. central sulcus.

28. Emotions involve the functioning of the cerebrum's:
    a. Broca's area.
    b. limbic system.
    c. reticular activating system.
    d. caudate nucleus.

29. The type of brain wave associated with deep sleep is:
    a. delta.
    b. beta.
    c. alpha.
    d. theta.

True or False

30. _____ The cerebellum is the second largest portion of the brain.

31. _____ Functions of the cerebellum include language, memory, and emotions.

32. _____ The vomiting reflex is mediated by the cerebellum.

33. _____ The shallow grooves of the cerebrum are called sulci.

34. _____ The islands of gray matter inside the hemispheres of the cerebrum are called the basal ganglia.

Labeling—label the following illustration of the left hemisphere of the cerebrum.

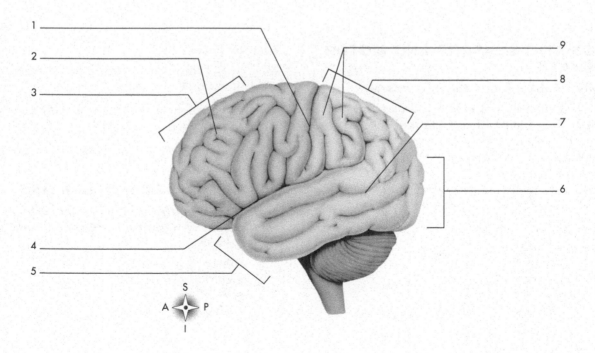

Labeling—label the functional areas of the cerebral cortex on the following illustration.

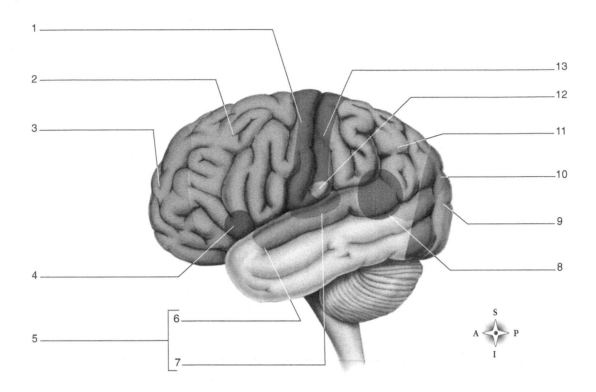

➜ *If you had difficulty with this section, review pages 445-464.*

V—SOMATIC SENSORY AND MOTOR PATHWAYS

Multiple Choice—select the best answer.

35. Which of the following is *not* a pathway that produces sensations of touch and pressure?
    a. medial lemniscal system
    b. spinothalamic pathway
    c. rubrospinal tract
    d. all of the above are pathways that produce sensations of touch and pressure.

36. Axons from the anterior gray horn of the spinal cord terminate in the:
    a. cerebral cortex.
    b. sensory receptors.
    c. skeletal muscle.
    d. none of the above.

37. Absence of reflexes is indicative of injury to:
    a. lower motor neurons.
    b. upper motor neurons.
    c. lower sensory neurons.
    d. upper sensory neurons.

True or False

38. _____ Poliomyelitis results in flaccid paralysis via destruction of anterior horn neurons.

39. _____ Extrapyramidal tracts are very simple pyramidal tracts.

➜ *If you had difficulty with this section, review pages 464-468.*

VI—MECHANISMS OF DISEASE

Matching—identify each disorder with its corresponding definition. Answer blanks are on page 137.

    a. Alzheimer disease
    b. cerebrovascular accident
    c. epilepsy
    d. Huntington disease

40. _____ an inherited form of dementia in which the symptoms first appear between 30 and 40 years of age

41. _____ a hemorrhage from or cessation of blood flow to the cerebral vessels, which destroys neurons

42. _____ a degenerative disease that affects memory, generally developing during the middle to late

adult years and causing characteristic lesions in the cortex

43. _____ recurring or chronic seizure episodes involving sudden bursts of abnormal neuron activity

➡ *If you had difficulty with this section, review pages 469-470.*

CROSSWORD PUZZLE

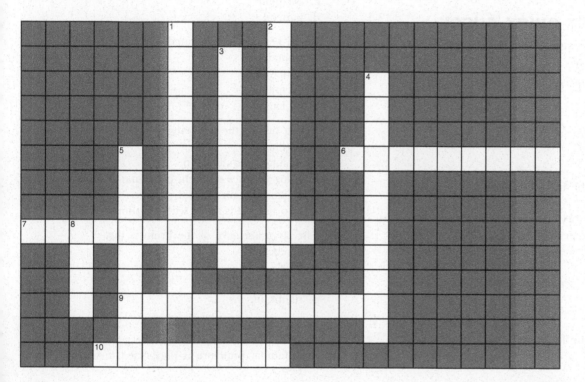

ACROSS
6. Black; tone; substance
7. Under or below; inner chamber
9. Together; roll; process
10. Membrane

DOWN
1. Between; within; head
2. Brain; small thing
3. Back of head; relating to
4. Pine; relating to; acorn (2 words)
5. Belly; little
8. Bridge

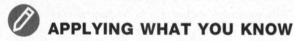

APPLYING WHAT YOU KNOW

44. Baby Dania was born with an excessive accumulation of CSF in the ventricles. A catheter was placed in the ventricle and the fluid was drained by means of a shunt into the circulating bloodstream. What condition does this medical history describe?

45. Julius is exhibiting loss of memory, increasingly limited attention span, deteriorating motor control, and changes in his personality. What is the general term that can be used to describe his condition? What specific condition may he be suffering from?

DID YOU KNOW?

- The short-term memory capacity for most people is between five and nine items or digits. This is one reason that phone numbers were kept to seven digits (not including the area code).
- The soft mass of the adult brain is motionless. Though it consumes up to 24% of the blood's oxygen supply, it does not grow, divide, or contract.
- The longest living cells in the body are brain cells, which can live an entire lifetime.

ONE LAST QUICK CHECK

Multiple Choice—select the best answer.

46. The portion of the brain stem that joins the spinal cord to the brain is the:
    a. pons.
    b. cerebellum.
    c. diencephalon.
    d. hypothalamus.
    e. medulla.

47. Which one of the following is *not* a function of the brain stem?
    a. conducts sensory impulses from the spinal cord to the higher centers of the brain
    b. conducts motor impulses from the cerebrum to the spinal cord
    c. controls heartbeat, respiration, and blood vessel diameter
    d. contains centers for speech and memory

48. Which one of the following is *not* part of the diencephalon?
    a. cerebrum
    b. thalamus
    c. hypothalamus
    d. pineal gland

49. Which one of the following parts of the brain helps in the association of sensations with emotions, as well as aiding in the arousal or alerting mechanism?
    a. pons
    b. hypothalamus
    c. cerebellum
    d. thalamus
    e. none of the above is correct

50. Which one of the following is *not* a function of the cerebrum?
    a. language
    b. consciousness
    c. memory
    d. conscious awareness of sensations
    e. all of the above are functions of the cerebrum

51. The area of the cerebrum responsible for the perception of sound lies in the _____ lobe.
    a. frontal
    b. temporal
    c. occipital
    d. parietal

52. Visual perception is located in the _____ lobe.
    a. frontal
    b. temporal
    c. occipital
    d. parietal

53. Which one of the following is *not* a function of the cerebellum?
    a. maintains equilibrium
    b. helps produce smooth, coordinated movements
    c. helps maintain normal posture
    d. associates sensations with emotions

54. The largest section of the brain is the:
    a. cerebellum.
    b. pons.
    c. cerebrum.
    d. midbrain.

55. Which statement is *false*?
    a. The spinal cord performs two general functions.
    b. A lumbar puncture is performed to withdraw CSF.
    c. The cardiac, vasomotor, and respiratory control centers are called the *vital centers*.
    d. The meninges end at L1 in a tapered cone called the *cauda equina*.

56. Which of the following is *not* a function of the hypothalamus?
    a. major relay station between the cerebral cortex and lower autonomic centers
    b. serves as a higher autonomic center
    c. plays an essential role in maintaining the waking state
    d. regulates voluntary motor functions
    e. part of the mechanism for regulating appetite

CHAPTER 21
Peripheral Nervous System

Twelve pairs of cranial nerves attach to the ventral surface of the brain. The cranial nerves are identified by both name and number. The name indicates the structures innervated by the nerve (e.g., facial, optic) or may refer to the function of the nerve (e.g., oculomotor). The number is designated by Roman numerals. These numbers indicate the order of the nerves as they are positioned from anterior to posterior on the brain.

Cranial nerves may be further classified by function into three categories: *mixed* cranial nerves, *sensory* cranial nerves, and *motor* cranial nerves. These distinctions refer to the bundles of axons that make up the nerves: mixed (axons of sensory and motor neurons), sensory (sensory axons only), and motor (mainly motor axons.)

Thirty-one pairs of spinal nerves are grouped into five regions of the vertebral column. They are the cervical, thoracic, lumbar, sacral, and coccygeal. Although they are not named individually, they are numbered according to the area of the vertebral column from which they emerge. Each spinal nerve is a mixed nerve consisting of both sensory and motor fibers. The fibers separate near the attachment of the nerve to the spinal cord, producing two "roots." The dorsal root is composed of the sensory fibers and is easily identified by a swelling known as the *dorsal root ganglion* (spinal ganglion). The ventral root is made up of motor fibers that carry information from the CNS toward effectors for appropriate response.

I—SPINAL NERVES

Multiple Choice—select the best answer.

1. Which of the following is an *incorrect* statement?
   a. There are 7 cervical nerve pairs.
   b. There are 12 thoracic nerve pairs.
   c. There are 5 lumbar nerve pairs.
   d. All of the above are correct statements.

2. The spinal root that has a noticeable swelling is the:
   a. ventral root.
   b. anterior root.
   c. dorsal root.
   d. none of the above.

3. The dorsal root ganglion contains:
   a. sensory neuron cell bodies.
   b. motor neuron cell bodies.
   c. both sensory neuron and motor neuron cell bodies.
   d. motor neuron fibers.

4. The phrenic nerve innervates the:
   a. spleen.
   b. diaphragm.
   c. chest muscles.
   d. none of the above.

5. The femoral nerve arises from the:
   a. lumbar plexus.
   b. sacral plexus.
   c. coccygeal plexus.
   d. brachial plexus.

True or False

6. _____ The lower end of the spinal cord is called the *cauda equina*.

7. _____ There are 31 pairs of spinal nerves, all of which are composed of both motor and sensory fibers.

8. _____ Herpes zoster is a unique bacterial infection that almost always affects the skin of a single dermatome.

9. _____ *Dermatome* is a term referring to a skeletal muscle group innervated by motor neuron axons from a given spinal nerve.

10. _____ The brachial plexus is found deep within the shoulder.

Labeling—match each term with its corresponding number on the following illustration of spinal nerves.

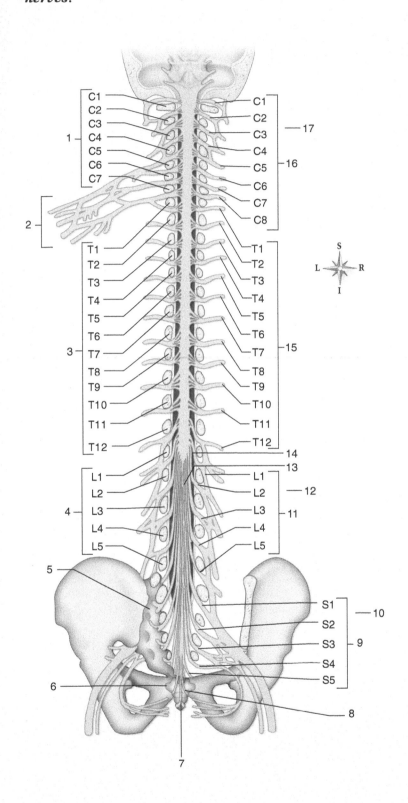

_____	cervical plexus
_____	filum terminale
_____	brachial plexus
_____	thoracic vertebrae
_____	coccyx
_____	lumbar plexus
_____	coccygeal nerve
_____	cervical vertebrae
_____	sacral nerves
_____	lumbar vertebrae
_____	cervical nerves
_____	cauda equina
_____	thoracic nerves
_____	lumbar nerves
_____	sacral plexus
_____	sacrum
_____	dura mater

➔ *If you had difficulty with this section, review pages 480-489.*

II—CRANIAL NERVES

Matching—identify each cranial nerve with its corresponding function.

a. olfactory
b. optic
c. oculomotor
d. trochlear
e. trigeminal
f. abducens
g. facial
h. vestibulocochlear
i. glossopharyngeal
j. vagus
k. accessory
l. hypoglossal

11. _____ facial expressions

12. _____ sense of smell

13. _____ peristalsis

14. _____ hearing and balance

15. _____ vision

16. _____ chewing

17. _____ swallowing

18. _____ regulation of pupil size

19. _____ innervation of the superior oblique muscle of the eye

20. _____ abduction of the eye

21. _____ tongue movements

22. _____ shoulder movements

Labeling—identify the cranial nerves by matching each term with its corresponding number in the following illustration.

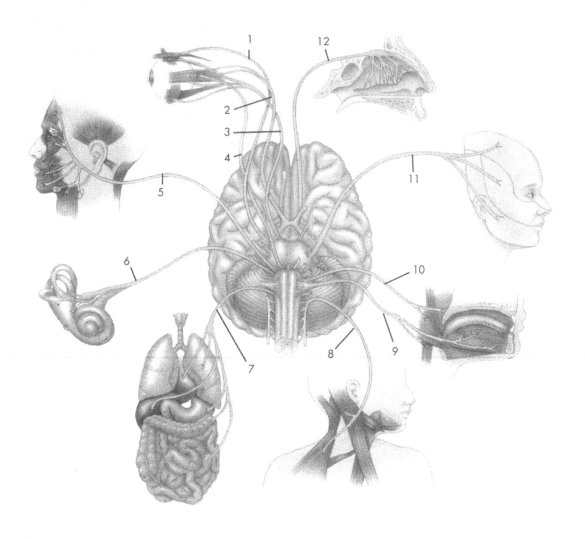

_____ glossopharyngeal nerve (IX)   _____ vagus nerve (X)   _____ facial nerve (VII)
_____ olfactory nerve (I)   _____ hypoglossal nerve (XII) _____ trochlear nerve (IV)
_____ abducens nerve (VI)   _____ trigeminal nerve (V)   _____ accessory nerve (XI)
_____ vestibulocochlear nerve (VIII) _____ oculomotor nerve (III) _____ optic nerve (II)

➡ *If you had difficulty with this section, review pages 489-494.*

III—SOMATIC MOTOR NERVOUS SYSTEM

Multiple Choice—select the best answer.

23. Somatic effectors are:
    a. smooth muscle.
    b. skeletal muscle.
    c. cardiac muscle.
    d. glands.

24. When the outer sole of the foot is stimulated, a normal infant will extend the great toe. This is called the:
    a. Babinski reflex.
    b. plantar reflex.
    c. tendon reflex.
    d. corneal reflex.

25. Which is the neurotransmitter in a somatic motor pathway?
    a. acetylcholine
    b. amines
    c. amino acids
    d. neuropeptides

Labeling—label the neural pathway involved in the patellar reflex on the following illustration.

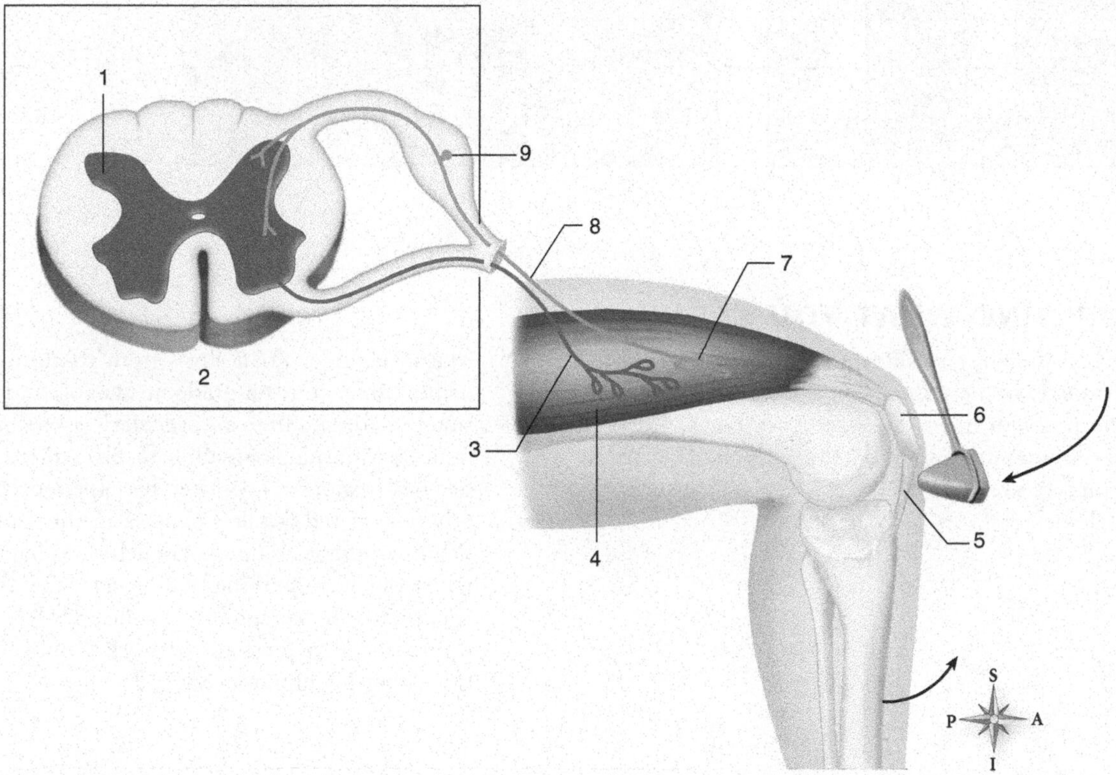

1. _____
2. _____
3. _____
4. _____
5. _____
6. _____
7. _____
8. _____
9. _____

➡ *If you had difficulty with this section, review pages 495-498.*

CROSSWORD PUZZLE

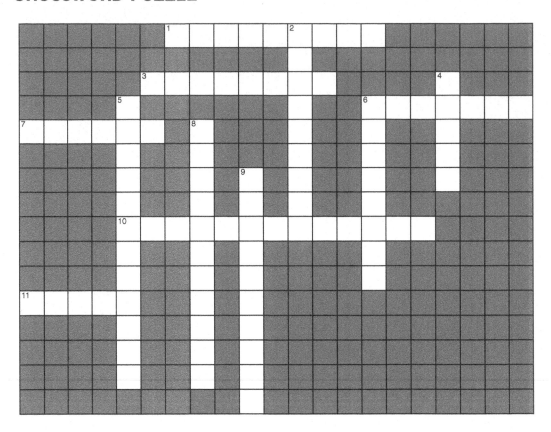

ACROSS
1. Skin; cut segment or region
3. Knot; unit
6. Hip joint; relating to
7. Again; bend
10. Body; relating to; again; bend (2 words)
11. Branch

DOWN
2. Pulley; relating to
4. Wanderer
5. Creep; girdle (2 words)
6. From; girdle
8. Tail; of a horse (2 words)
9. Three; twin or pair; relating to

 APPLYING WHAT YOU KNOW

26. Ethan had difficulty swallowing and he noticed his mouth was extremely dry. The doctor advised him that the problem may be related to a nerve. What two nerves might possibly be causing the problem? These nerves are mixed nerves. What is meant by that statement?

27. Mason is under great stress from trying to advance in his career, pursue graduate school, and raise two small children. After a particularly stressful event, he noticed a burning sensation in his axillary and pectoral regions. Days later he experienced an eruption of red swollen plaques in the same area. What condition is he experiencing? What is the name of the responsible pathogen? Why did he experience the symptoms that he did? What may be the reason that the pathogen was capable of breaching his immune system?

? DID YOU KNOW?

- The human brain continues sending out electrical wave signals for up to 37 hours after death.
- Your brain consists of approximately 100 billion neurons.
- The human brain is the fattest organ in the body and may consist of at least 60% fat.

✓ ONE LAST QUICK CHECK

Multiple Choice—select the best answer.

28. Which one of the following doesn't have a sensory function?
    a. abducens
    b. trigeminal
    c. facial
    d. vagus

29. Which nerve is a mixed nerve that arises from the medulla and is distributed to numerous organs?
    a. trochlear
    b. accessory
    c. hypoglossal
    d. vagus

30. Parasympathetic innervation of the heart is assisted by the:
    a. vagus nerve.
    b. facial nerve.
    c. trigeminal nerve.
    d. glossopharyngeal nerve.

31. Which nerve is involved in smiling and frowning?
    a. vagus
    b. trigeminal
    c. facial
    d. glossopharyngeal

Fill in the blanks.

32. The _____ nerve assists with balance or equilibrium.

33. Tic douloureux is damage to the _____ nerve.

34. The most common cause of peripheral nerve damage in the United States and Europe is _____ _____.

35. The somatic motor nervous system includes all of the _____ motor pathways outside the CNS.

36. Somatic reflexes are contractions of _____ muscle.

37. The _____ nerves supply the diaphragm. Any disease or injury to the spinal cord between the 3rd and 5th cervical segments may paralyze the _____ nerve and therefore the diaphragm as well.

Matching—select the best choice for the following words and insert the correct letter in the answer blank.

  a. cranial nerves
  b. spinal nerves

38. _____ 12 pairs

39. _____ dermatome

40. _____ vagus

41. _____ shingles

42. _____ 31 pairs

43. _____ optic

44. _____ C1

45. _____ plexus

46. _____ myotome

47. _____ accessory

CHAPTER 22

Autonomic Nervous System

While you concentrate on this chapter, your body is performing a multitude of functions. Fortunately for us, the beating of the heart, digestion of food, breathing, and most of our day-to-day processes do not require our supervision or thought. They function automatically, and the division of the nervous system that regulates these functions is known as the *autonomic nervous system*.

The autonomic nervous system is a division of the peripheral nervous system (PNS). There are two functional divisions of the PNS—the afferent (sensory) division and the efferent (motor) division. The efferent division is divided into the somatic nervous system, responsible for voluntary motor responses, and the autonomic nervous system, responsible for involuntary motor responses. The autonomic nervous system consists of two divisions called the *sympathetic system* and the *parasympathetic system*. The sympathetic system functions as an emergency system and prepares us for "fight or flight." The parasympathetic system dominates control of many visceral effectors under normal everyday conditions. Together, these two divisions regulate the body's automatic functions to help maintain homeostasis. Your understanding of this chapter will alert you to the functions and complexity of the peripheral nervous system and the "automatic pilot" of your body—the autonomic system.

I—STRUCTURES OF THE AUTONOMIC NERVOUS SYSTEM

Multiple Choice—select the best answer.

1. Somatic motor and autonomic pathways share all of the following *except*:
   a. direction of impulse conduction.
   b. effectors located outside the CNS.
   c. number of neurons between the CNS and effector.
   d. acetylcholine as a possible neurotransmitter.

2. Within the sympathetic chain ganglion, the preganglionic fiber may:
   a. synapse with a sympathetic postganglionic neuron.
   b. send an ascending branch through the sympathetic trunk.
   c. pass through chain ganglia and synapse in a collateral ganglion.
   d. all of the above.

3. Beta receptors bind with:
   a. acetylcholine.
   b. norepinephrine.
   c. toxin muscarine.
   d. none of the above.

4. Which of the following is *not* an example of sympathetic stimulation?
   a. decreased heart rate
   b. decreased secretion of the pancreas
   c. constriction of the urinary sphincters
   d. dilation of skeletal muscle blood vessels

5. "Fight or flight" physiologic changes include all of the following *except*:
   a. increased conversion of glycogen to glucose.
   b. constriction of respiratory airways.
   c. increased perspiration.
   d. dilation of blood vessels in skeletal muscles.

True or False

6. _____ The enteric nervous system is a specialized part of the ANS that controls visceral effectors in the gut wall.

7. _____ Many autonomic effectors are dually innervated.

8. _____ The sympathetic division is also called the *thoracolumbar division*.

9. _____ The sympathetic division is the dominant controller of the body at rest.

10. _____ Sympathetic responses are usually widespread, involving many organ systems at once.

Labeling—using the terms provided, label the following diagram of autonomic conduction paths.

sympathetic ganglion   axon of preganglionic sympathetic
postganglionic neuron's axon   neuron
collateral ganglion   axon of somatic motor neuron

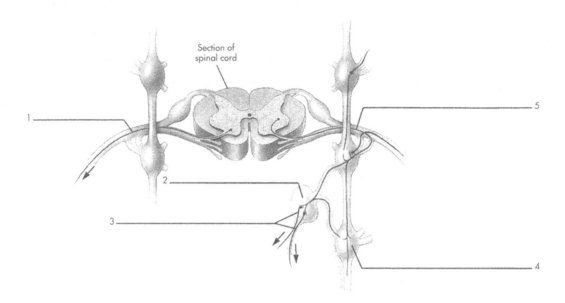

Fill in the blanks.

11. Each efferent autonomic pathway is made up of
    _____ _____, _____, and
    _____.

12. _____ neurons conduct impulses from
    the brain stem or spinal cord to an autonomic
    ganglion.

13. Sympathetic ganglia located a short distance from
    the spinal cord are known as _____ ganglia.

14. Some postganglionic axons return to a spinal nerve
    by way of a short branch called the *gray*
    _____.

15. Axon terminals of autonomic neurons release either
    acetylcholine or _____.

Circle the correct answer.

16. In the sympathetic division, preganglionic neurons
    are relatively (short or long) and postganglionic
    neurons are relatively (short or long).

17. Norepinephrine affects visceral effectors by first
    binding to (cholinergic or adrenergic) receptors in
    their plasma membranes.

18. The effect of a neurotransmitter on any postsynaptic
    cell is determined by the (characteristics of the
    receptor or neurotransmitter).

19. A (nicotinic or beta) receptor is a main type of
    cholinergic receptor.

20. The action of acetylcholine is (slowly or quickly)
    terminated when hydrolyzed by the enzyme
    acetylcholinesterase.

➡ *If you had difficulty with this section, review pages 504-516.*

II—FUNCTIONS OF THE AUTONOMIC NERVOUS SYSTEM

True or False

21. _____ Both sympathetic and parasympathetic
    divisions are tonically active, meaning they
    continually conduct impulses to autonomic effectors.

22. _____ Sympathetic impulses inhibit effectors and
    parasympathetic impulses stimulate effectors.

23. _____ Autonomic centers function in a hierarchy
    in their control of the ANS, with the highest ranking
    being the autonomic centers in the cerebral cortex.

24. _____ The sympathetic system plays a crucial role
    in maintaining blood pressure.

25. _____ The sympathetic system dominates during
    "rest and repair."

➡ *If you had difficulty with this section, review pages 512-517.*

23
Physiology of Sensation

Millions of sense organs called *sensory receptors* help us to respond to and enjoy life to its fullest. Sensory receptors are structures that transmit information about changes in both our internal and external environment. The receptors monitor these environments and transmit peripheral signals to the CNS for processing.

These receptors may be classified according to the location, the stimulus detected, or by structure or function. In addition to vision, smell, hearing, taste, and equilibrium, they are receptors for pain, temperature, discriminative touch, and several other tactile sensations. This chapter describes the importance of sensory receptors in the body and the critical role they play in our survival.

I—SENSORY RECEPTORS

Multiple Choice—select the best answer.

1. Which of the following is *not* a general sense?
   a. touch
   b. taste
   c. temperature
   d. pain

2. Which of the following is *not* a true statement?
   a. Mechanoreceptors are activated by stimuli that "deform" the receptor.
   b. Taste and smell are examples of chemoreceptors.
   c. Photoreceptors respond to light stimuli.
   d. Thermoreceptors are activated by pressure.

3. Which of the following structures is a disc-shaped nerve ending that is responsible for discerning light touch?
   a. Merkel disks
   b. Pacini corpuscles
   c. nociceptors
   d. Golgi tendon receptors

4. Which of the following is *not* a proprioceptor?
   a. muscle spindle
   b. root hair plexus
   c. Golgi tendon receptor
   d. all of the above are proprioceptors

5. Proprioceptors:
   a. function in relation to movements and body position.
   b. are superficial.
   c. are receptors for touch, pain, heat, and cold.
   d. are widely distributed throughout the skin.

True or False

6. _____ Mechanoreceptors are activated by a change in temperature.

7. _____ Free nerve endings are the simplest, most common, and most widely distributed sensory receptors.

8. _____ Somatic sense receptors located in muscles and joints are called *visceroreceptors*.

9. _____ Golgi tendon receptors are stimulated by excessive muscle contraction.

10. _____ Exteroceptors are often called *cutaneous receptors* because of their placement in the skin.

➡ *If you had difficulty with this section, review pages 520-527.*

II—SENSE OF PAIN

Fill in the blanks.

11. The term_____ describes the free nerve endings that serve as the primary sensory receptors for pain.

12. "Take your breath away" fast pain is also known as _____ pain.

13. Deep pain that develops slowly over time and travels over B fibers is also called _____ _____ pain.

14. The inability of diabetics to sense pain on certain areas of the body surface is known as diabetic _____.

15. The primary mechanism of _____ appears to be an abnormal amplification of pain information processed in the CNS causing chronic and widespread musculoskeletal pain.

➡ *If you had difficulty with this section, review pages 523-525.*

III—SENSE OF TEMPERATURE, TOUCH, AND PROPRIOCEPTION

Matching—select the best answer.

a. light touch
b. Pacini corpuscle
c. Meissner corpuscle
d. thermoreceptor
e. proprioceptors
f. brain
g. itch
h. histamine
i. Krause end bulb
j. tickle

16. _____ mediates sensations of heat and cold

17. _____ tactile sensation mediated by free nerve endings

18. _____ Golgi tendon organs

19. _____ tactile stimulation of the skin by someone else

20. _____ mediated by a free nerve ending called a "Merkel disk"

21. _____ encapsulated tactile end organs

22. _____ variant of Meissner corpuscle that acts as a mechanoreceptor

23. _____ found in the deep dermis of the skin and responds quickly to sensations of deep pressure

24. _____ incapable of feeling painful stimuli

25. _____ release occurs during allergic reaction

→ *If you had difficulty with this section, review pages 525-528.*

CROSSWORD PUZZLE

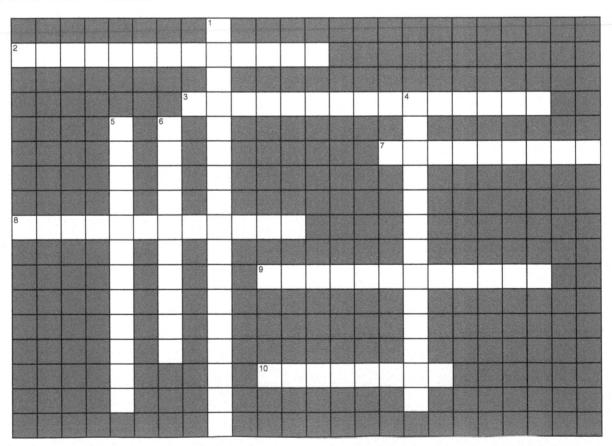

ACROSS
2. One's own; receive; agent
3. Machine; receive; agent
7. Feel; process
8. Outside; receive; agent
9. Inward; receive; agent
10. Adjust; process

DOWN
1. Receive agent; power; relating to (2 words)
4. Chemical; receive; agent
5. Push; receive; agent
6. To harm; receive; agent

APPLYING WHAT YOU KNOW

26. Sean was 35 and started noticing some visual symptoms, frequent bouts of imbalance, and memory loss. He hesitates to go to the doctor because he has no pain and thinks that the symptoms will probably "go away soon." What is wrong with Sean's attitude towards these symptoms?

27. Dick is a diabetic. He has been complaining of numbness in his feet. The doctor took great time and care to use cold and warm probes and methodically check areas of his feet repeatedly. Is this necessary?

 DID YOU KNOW?

- The skin contains approximately 640,000 sense receptors, scattered unevenly over the body's surface. These receptors are most abundant in the ridges of the fingertips, in the lips, at the tip of the tongue, in the palms, on the soles of the feet, and in the genitals.
- Humans smell "in stereo." Scent signals from each nostril travel to different regions in the brain. This may help a person determine the direction the odor is coming from.
- The first sense to develop in utero is the sense of touch.

 ONE LAST QUICK CHECK

Fill in the blanks.

28. General (somatic) sensory receptors may be classified anatomically as either free nerve endings or _____ _____ _____.

29. Pain that is perceived as being superficial but is actually caused by an underlying organ is called _____ pain.

30. Visceroceptors are located in the _____ _____.

31. Somatic senses enable sensation of _____, _____, and _____.

32. Intense stimuli, of any type, that results in tissue damage will activate _____.

33. The receptors responsible for sensing deep pressure and continuous touch are the _____ corpuscles.

34. _____ function in relation to movement and position.

35. _____ _____ _____ are receptors found in most body tissues.

36. As you wear a new engagement ring, you lose the constant feeling of its presence on your hand; this is _____.

Matching—select the best answer.

a. chemoreceptors
b. mechanoreceptors
c. thermoreceptors
d. photoreceptors
e. osmoreceptors
f. nociceptors

37. ____ found only in the eye

38. ____ activated by changes in temperature

39. ____ concentrated in the hypothalamus

40. ____ sensation is one of pain that may be caused by a toxic chemical

41. ____ activated for sense of taste and smell

42. ____ activated by stimuli that "deform" or change the position of the receptor

True or False

43. ____ A receptor potential is a graded response that is graded to the strength of the stimulus.

44. ____ If we not only remain aware of a particular sensation over time but also interpret what that sensation means in a larger context, the process is called *adaptation*.

45. ____ Special sense receptors are grouped into localized areas.

46. ____ A procedure to determine the density and distribution of general sense receptors is known as the *three-point discrimination test*.

47. ____ Proprioception tells us at each moment the level of contraction and stretch in each of our skeletal muscles.

CHAPTER 24
Sense Organs

Consider this scene for a moment. You are walking along a beautiful beach watching the sunset. You notice the various hues and are amazed at the multitude of shades that cover the sky. The waves are melodious as they splash along the shore, and you wiggle your feet with delight as you sense the warm, soft sand trickling between your toes. You sip on a soda and then inhale the fresh salt air as you continue your stroll along the shore.

It is a memorable scene, but one that would not be possible without the assistance of your sense organs. The sense organs pick up messages that are sent over nerve pathways to specialized areas in the brain for interpretation. They make communication with and enjoyment of the environment possible. The visual, auditory, tactile, olfactory, and gustatory sense organs not only protect us from danger but also add an important dimension to our daily pleasures of life. Your study of this chapter will give you an understanding of another of the systems necessary for homeostasis and survival.

I—THE SENSE OF SMELL AND THE SENSE OF TASTE

Multiple Choice—select the best answer.

1. Olfactory receptors and taste buds are:
   a. thermoreceptors.
   b. chemoreceptors.
   c. nociceptors.
   d. mechanoreceptors.

2. Olfactory epithelium consists of:
   a. epithelial support cells.
   b. basal cells.
   c. cilia.
   d. all of the above.

3. All of the following are primary taste sensations *except*:
   a. sweet.
   b. sour.
   c. spicy.
   d. bitter.

4. Nerve impulses responsible for the sensation of taste are carried in all of the following cranial nerves *except*:
   a. VII.
   b. VIII.
   c. IX.
   d. X.

True or False

5. _____ Olfaction requires the chemical response of a dissolved substance for a stimulus.

6. _____ The olfactory receptor cells lie in an excellent position functionally to smell delicate odors.

7. _____ The transmission pathway for olfactory sensations is as follows: olfactory cilia, olfactory bulb, olfactory tract, thalamic and olfactory centers of the brain.

8. _____ The tip of the tongue reacts best to bitter taste.

Labeling—label the midsagittal section of the nasal area on the following illustration.

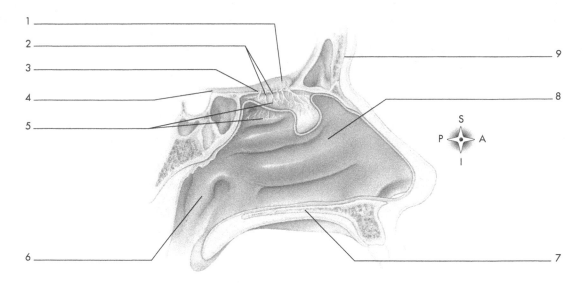

➡️ *If you had difficulty with this section, review pages 532-536.*

II—THE EAR: SENSE OF HEARING AND BALANCE

Multiple Choice—select the best answer.

9. Which of the following is a structure of the middle ear?
   a. incus
   b. oval window
   c. cranial nerve VII
   d. vestibule

10. The auditory tube connects the:
    a. inner ear and cranial nerve VIII.
    b. middle ear and the auditory ossicles.
    c. middle ear and the nasopharynx.
    d. oval window and the round window.

11. The only structure of the inner ear concerned with hearing is the:
    a. utricle.
    b. saccule.
    c. semicircular canals.
    d. cochlear duct.

12. Otoliths are:
    a. responsible for tinnitus.
    b. responsible for the "righting reflex."
    c. responsible for excess ear wax.
    d. ear stones.

13. The neuronal pathway of hearing begins at the:
    a. vestibular nerve.
    b. cochlear nerve.
    c. vestibulocochlear nerve.
    d. cranial nerve VII.

14. Dynamic equilibrium depends on the functioning of the:
    a. organ of Corti.
    b. crista ampullaris.
    c. macula.
    d. tectorial membrane.

15. The sense organ(s) responsible for the sense of balance is/are located in the:
    a. vestibule.
    b. cochlea.
    c. semicircular canals.
    d. both a and c.

True or False

16. _____ The membranous labyrinth is filled with endolymph.

17. _____ The correct order of the auditory ossicles from deep to the tympanic membrane is incus, malleus, and stapes.

18. _____ If the hairs of the organ of Corti are damaged, nerve deafness results—even if the vestibulocochlear nerve is healthy.

19. _____ Movement of the tympanic membrane from sound waves initiates vibration of the auditory ossicles.

20. _____ Vertigo essentially means "fear of heights."

Labeling—identify the structures of the ear by matching each term with its corresponding number on the following illustration.

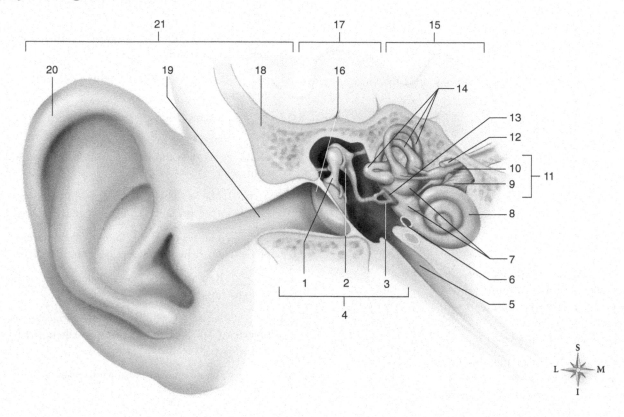

_____ auditory tube	_____ external ear	_____ oval window
_____ stapes	_____ middle ear	_____ incus
_____ cochlea	_____ inner ear	_____ vestibule
_____ semicircular canals	_____ auditory ossicles	_____ temporal bone
_____ facial nerve	_____ malleus	_____ cochlear nerve
_____ external acoustic meatus	_____ round window	_____ tympanic membrane
_____ vestibulocochlear (acoustic) nerve	_____ auricle (pinna)	
	_____ vestibular nerve	

 If you had difficulty with this section, review pages 536-542.

III—VISION: THE EYE

Multiple Choice—select the best answer.

21. From superficial to deep, the three layers of tissue that compose the eyeball are:
    a. sclera, retina, choroid.
    b. choroid, sclera, retina.
    c. sclera, choroid, retina.
    d. retina, choroid, sclera.

22. The anterior portion of the sclera is called the:
    a. cornea.
    b. iris.
    c. lens.
    d. conjunctiva.

23. The neurons of the retina, in the order in which they conduct impulses, are:
    a. photoreceptor neurons, bipolar neurons, ganglion neurons.
    b. photoreceptor neurons, ganglion neurons, bipolar neurons.
    c. bipolar neurons, photoreceptor neurons, ganglion neurons.
    d. bipolar neurons, ganglion neurons, photoreceptor neurons.

24. All of the axons of ganglion neurons extend back to an area of the posterior eyeball called the:
    a. fovea centralis.
    b. macula lutea.
    c. canal of Schlemm.
    d. optic disk.

25. Which of the following spaces contains the vitreous body?
    a. anterior chamber
    b. posterior chamber
    c. anterior cavity
    d. posterior cavity

26. The white of the eye is called the:
    a. sclera.
    b. choroid.
    c. retina.
    d. cornea.

27. The function of the lacrimal gland is to:
    a. secrete aqueous humor.
    b. secrete vitreous humor.
    c. secrete tears.
    d. none of the above.

28. Accommodation of the lens for near vision necessitates:
    a. increased curvature of the lens.
    b. relaxation of the ciliary muscle.
    c. contraction of the suspensory ligament.
    d. dilation of the pupil.

29. People whose acuity is worse than 20/200 after correction are considered to be:
    a. nearsighted.
    b. farsighted.
    c. legally blind.
    d. none of the above.

30. An intrinsic eye muscle is the:
    a. iris.
    b. pupil.
    c. sclera.
    d. retina.

True or False

31. _____ Mucous membrane, called *canthus*, lines each eyelid.

32. _____ All the muscles associated with the eye are smooth or involuntary.

33. _____ Conjunctivitis is a highly contagious infection.

34. _____ Corneal tissue is avascular.

35. _____ Deficiency of the blue-sensitive photopigments is the most common form of color blindness.

36. _____ The opening and separation of opsin and retinal in the presence of light is called *bleaching*.

37. _____ The retina is the incomplete innermost coat of the eyeball in that it has no anterior portion.

38. _____ Refraction means "the deflection or bending of light rays."

39. _____ A person with a 20/100 vision can see objects at 100 feet that a person with normal vision can see at 20 feet.

40. _____ A person with strabismus usually has double vision.

Labeling—using the terms provided, label the horizontal section through the eyeball on the following illustration.

sclera
pupil
ciliary body
optic nerve
posterior chamber
optic disk

central artery and vein
fovea centralis
lens
cornea (transparent)
lacrimal caruncle
iris

macula
choroid
retina
lower (inferior) lid
anterior chamber

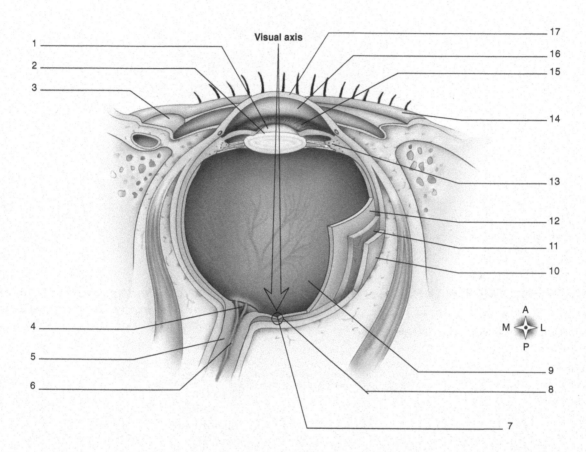

Labeling—label the extrinsic muscles of the right eye on the following illustration.

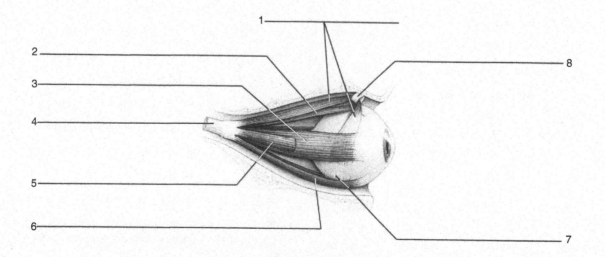

Labeling—label the structures of the lacrimal apparatus on the following illustration.

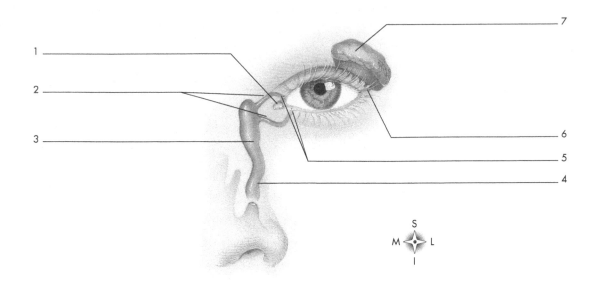

→ *If you had difficulty with this section, review pages 542-553 and page 555.*

IV—MECHANISMS OF DISEASE

Matching—identify the best answer from the choices given and insert the letter in the answer blank.

a. tinnitus
b. presbycusis
c. otosclerosis
d. otitis media
e. vertigo
f. Ménière disease

41. _____ inherited bone disorder that impairs conduction by causing structural irregularities in the stapes

42. _____ "ringing in the ear"

43. _____ middle ear infection

44. _____ sensation of spinning

45. _____ progressive hearing loss associated with aging

46. _____ chronic inner ear disease characterized by progressive nerve deafness and vertigo

Matching—select the best answer from the choices given and insert the letter in the answer blank.

a. trachoma
b. retinopathy
c. myopia
d. glaucoma
e. astigmatism
f. conjunctivitis
g. nyctalopia
h. hyperopia
i. scotoma
j. cataracts

47. _____ nearsightedness

48. _____ an irregularity in the cornea

49. _____ "pink-eye"

50. _____ chlamydial conjunctivitis

51. _____ cloudy spots in the eye's lens

52. _____ often caused by diabetes mellitus

53. _____ farsightedness

54. _____ "night blindness"

55. _____ loss of only the center of the visual field

56. _____ excessive intraocular pressure caused by abnormal accumulation of aqueous humor

→ *If you had difficulty with this section, review pages 553-555.*

CROSSWORD PUZZLE

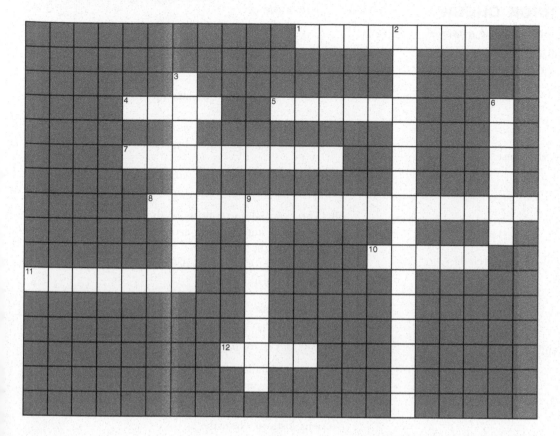

ACROSS
1. Gray or silver; tumor
4. Lentil
5. Ear; inflammation
7. Red; vision; substance
8. Drum; relating to; thin skin (2 words)
10. Doll; little
11. Ear; stone
12. Rainbow

DOWN
2. Ridge; flask; little; relating to; thing (2 words)
3. Within; water
6. Net; relating
9. Hear; relating to

 APPLYING WHAT YOU KNOW

57. Jada became ill repeatedly with throat infections during her first few years of school. Lately she has noticed that whenever she has a throat infection, her ears become very sore also. What might be the cause of this additional problem?

58. Deb is a woman with unusually poor vision. Without glasses, she needs to stand 20 feet away from an object to see it, whereas a person with normal vision could see that same object from 400 feet. How would you quantify her visual acuity? What must she score in a visual acuity exam after correction with glasses to avoid being designated as legally blind? With which type of refraction disorder is she afflicted? What shape lenses would be required to focus a clear image on her retina?

 DID YOU KNOW?

- Synesthesia is a rare condition in which the senses are combined. Synesthetes see words, taste colors and shapes, and feel flavors.
- A human can taste one gram of salt in 500 liters of water (0.0001 M).
- Men can read smaller print than women; women can hear better than men.

ONE LAST QUICK CHECK

Multiple Choice—select the best answer.

59. Where are the specialized mechanoreceptors of hearing and balance located?
    a. inner ear
    b. malleus
    c. helix
    d. all of the above

60. The organ of Corti is the sense organ of what sense?
    a. sight
    b. hearing
    c. pressure
    d. taste

61. Where are taste sensations interpreted?
    a. cerebral cortex
    b. nasal cavity
    c. area of stimulation
    d. none of the above

62. An eye physician is an:
    a. oculist.
    b. optometrist.
    c. ophthalmologist.
    d. none of the above.

63. Which of the following statements about the sclera is true?
    a. It is a mucous membrane.
    b. It is called the *white of the eye*.
    c. It lies behind the iris.
    d. All of the above are true.

64. Which of the following is activated by chemoreceptors?
    a. rods and cones
    b. gustatory cells
    c. organ of Corti
    d. cristae ampullares

65. The retina contains microscopic receptor cells called:
    a. mechanoreceptors.
    b. chemoreceptors.
    c. olfactory receptors.
    d. rods and cones.

66. Which two involuntary muscles make up the front part of the eye?
    a. malleus and incus
    b. iris and ciliary muscle
    c. retina and pacinian muscle
    d. sclera and iris

67. Which of the following statements about gustatory sense organs is true?
    a. They are called *taste buds*.
    b. They are innervated by cranial nerves VII and IX.
    c. They work together with the olfactory senses.
    d. All of the above are true.

68. The external ear consists of the:
    a. auricle and external acoustic meatus.
    b. labyrinth.
    c. organ of Corti and cochlea.
    d. none of the above.

True or False

69. _____ The tympanic membrane separates the middle ear from the external ear.

70. _____ Glaucoma may result from a blockage of flow of the vitreous body.

71. _____ With the condition of presbyopia, the eye lens loses its elasticity.

72. _____ The crista ampullaris is located in the nasal cavity.

73. _____ Myopia occurs when images are focused in front of the retina rather than on it.

74. _____ Light enters through the pupil, and the size of the pupil is regulated by the iris.

75. _____ The retina is the innermost layer of the eye and contains structures called *rods*.

76. _____ The olfactory receptors are chemical receptors.

77. _____ Meissner's corpuscle is a tactile corpuscle.

78. _____ The macula provides information related to head position or acceleration.

CHAPTER 25
Endocrine Regulation

The endocrine system is a system of communication, regulation, and control. It differs from the nervous system in that hormones provide a slower, longer-lasting effect than do nerve stimuli and responses. It is a ductless system that releases hormones into the bloodstream to help regulate body functions. The pituitary gland stimulates many of the endocrine glands to secrete their powerful hormones. All hormones, whether stimulated in this manner or by other control mechanisms, are interdependent. A change in the level of one hormone may affect the level of many other hormones.

Hormones may be classified in many ways, but one of the most commonly accepted ways is simply as *steroid* or *nonsteroid* hormones. Steroid hormones are manufactured by endocrine cells from cholesterol, and nonsteroid hormones are synthesized primarily from amino acids. Steroid hormones such as estrogen and testosterone enter target cells and directly interact with the DNA in the nucleus. Nonsteroid hormones such as adrenaline generally do not enter the target cell but instead bind to a receptor protein found on external cell membranes. This then causes a succession of metabolic effects.

In addition to the endocrine glands, prostaglandins, or "tissue hormones," are powerful substances similar to hormones that have been found in a variety of body tissues. These hormones are often produced in a tissue and diffuse only a short distance to act on cells within that area. Eicosanoids influence respiration, blood pressure, gastrointestinal secretions, and the reproductive system and may one day play an important role in the treatment of diseases such as hypertension, asthma, and ulcers.

As you review the endocrine system, you will be struck by the critical role that this system plays in our daily lives. Understanding the "system of hormones" will alert you to one of the mechanisms of our emotions, response to stress, growth, chemical balances, and many other body functions.

I—THE ENDOCRINE SYSTEM AND HORMONES

Multiple Choice—select the best answer.

1. The chemical messengers of the endocrine system are:
   a. hormones.
   b. neurotransmitters.
   c. target tissues.
   d. target organs.

2. Which of the following statements is true of the endocrine system?
   a. The cells secreting the chemical messengers are called *neurons*.
   b. The distance traveled by the chemical messengers is short (across a microscopic synapse).
   c. Its effects are slow to appear, yet long-lasting.
   d. None of the above.

3. Which of the following is *not* an endocrine gland?
   a. pineal
   b. placenta
   c. parathyroid
   d. intestines

4. The neuroendocrine system performs all of the following functions *except*:
   a. communication.
   b. control.
   c. conduction.
   d. integration.

5. The many hormones secreted by endocrine tissues can be classified simply as:
   a. steroid or nonsteroid hormones.
   b. anabolic or catabolic hormones.
   c. sex or nonsex hormones.
   d. tropic or hypotropic hormones.

6. Nonsteroid hormones include:
   a. proteins.
   b. peptides.
   c. glycoproteins.
   d. all of the above.

7. Anabolic hormones:
   a. target other endocrine glands and stimulate their growth and secretion.
   b. target reproductive tissue.
   c. stimulate anabolism in their target cells.
   d. stimulate catabolism in their target cells.

8. The second messenger often involved in nonsteroid hormone action is:
   a. cAMP.
   b. mRNA.
   c. ATP.
   d. GTP.

9. The control of hormone secretion is:
   a. usually part of a negative feedback loop.
   b. rarely part of a positive feedback loop.
   c. both a and b.
   d. none of the above.

10. When a small amount of hormone allows a second hormone to have its full effect on a target cell, the phenomenon is called:
    a. synergism.
    b. permissiveness.
    c. antagonism.
    d. combination.

True or False

11. _____ The nervous system functions at a much greater speed than the endocrine system.

12. _____ The most widely used method of hormone classification is by chemical structure.

13. _____ Steroid hormone receptors are usually attached in the plasma membrane of a target cell.

14. _____ Production of too much hormone of a diseased gland is termed *hyposecretion*.

15. _____ Input from the nervous system influences secretion of hormones.

Labeling—label the locations of the major endocrine glands on the following illustration.

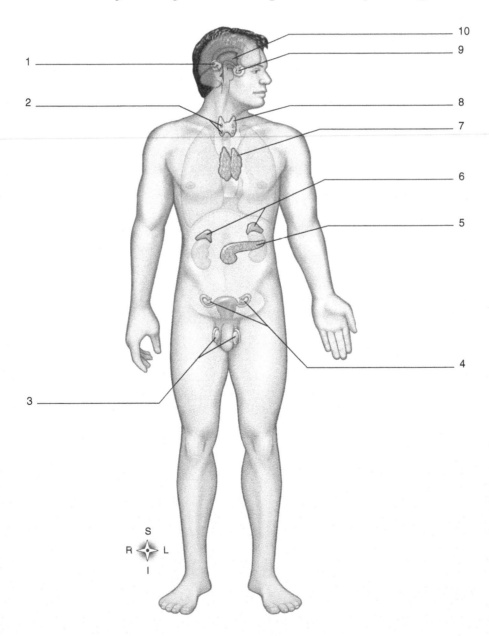

➜ *If you had difficulty with this section, review pages 562-571 and page 574.*

Matching—select the best choice for the following and insert the correct letter in the blanks.

a. Steroid hormone
b. Nonsteroid hormone

16. _____ Binds to specific plasma membrane receptor

17. _____ Response time is usually 1 hour to several days

18. _____ Receptor is mobile in the cytoplasm or nucleus

19. _____ Lipid

20. _____ Regulates gene activity

21. _____ Stored in secretory vesicles before release

22. _____ One or more amino acids

23. _____ Response time is usually several seconds to a few minutes

➡ *If you had difficulty with this section, review pages 569-572.*

II—EICOSANOIDS

Multiple Choice—select the best answer.

24. Eicosanoids are referred to as:
    a. growth hormones.
    b. tissue hormones.
    c. target cells.
    d. thyroxins.

25. Which of the following is *false*?
    a. Eicosanoids tend to integrate activities of neighboring cells.
    b. The first prostaglandin was discovered in semen.
    c. Aspirin produces some of its effects by increasing PGE synthesis.
    d. PGFs have been used to induce labor and accelerate delivery of a baby.

Fill in the blanks.

26. _____ hormones are hormones that regulate activity in nearby cells within the same tissue as their source.

27. _____ hormones regulate activity in the secreting cell itself.

28. The _____ _____ of the male reproductive system secretes prostaglandin in the semen.

29. Leukotrienes are regulators of _____.

30. PGFs are required for normal _____ to occur in the digestive tract.

➡ *If you had difficulty with this section, review pages 572-574.*

Labeling—using the terms provided, label the location and structure of the target cell concept.

capillary
hormone

target cells
receptors

nontarget cells

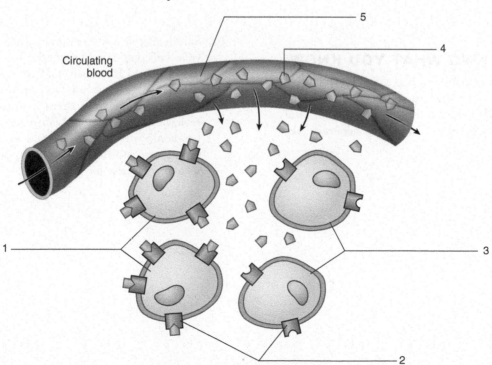

CROSSWORD PUZZLE

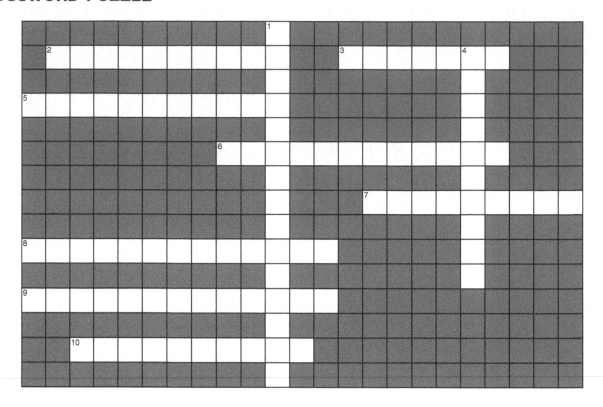

ACROSS
2. Extremities; great; state
3. Excite
5. Clot; oxygen; chemical
6. Self; free; state
7. Together; work; condition of (2 words)
8. Turn or change; relating to; excite (2 words)
9. Before; set or place; acorn; substance
10. Against; struggle; condition of

DOWN
1. Excessive shield; like; condition
4. Not; solid; like

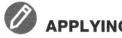 **APPLYING WHAT YOU KNOW**

31. India was pregnant and was 2 weeks past her due date. Her doctor suggested that she enter the hospital and he would induce labor. What local hormone might he give India to encourage labor?

32. Susie suffered a severe sprain while playing volleyball one day. She noticed her leg was swollen, red, warm to the touch, and very painful. X-rays indicated that there was no fracture, but, nonetheless, she was extremely uncomfortable. After reviewing the x-rays and lab reports, the doctor sent her home with instructions and suggested that she simply take aspirin for pain. Why did he make this recommendation for pain?

DID YOU KNOW?

- People with dwarfism almost always have normal-sized children, even if both parents have dwarfism.
- The pituitary weighs little more than a small paper clip.

ONE LAST QUICK CHECK

Fill in the blanks.

33. Responses that result from the operation of feedback loops within the endocrine system are called _____ _____.

34. Unused hormones circulating in the blood are excreted by the _____.

35. In _____, one hormone produces the opposite effect of another hormone.

36. In second messenger systems, the hormone-receptor complexes may be taken into the cell by means of _____.

37. The _____ of steroid hormone present determines the magnitude of a target cell's response.

Circle the correct answer.

38. Endocrine target cells must have the appropriate receptor to be influenced by the signaling chemical—a process called (signal transduction or signal induction).

39. If too little hormone is produced, the condition is called (hypersecretion or hyposecretion).

40. Many nonsteroid hormones seem to use cAMP as the (first messenger or second messenger).

41. Some hormones produce their effects by triggering the opening of (calcium or potassium) channels.

42. The (pituitary or parathyroids) regulate(s) the thyroid by producing thyroid-stimulating hormone (TSH).

Matching—select the best choice for the following and insert the correct letter in the blanks.

a. tissue hormone
b. eicosanoids
c. ibuprofen
d. thromboxane
e. leukotrienes

43. _____ blood regulator important in blood clotting

44. _____ immunity regulator

45. _____ local hormone

46. _____ lipid molecules

47. _____ inhibits PGE synthesis

Multiple Choice—select the best answer.

48. If norepinephrine diffuses into the blood and then binds to an adrenergic receptor in a distant target cell, it is known as a:
a. hormone.
b. neurotransmitter.
c. second messenger.
d. none of the above.

49. All steroid hormones are derived from which common molecule?
a. amino acid
b. peptide
c. cholesterol
d. protein

50. Which of the following is *not* a peptide?
a. antidiuretic hormone (ADH)
b. oxytocin (OT)
c. melanocyte-stimulating hormone (MSH)
d. testosterone

51. Combinations of hormones will have a greater effect on a target cell than the sum of the effects that each would have if acting alone. This phenomenon is called:
a. permissiveness.
b. synergism.
c. antagonism.
d. transduction.

52. The target cell concept is an example of the _____ model of chemical reactions.
a. lock-and-key
b. signal transduction
c. mobile-receptor
d. nuclear-receptor

CHAPTER 26
Endocrine Glands

The endocrine system has often been compared to a fine concert symphony. When all instruments are playing properly, the sound is melodious. If one instrument plays too loud or too soft, however, it affects the overall quality and enjoyment of the entire performance.

The endocrine system is a ductless system that releases hormones into the bloodstream to help regulate body functions. The pituitary gland may be considered the conductor of the orchestra because it stimulates many of the endocrine glands to secrete their powerful hormones. As mentioned in the previous chapter, all hormones, whether stimulated in this manner or by other control mechanisms, are interdependent. A change in the level of one hormone may affect the level of many other hormones. This fact makes the treatment of diseases or disorders of this system often very challenging. A hypersecretion of one gland may influence the secretion of another gland. It is therefore not uncommon for someone to have multiple disorders of the endocrine system.

This chapter reviews the individual glands and structures of the endocrine system and the effect that each has on the body individually and collectively. Your study of the "system of hormones" will result in a real appreciation for the critical role that the endocrine system plays in homeostasis and survival.

I—PITUITARY GLAND

Multiple Choice—select the best answer.

1. The pituitary is attached to the hypothalamus by a stalk called the:
   a. physis.
   b. infundibulum.
   c. pars intermedia.
   d. none of the above.

2. The vascular link between the hypothalamus and the adenohypophysis is called the:
   a. hypophyseal portal system.
   b. hepatic portal system.
   c. releasing hormone portal system.
   d. both a and c.

3. Which of the following links the nervous system with the endocrine system?
   a. pituitary
   b. pineal gland
   c. thalamus
   d. hypothalamus

4. Hypersecretion of prolactin can cause:
   a. insufficient milk production in nursing women.
   b. atrophy of breast tissue in non-nursing women.
   c. impotence in men.
   d. both a and b.

5. Psychosomatic and somatopsychic relationships between human body systems and the brain:
   a. are not believed to exist.
   b. are a real phenomenon.
   c. have a minimal effect on human physiology.
   d. none of the above.

Matching—identify each hormone with its corresponding function or description.

   a. adrenocorticotropic hormone (ACTH)
   b. antidiuretic hormone (ADH)
   c. follicle-stimulating hormone (FSH)
   d. growth hormone (GH)
   e. luteinizing hormone (LH)
   f. tropic hormone
   g. oxytocin (OT)
   h. prolactin (PRL)
   i. thyroid-stimulating hormone (TSH)

6. _____ promotes development and secretion in the adrenal cortex

7. _____ promotes growth by stimulating protein anabolism and fat mobilization

8. _____ promotes development of ovarian follicles in females and sperm in males

9. _____ triggers ovulation in females and production of testosterone in males

10. _____ promotes milk secretion

11. _____ stimulates uterine contractions and milk ejection into mammary ducts

12. _____ stimulates the synthesis and secretion of target hormones

13. _____ stimulates development and secretion in the thyroid gland

14. _____ promotes water retention in kidney tubules

Labeling—using the terms provided, label the location and structure of the pituitary gland on the following illustration. Some terms may be used more than once.

pineal gland
adenohypophysis
nasal cavity
infundibulum
pituitary (hypophysis)
hypothalamus

third ventricle
thalamus
pars anterior
optic chiasma
neurohypophysis

pars intermedia
sella turcica (of sphenoid bone)
brainstem
mammillary body
pituitary diaphragm

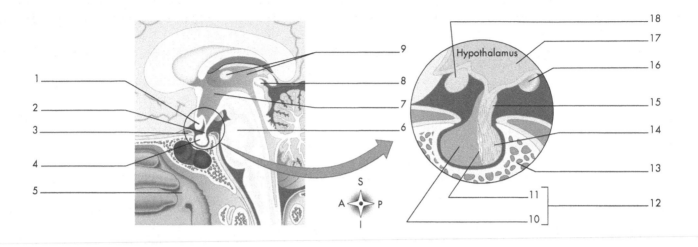

 If you had difficulty with this section, review pages 580-586.

II—PINEAL, THYROID, AND PARATHYROID GLANDS

Multiple Choice—select the best answer.

15. Which thyroid hormone is released in greatest quantity?
    a. T_3
    b. T_4
    c. triiodothyronine
    d. calcitonin

16. The principal thyroid hormone is:
    a. thyroxine.
    b. triiodothyronine.
    c. T_4.
    d. both a and c.

17. The two lobes of the thyroid are connected by the:
    a. infundibulum.
    b. isthmus.
    c. peninsula.
    d. islet.

18. High blood calcium levels can cause all of the following *except*:
    a. constipation.
    b. muscle spasms.
    c. lethargy.
    d. coma.

19. PTH increases calcium absorption in the intestines by activating:
    a. vitamin A.
    b. vitamin C.
    c. vitamin D.
    d. iron.

True or False

20. _____ Calcitonin in humans does not seem to have a great effect.

21. _____ The parathyroid glands are located on the anterior surface of the thyroid gland.

22. _____ Hypersecretion of thyroid hormone can cause Graves disease.

23. _____ The pineal gland functions to support the body's biological clock.

24. _____ The structural units of thyroid tissue are called *colloids*.

Labeling—label the following illustration showing the structure of the thyroid and parathyroid glands.

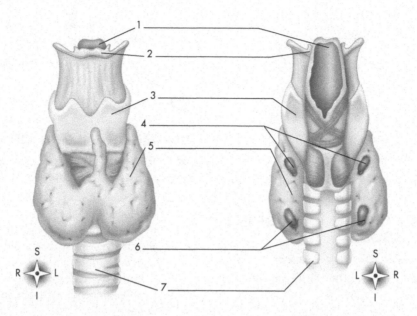

➜ *If you had difficulty with this section, review pages 586-592.*

III—ADRENAL GLANDS

Multiple Choice—select the best answer.

25. Which of the following hormones is *not* secreted by the adrenal cortex?
    a. aldosterone
    b. epinephrine
    c. adrenal androgens
    d. adrenal estrogens

26. Which of the following hormones is *not* secreted by the adrenal medulla?
    a. epinephrine
    b. norepinephrine
    c. adrenaline
    d. all of the above are secreted by the adrenal medulla

27. The most physiologically important mineralocorticoid is:
    a. aldosterone.
    b. angiotensin II.
    c. renin.
    d. angiotensin I.

True or False

28. _____ The outer portion of the adrenal gland is called the *adrenal cortex*.

29. _____ Hypersecretion of cortisol from the adrenal cortex produces a collection of symptoms called *Addison disease*.

30. _____ The renin-angiotensin-aldosterone mechanism is a negative feedback mechanism that helps maintain homeostasis of blood pressure.

➜ *If you had difficulty with this section, review pages 592-595.*

IV—PANCREATIC ISLETS

Multiple Choice—select the best answer.

31. Glucagon functions to:
    a. promote the entry of glucose into cells.
    b. convert glucose into glycogen.
    c. increase blood glucose concentration.
    d. decrease blood glucose concentration.

32. Insulin functions to:
    a. decrease blood concentration of glucose, amino acids, and fatty acids.
    b. increase blood concentration of glucose, amino acids, and fatty acids.
    c. inhibit the secretion of growth hormone.
    d. both a and c.

True or False

33. _____ Somatostatin has the primary role of inhibiting the secretion of pancreatic hormones.

34. _____ Pancreatic polypeptide is the dominant pancreatic hormone in the regulation of blood glucose homeostasis.

Matching—identify each pancreatic islet cell type with its appropriate hormone secretion.

  a. alpha cells
  b. beta cells
  c. delta cells
  d. pancreatic polypeptide cells

35. _____ insulin

36. _____ somatostatin

37. _____ glucagon

38. _____ pancreatic polypeptide

➔ *If you had difficulty with this section, review pages 595-597.*

V—GONADS AND OTHER ENDOCRINE GLANDS AND TISSUES

Multiple Choice—select the best answer.

39. The major hormone produced by the corpus luteum is:
  a. progesterone.
  b. estrogen.
  c. human chorionic gonadotropin (hCG).
  d. none of the above.

40. Testosterone is produced by:
  a. seminiferous tubules.
  b. interstitial cells.
  c. LH.
  d. the scrotum.

41. The hormone that can be detected during the early part of a woman's pregnancy with an over-the-counter kit is:
  a. LH.
  b. estrogen.
  c. hCG.
  d. atrial natriuretic hormone (ANH).

True or False

42. _____ Thymosin is a major digestive hormone.

43. _____ ANH aids in the homeostasis of blood volume and blood pressure.

44. _____ Secretin plays a major regulatory role in the digestive process.

➔ *If you had difficulty with this section, review pages 598-600.*

VI—MECHANISMS OF DISEASE

Matching—identify the disease with its appropriate description.

  a. hypersecretion of ACTH
  b. lack of iodine
  c. hypersecretion of thyroid hormone
  d. hypersecretion of melatonin
  e. hypersecretion of GH (adults)
  f. extreme hyposecretion of thyroid (adult)
  g. hyposecretion of estrogen in postmenopausal women
  h. hyposecretion of adrenal cortex

45. _____ acromegaly

46. _____ Addison disease

47. _____ Cushing disease

48. _____ Graves disease

49. _____ myxedema

50. _____ osteoporosis

51. _____ simple goiter

52. _____ winter depression

➔ *If you had difficulty with this section, review pages 601-602.*

CROSSWORD PUZZLE

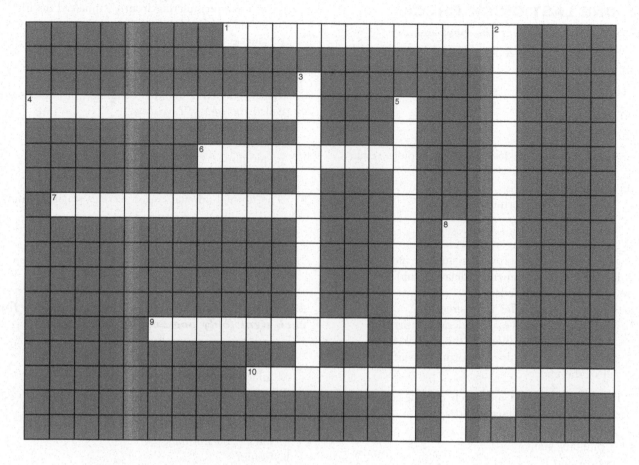

ACROSS
1. Toward; kidney; relating to; acorn (2 words)
4. Muscle; disease; combining form; study of; activity
6. Shield; oxygen; chemical
7. Aldehyde; solid or steroid derivative; chemical
9. Great; condition
10. Belt; having little bundles (2 words)

DOWN
2. Siphon; honey sweet (2 words)
3. Under or below; separate; process
5. Gland; under or below; growth
8. Idiot; condition

 ## APPLYING WHAT YOU KNOW

53. After a visit with the doctor, Amanda and Bill were elated to learn of the high levels of hCG in Amanda's urine. Why would this couple be so delighted? Which organ produced this hormone in her body and what is its function?

54. Dania has been experiencing excessive thirst, hunger, and copious urination. Which endocrine system syndrome may she be experiencing? What are the actual physiologic mechanisms that are causing her symptoms? How is she most likely to be treated?

 ## DID YOU KNOW?

- The total daily output of the pituitary gland is less than 1/1,000,000 of a gram, yet this small amount is responsible for stimulating the majority of all endocrine functions.
- The endocrine system is one of the primary means by which the body translates emotions into physical responses, such as love.

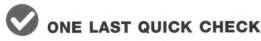 **ONE LAST QUICK CHECK**

Multiple Choice—select the best answer.

55. What does the outer zone of the adrenal cortex secrete?
    a. mineralocorticoids
    b. sex hormones
    c. glucocorticoids
    d. epinephrine

56. From what condition does diabetes insipidus result?
    a. low insulin levels
    b. high glucagon levels
    c. low antidiuretic hormone levels
    d. high steroid levels

57. Which of the following statements is true regarding a young child whose growth is stunted, metabolism is low, sexual development is delayed, and mental development is retarded?
    a. The child may suffer from cretinism.
    b. The child may have an underactive thyroid.
    c. Profound manifestations of the described condition may result in deformed dwarfism.
    d. all of the above

58. What can result when too much growth hormone is produced by the pituitary gland?
    a. hyperglycemia
    b. a pituitary giant
    c. both a and b
    d. none of the above

59. Which of the following glands is/are *not* regulated by the pituitary?
    a. thyroid
    b. ovaries
    c. adrenals
    d. thymus

60. Which of the following statements about the antidiuretic hormone is true?
    a. It is released by the posterior lobe of the pituitary.
    b. It causes diabetes insipidus when produced in insufficient amounts.
    c. It decreases urine volume.
    d. all of the above

61. What controls the development of the body's immune system?
    a. pituitary
    b. thymus
    c. pineal body
    d. thyroid

62. Administration of which of the following would best treat a person suffering from rheumatoid arthritis?
    a. gonadocorticoids
    b. glucagon
    c. mineralocorticoids
    d. glucocorticoids

63. Which endocrine gland is composed of cell clusters called the *islets of Langerhans*?
    a. adrenals
    b. thyroid
    c. pituitary
    d. pancreas

64. The normal adrenal cortex secretes small amounts of _____.
    a. epinephrine
    b. androgens
    c. ADH
    d. hCG

Matching—select the most correct answer for each item (only one answer is correct).

    a. glucocorticoid hormones
    b. antidiuretic hormone
    c. mineralocorticoid
    d. oxytocin
    e. growth hormone
    f. placenta
    g. luteinizing hormone
    h. insulin
    i. prolactin
    j. thyroid hormones

65. _____ goiter

66. _____ ovulation

67. _____ diabetes mellitus

68. _____ lactation

69. _____ diabetes insipidus

70. _____ human chorionic gonadotropin

71. _____ Cushing syndrome

72. _____ labor

73. _____ acromegaly

74. _____ aldosterone

CHAPTER 27

Blood

Blood, the river of life, is the body's primary means of transportation. Although the respiratory system provides oxygen for the body, the digestive system provides nutrients, and the urinary system eliminates wastes, none of these functions could be provided for the individual cells without the blood. In less than 1 minute, a drop of blood will complete a trip through the entire body, distributing nutrients and collecting the wastes of metabolism.

Blood is divided into plasma (the liquid portion of blood) and the formed elements (the blood cells). There are three types of blood cells: red blood cells, white blood cells, and platelets. Together these cells and plasma provide a means of transportation that delivers the body's daily necessities.

Although all of us have red blood cells that are similar in shape, we have different blood types. Blood types are identified by the presence of certain antigens in the red blood cells. Every person's blood belongs to one of four main blood groups: type A, B, AB, or O. Any one of the four groups, or "types," may or may not have the Rh factor present in the red blood cells. If an individual has a specific antigen called the *Rh factor* present in his or her blood, the blood is Rh positive. If this factor is missing, the blood is Rh negative. Approximately 85% of the population have the Rh factor (Rh positive), while 15% do not have the Rh factor (Rh negative).

Your understanding of this chapter is necessary to prepare a proper foundation for the study of the circulatory system.

I—COMPOSITION OF BLOOD, PLASMA, AND RED BLOOD CELLS

Multiple Choice—select the best answer.

1. The composition of blood is:
   a. 55% plasma, 45% formed elements.
   b. 45% plasma, 55% formed elements.
   c. 50% plasma, 50% formed elements.
   d. none of the above

2. A hematocrit of 45% means that in every 100 mL of whole blood:
   a. there are 45 mL of red blood cells and 55 mL of plasma.
   b. there are 45 mL of plasma and 55 mL of red blood cells.
   c. 45% of the formed elements are red blood cells.
   d. plasma is 45% of the circulating whole blood.

3. Reduced red blood cell numbers cause:
   a. polycythemia.
   b. buffy coat.
   c. anemia.
   d. both a and c.

4. Which of the following formed elements carry oxygen?
   a. leukocytes
   b. erythrocytes
   c. thrombocytes
   d. monocytes

5. All formed elements arise from which stem cell?
   a. proerythroblast
   b. megakaryoblast
   c. lymphoblast
   d. hemocytoblast

True or False

6. _____ *Hematocrit* and *packed cell volume (PCV)* are synonymous terms.

7. _____ A reticulocyte count can indicate to a physician the rate of leukocyte formation.

8. _____ Oxygen deficiency increases RBC numbers by increasing the secretion of erythropoietin by the kidneys.

9. _____ The life span of circulating RBCs is about 10 to 12 days.

10. _____ Heme is broken down into iron and amino acids for use in the synthesis of new RBCs.

11. _____ Plasma is a pale yellow fluid that accounts for more than half of the blood volume.

12. _____ Scrum is whole blood minus the clotting elements.

13. _____ Synthesis of plasma proteins occurs in the spleen.

14. _____ The mature erythrocyte does not contain ribosomes, mitochondria, and other organelles typical of most body cells.

15. _____ The final step in RBC formation is called *erythropoiesis*.

➡ *If you had difficulty with this section, review pages 611-618.*

II—BLOOD TYPES

Multiple Choice—select the best answer.

16. A person with antibody A in his or her plasma would have which blood type?
   a. type A
   b. type B
   c. type AB
   d. type O

17. People with type O blood are considered to be universal donors because their blood contains:
   a. neither A nor B antigens on their RBCs.
   b. both A and B antigens in their blood plasma.
   c. the Rh antigen on their RBCs.
   d. none of the above

18. A blood type and crossmatch is performed prior to transfusion. If this procedure is *not* completed:
   a. the blood may agglutinate.
   b. blood lysis may occur.
   c. a transfusion reaction may occur.
   d. all of the above

Fill in the blanks.

19. _____ _____ blood is considered to be the universal recipient.

20. Type AB blood contains both the A and B _____ on the RBC membrane.

21. Blood does not normally contain the anti-Rh _____, but they may appear in the blood of an Rh-negative mother during certain circumstances.

➡ *If you had difficulty with this section, review pages 617-621.*

Blood Typing—using the key below, draw the appropriate reaction with the donor's blood in the circles.

Recipient's blood		Reactions with donor's blood			
RBC antigens	Plasma antibodies	Donor type O	Donor type A	Donor type B	Donor type AB
None (Type O)	Anti-A Anti-B	◯	◯	◯	◯
A (Type A)	Anti-B	◯	◯	◯	◯
B (Type B)	Anti-A	◯	◯	◯	◯
AB (Type AB)	(none)	◯	◯	◯	◯

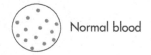 Normal blood

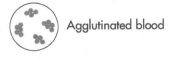 Agglutinated blood

III—WHITE BLOOD CELLS AND PLATELETS

Matching—identify each term with its corresponding description.

a. agranulocytes
b. basophils
c. eosinophils
d. granulocytes
e. leukocytes
f. lymphocytes
g. megakaryocytes
h. monocytes
i. neutrophils
j. platelets

22. _____ classification of leukocytes that contain cytoplasmic granules

23. _____ most numerous leukocytes

24. _____ granulocytes that release heparin and histamine

25. _____ granulocytes that protect against infections from parasitic worms and allergic reactions

26. _____ agranulocytes that produce antibodies

27. _____ agranulocytes that can enter tissue spaces as macrophages

28. _____ cell fragments that function in blood clotting and hemostasis

29. _____ cells from which platelets are formed

30. _____ classification of leukocytes without cytoplasmic granules

31. _____ classification of formed elements that are nucleated cells lacking hemoglobin

→ *If you had difficulty with this section, review pages 621-624.*

Human Blood Cells

Fill in the missing areas of the table.

BODY CELL	FUNCTION

IV—HEMOSTASIS

Multiple Choice—select the best answer.

32. Which of the following is *not* a critical component of coagulation?
    a. thrombin
    b. fibrinolysis
    c. fibrinogen
    d. fibrin

33. For prothrombin to be synthesized by the liver, an adequate amount of which vitamin is required?
    a. vitamin A
    b. vitamin C
    c. vitamin D
    d. vitamin K

34. Which of the following does *not* hasten clotting?
    a. rough spot in the endothelium
    b. abnormally slow blood flow
    c. heparin
    d. all of the above hasten clotting

→ *If you had difficulty with this section, review pages 624-629.*

V—MECHANISMS OF DISEASE

Fill in the blanks.

35. _____ is an excess of RBCs.

36. _____ _____ often results from the destruction of bone marrow by drugs, toxic chemicals, or radiation.

37. An anemia resulting from a dietary deficiency of vitamin B_{12} is _____ _____.

38. An example of a hemolytic anemia is _____ _____ _____.

39. _____ refers to an abnormally low WBC count.

40. A(n) _____ is a stationary clot.

41. A circulating clot is a(n) _____.

42. _____ is a type of X-linked inherited disorder that results from a failure to form blood-clotting factor VIII, IX, or XI.

→ *If you had difficulty with this section, review pages 629-631.*

CROSSWORD PUZZLE

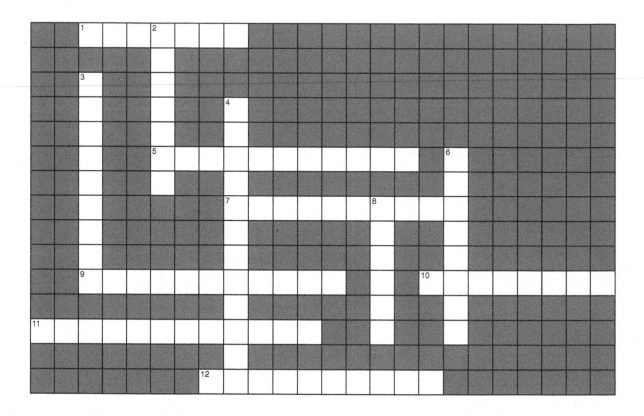

ACROSS
1. Liver; substance
5. Red; cell
7. Chemical; movement or reaction
9. Electricity; loosening
10. Clot
11. Fiber; loosening
12. Blood; love; condition

DOWN
2. Against; produce
3. White; cell
4. Net; relating to; little; cell
6. Foundation; love
0. Without; blood; condition

APPLYING WHAT YOU KNOW

43. Pepper is an elite competitive cyclist who wanted to gain a physiologic advantage over his competitors. He decided to have his own blood drawn and stored so that it could be infused into him prior to competition. What is the theory behind this practice? How effective is this procedure?

44. Mrs. Shearer's blood type is O positive. Her husband's type is O negative. Her newborn baby's blood type is O negative. Is there any need for concern with this combination?

45. After Mrs. Wiedeke's baby was born, the doctor applied a gauze dressing for a short time on the umbilical cord. He also gave the baby a dose of vitamin K. Why did the doctor perform these two procedures?

DID YOU KNOW?

- In the second it takes to turn the page of a book, you will lose about 3 million red blood cells. During that same second, your bone marrow will have produced the same number of new ones.
- There is enough iron in a human to make a small nail.

ONE LAST QUICK CHECK

Multiple Choice—select the best answer.

46. Which of the following statements is *false*?
    a. Sickle cell anemia is caused by a genetic defect.
    b. Leukemia is characterized by a low number of WBCs.
    c. Polycythemia is characterized by an abnormally high number of erythrocytes.
    d. Pernicious anemia is caused by a lack of vitamin B_{12}.

47. Deficiency in the number or function of erythrocytes is called:
    a. leukemia.
    b. anemia.
    c. polycythemia.
    d. leukopenia.

48. Which of the following statements does *not* describe a characteristic of leukocytes?
    a. They are disc-shaped cells that do not contain a nucleus.
    b. They have the ability to fight infection.
    c. They provide defense against certain parasites.
    d. They provide immune defense.

49. Which of the following substances is *not* found in serum?
    a. clotting factors
    b. water
    c. hormones
    d. all of the above are found in serum

50. Which of the following substances is *not* found in blood plasma?
    a. water
    b. oxygen
    c. hormones
    d. all of the above are found in blood plasma

51. An allergic reaction may increase the number of:
    a. eosinophils.
    b. neutrophils.
    c. lymphocytes.
    d. monocytes.

52. What is a blood clot that is moving through the body called?
    a. embolism
    b. fibrosis
    c. heparin
    d. thrombosis

53. When could difficulty with the Rh blood factor arise?
    a. Rh-negative man and woman produce a child.
    b. Rh-positive man and woman produce a child.
    c. Rh-positive woman and an Rh-negative man produce a child.
    d. Rh-negative woman and an Rh-positive man produce a child.

54. What is the primary function of hemoglobin?
    a. fight infection
    b. produce blood clots
    c. carry oxygen
    d. transport hormones

55. Are any of the following steps *not* involved in blood clot formation?
    a. A blood vessel is injured and platelet factors are formed.
    b. Thrombin is converted into prothrombin.
    c. Fibrinogen is converted into fibrin.
    d. All of the above are involved in blood clot formation.

Matching—select the most correct answer for each item.

a. heparin
b. contains anti-A and anti-B antibodies
c. clotting
d. immunity
e. erythroblastosis fetalis
f. anemia
g. cancer
h. contains A and B antigens
i. thin, white layer of leukocytes and platelets
j. phagocytosis
k. volume percent of RBCs in whole blood
l. decrease in WBCs
m. diapedesis

56. _____ lymphocytes

57. _____ erythrocyte disorder

58. _____ type AB

59. _____ basophils

60. _____ leukemia

61. _____ platelets

62. _____ type O

63. _____ Rh factor

64. _____ buffy coat

65. _____ neutrophils

66. _____ leukopenia

67. _____ hematocrit

68. _____ neutrophils

CHAPTER 28
The Heart

The heart is actually two pumps—one moves blood to the lungs, the other pushes it out into the body. These two functions seem rather elementary in comparison to the complex and numerous functions performed by most of the other body organs, and yet if this pump stops, within a few short minutes, life ceases.

The heart is divided into two upper compartments called *atria*, or receiving chambers, and two lower compartments, or discharging chambers, called *ventricles*. By age 45, approximately 300,000 tons of blood will have passed through these chambers to be circulated to the blood vessels. This closed system of circulation provides distribution of blood to the entire body (systemic circulation) and to specific regions, such as the pulmonary circulation or coronary circulation.

The beating of the heart must be coordinated in a rhythmic manner if the heart is to pump effectively. That is achieved by electrical impulses that are stimulated by specialized structures embedded in the walls of the heart. The sinoatrial (SA) node, atrioventricular (AV) node, bundle of His, and Purkinje fibers combine efforts to produce the tiny electrical currents necessary to contract the heart. A healthy heart is necessary to pump blood throughout the body to nourish and oxygenate cells continuously. Any interruption or failure of this system may result in serious pathology. Your review of the heart will give you an understanding and appreciation of how quickly all life can cease when the heart is not functioning properly.

I—HEART

Multiple Choice—select the best answer.

1. The visceral pericardium is found:
   a. inside the fibrous pericardium.
   b. adhering to the surface of the heart.
   c. lining the inside of the chambers of the heart.
   d. comprising the bulk of the heart tissue.

2. The correct layers of the heart, from superficial to deep, are:
   a. myocardium, pericardium, endocardium.
   b. epicardium, myocardium, pericardium.
   c. epicardium, myocardium, endocardium.
   d. endocardium, myocardium, epicardium.

3. The atrioventricular valves are also called:
   a. cuspid valves.
   b. semilunar valves.
   c. aortic valves.
   d. pulmonary valves.

4. Respectively, the right and left atrioventricular valves are also referred to as:
   a. tricuspid, mitral.
   b. bicuspid, tricuspid.
   c. mitral, bicuspid.
   d. bicuspid, mitral.

5. Semilunar valves prevent backflow of blood into the:
   a. atria.
   b. lungs.
   c. vena cava.
   d. ventricles.

6. The most abundant blood supply goes to the:
   a. right atrium.
   b. right ventricle.
   c. left atrium.
   d. left ventricle.

7. Branching of an artery as it progresses from proximal to distal is called:
   a. ischemia.
   b. infarction.
   c. anastomosis.
   d. both a and c.

8. The cavity of the heart that normally has the thickest wall is the:
   a. right atrium.
   b. right ventricle.
   c. left atrium.
   d. left ventricle.

9. Which of the following is a semilunar valve?
   a. aortic
   b. pulmonary
   c. mitral
   d. both a and b

10. The pacemaker of the heart is/are the:
    a. AV bundle.
    b. SA node.
    c. bundle of His.
    d. Purkinje fibers.

Labeling

11. Trace the blood flow through the heart by numbering the following structures in the correct sequence. Start with number 1 for the right atrium and proceed until you have numbered all the structures.

_____ right atrioventricular (tricuspid) valve
_____ pulmonary veins
_____ pulmonary arteries

_____ pulmonary semilunar valve
_____ left atrioventricular (mitral) valve
_____ left ventricle
_____ right atrium
_____ right ventricle
_____ left atrium
_____ aorta
_____ aortic semilunar valve

Labeling—using the terms provided, label the following illustration of the heart. Some terms may be used more than once.

openings to coronary arteries
aorta
right atrium
pulmonary veins
right AV (tricuspid) valve

left AV (mitral) valve
left ventricle
right ventricle
interventricular septum
aortic (SL) valve

chordae tendineae
papillary muscle
pulmonary trunk
superior vena cava
left atrium

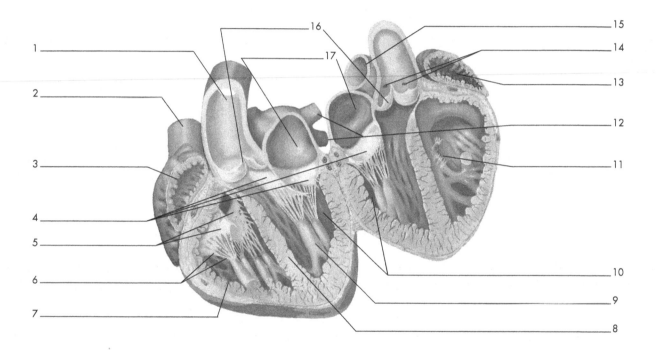

Fill in the blanks.

12. Rhythmic compressions of the heart combined with effective artificial respiration in cases of cardiac arrest are known as _____ _____ _____.

13. Increased serum levels in the blood often indicate a recent myocardial infarction. These levels are often monitored by a blood test called _____ and a blood marker known as _____ _____ _____.

14. Because cardiac muscles are capable of contracting on their own in a slow, steady rhythm, they are considered _____.

15. The free edges of the cuspid flaps are anchored to the papillary muscles of the ventricles by several tendinous cords that are more commonly referred to as _____ _____.

➡ _If you had difficulty with this section, review pages 638-649._

II—THE HEART AS A PUMP

16. A tiny bump at the end of a T wave is usually:
    a. an indicator of an imminent cardiac attack.
    b. a U wave.
    c. indicative of a murmur.
    d. a sign of hyperkalemia.

17. The normal pattern of impulse conduction through the heart is:
    a. AV node, SA node, AV bundle, Purkinje fibers.
    b. SA node, AV node, AV bundle, Purkinje fibers.
    c. AV bundle, AV node, SA node, Purkinje fibers.
    d. AV node, SA node, Purkinje fibers, AV bundle.

18. An ECG P wave represents:
    a. depolarization of the atria.
    b. repolarization of the atria.
    c. depolarization of the ventricles.
    d. repolarization of the ventricles.

19. Repolarization of the atria is:
    a. clearly depicted by the QRS complex.
    b. masked by the massive ventricular depolarization.
    c. masked by the massive ventricular repolarization.
    d. none of the above.

20. Contraction of the ventricles produces:
    a. the first heart sound (lub).
    b. the second heart sound (dupp).
    c. both of these.
    d. none of these.

True or False

21. _____ The contraction phase of the cardiac cycle is referred to as *systole*.

22. _____ Vagus fibers to the heart serve as accelerator nerves.

23. _____ The QRS complex represents repolarization of the ventricles.

24. _____ Rapid ejection is characterized by a marked increase in ventricular and aortic pressure and in aortic blood flow.

25. _____ Isovolumetric ventricular contraction occurs between the start of ventricular systole and the opening of the semilunar valves.

Fill in the blanks.

26. _____ _____ are also known as *Purkinje fibers*.

27. Pacemakers other than the SA node are abnormal and are usually _____ _____.

28. A complete heartbeat is referred to as a _____ _____.

29. A considerable quantity of blood, called the _____ _____, normally remains in the ventricles at the end of the ejection period.

30. A "swishing" abnormal heart sound indicating an incomplete closing of the vales or a stenosis of them is known as a _____ _____.

Labeling—label the following ECG deflection waves.

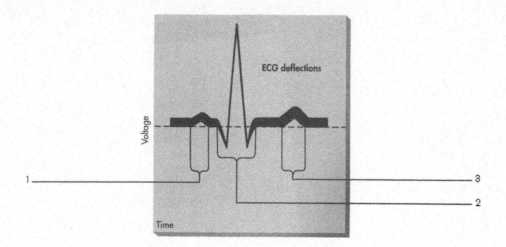

➔ *If you had difficulty with this section, review pages 649-656.*

III—MECHANISMS OF DISEASE

Matching—identify the term with the proper selection

a. cardiac tamponade
b. pericardiocentesis
c. aortic regurgitation
d. coronary artery disease
e. angina pectoris
f. congestive heart failure
g. cardiomyopathy
h. heart block
i. extrasystoles
j. atrial fibrillation
k. beta-adrenergic blockers
l. tissue plasminogen

31. _____ severe chest pain that occurs when the myocardium is deprived of adequate oxygen

32. _____ describes a number of different types of heart diseases that result in abnormal enlargement

33. _____ premature contractions

34. _____ impulses are blocked from getting through to the ventricular myocardium, resulting in the ventricles contracting at a much slower rate than normal

35. _____ serious compression of the heart that can be caused by pericardial effusion

36. _____ medication that blocks norepinephrine receptors and thus reduces the strength and rate of heartbeats.

37. _____ pericardial draining

38. _____ left-sided heart failure

39. _____ condition in which blood not only ejects forward into the aorta but also flows back into the ventricle because of a leaky aortic semilunar valve

40. _____ caused by a reduction in the flow of blood to the vital myocardial tissue

41. _____ sometimes the result of "extra beats" originating in the pulmonary veins

42. _____ helps dissolve clots

➔ *If you had difficulty with this section, review pages 656-660.*

CROSSWORD PUZZLE

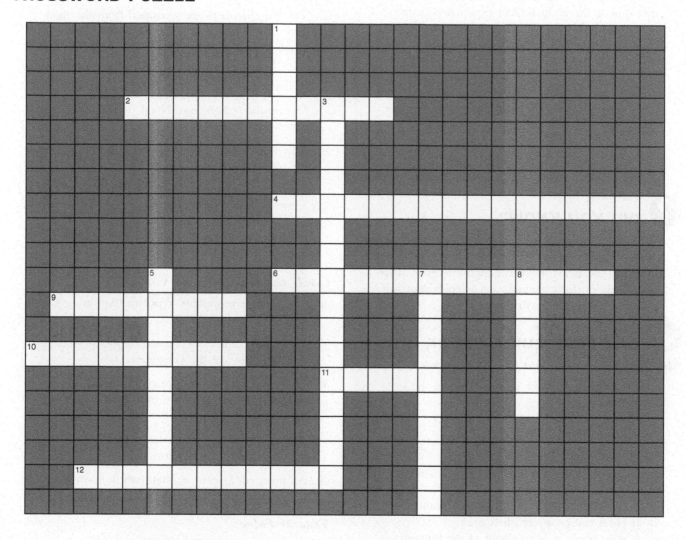

ACROSS
2. Within; heart; thing
4. Heart; relating to; plug; process (2 words)
6. Heart; muscle; disease; state
9. Hold back; blood; condition
10. Belly; little
11. Lifted; thing
12. Disordered; rhythm; condition

DOWN
1. Bishop's hat; relating to
3. Lower; quality; vein; hollow (3 words)
5. Half; moon
7. Muscle; heart; thing
8. Entrance courtyard

 APPLYING WHAT YOU KNOW

43. Mr. Shearer was admitted to the emergency department with severe swelling in his extremities, difficulty breathing, and elevated blood pressure. His doctor advised him that he had "left-sided heart failure." What is the other name for this condition, and could you elaborate on the possible serious outcome of this diagnosis if Mr. Shearer does not respond to this treatment?

44. Else was experiencing angina pectoris. Her doctor suggested a surgical procedure that would require the removal of a vein from another region of her body. What is the name of this surgical procedure?

45. Mr. Wertz called his doctor and informed him that during the night he had experienced some "heartburn" and "night sweats." His wife had insisted that he call the doctor even though he felt better. Mr. Wertz's doctor ordered blood work to be done and was not surprised when the serum levels of CRP and the troponins test came back elevated. How would you explain this elevation in blood serum levels?

 DID YOU KNOW?

- Your heart pumps more than 5 quarts of blood every minute. That's 2000 gallons a day!
- Every day the heart creates enough energy to drive a truck 20 miles. In a lifetime, that is equivalent to driving to the moon and back.

 ONE LAST QUICK CHECK

Multiple Choice—select the best answer.

46. The superior vena cava carries blood to the:
    a. left ventricle.
    b. coronary arteries.
    c. right atrium.
    d. pulmonary veins.

47. Which of the following statements is *false* regarding pericarditis?
    a. It may be caused by infection or trauma.
    b. It often causes severe chest pain.
    c. It may result in impairment of the pumping action of the heart.
    d. All of the above statements are true.

48. The outside covering that surrounds and protects the heart is called the:
    a. endocardium.
    b. myocardium.
    c. pericardium.
    d. ectocardium.

49. A valve that permits blood to flow from the right ventricle into the pulmonary artery is called the:
    a. tricuspid.
    b. mitral.
    c. aortic semilunar.
    d. pulmonary semilunar.

50. A common type of vascular disease that occludes arteries by lipids and other substances is:
    a. an aneurysm.
    b. atherosclerosis.
    c. varicose veins.
    d. thrombophlebitis.

Fill in the blanks.

51. The left chambers are separated from the right chambers by an extension of the heart wall called the _____.

52. _____ return blood from various tissues to the heart.

53. Myocardial cells receive blood by way of two small vessels, the right and left _____ _____.

54. The death of ischemic heart muscle that is usually the result of a blood clot to one of the larger coronary artery branches is known as _____ _____.

55. The cardiac veins drain into the right atrium through a common venous channel called the _____ _____.

Circle the best answer.

56. The P wave represents (repolarization or depolarization) of the atria.

57. The QRS complex represents (repolarization or depolarization) of the ventricles.

58. At the same time that the ventricles are depolarizing, the atria are (repolarizing or depolarizing).

59. The T wave reflects (repolarization or depolarization) of the ventricles.

60. An inverted T wave is often seen following a (myocardial infarction or pericarditis).

True or False

61. _____ Ventricular diastole begins with the isovolumetric ventricular relaxation period of the cardiac cycle.

62. _____ A stenosed valve is narrower than normal.

63. _____ MVP is a condition affecting the bicuspid valve.

64. _____ Atherosclerosis is a buildup of primarily lipids within the walls of blood vessels, making them hard and brittle.

65. _____ Tachycardia is a slow heart rhythm—below 60 beats/min.

CHAPTER 29
Blood Vessels

One hundred thousand miles of blood vessels make up the elaborate transportation system that circulates materials for energy, growth, and repair and eliminates wastes from your body. These vessels are called *arteries, veins,* and *capillaries* (which are exchange vessels, or connecting links, between the arteries and veins). The pumping action of the heart keeps blood moving through the closed system of vessels. This closed system of circulation provides distribution of blood to the entire body and to specific regions such as the pulmonary circulation or hepatic portal circulation. Your review of blood vessels will provide you with an understanding of the complex transportation mechanism necessary to provide oxygen and nutrients to our tissues.

I—BLOOD VESSEL TYPES

Matching—identify the term with the proper selection.

a. smooth muscle cells that guard the entrance to capillaries
b. carry blood to the heart
c. carry blood into the venules
d. carry blood away from the heart
e. outermost layers of arteries and veins
f. capillary that has a large lumen and more tortuous course than other capillary vessels
g. endothelium

1. _____ arteries

2. _____ capillaries

3. _____ tunica externa

4. _____ tunica intima

5. _____ sinusoid

6. _____ veins

7. _____ precapillary sphincters

True or False

8. _____ Veins are the only blood vessels to contain semilunar valves.

9. _____ The walls of veins are much thicker than those of arteries.

10. _____ Arteries become progressively smaller as blood flows away from the heart and into branches feeding other areas of the body.

11. _____ Arteries are often referred to as *capacitance vessels.*

Labeling—using the numbers provided, identify the structures of the blood vessels depicted in the following diagram. Some numbers may be used more than once.

_____ internal elastic membrane
_____ valve
_____ endothelium (tunica intima)
_____ fibrous connective tissue (tunica externa)
_____ basement membrane (tunica intima)
_____ smooth muscle (tunica media)

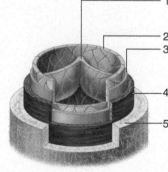

Vein.

Artery.

 If you had difficulty with this section, review pages 666-670.

II—CIRCULATION ROUTES AND MAJOR BLOOD VESSELS

Multiple Choice—select the best answer.

12. The aorta carries blood out of the:
    a. right atrium.
    b. right ventricle.
    c. left atrium.
    d. left ventricle.

13. The superior vena cava returns blood to the:
    a. left atrium.
    b. left ventricle.
    c. right atrium.
    d. right ventricle.

14. Blood returns from the lungs during pulmonary circulation via the:
    a. pulmonary artery.
    b. pulmonary veins.
    c. aorta.
    d. inferior vena cava.

15. The hepatic portal circulation serves the body by:
    a. removing excess glucose and storing it in the liver as glycogen.
    b. detoxifying blood.
    c. assisting the body to maintain proper blood glucose.
    d. all of the above.

16. Which of the following is *not* an artery?
    a. femoral
    b. popliteal
    c. coronary
    d. inferior vena cava

Fill in the blanks.

17. Blood flow from the heart to all parts of the body and back again is known as _____ _____.

18. Small vessels join the anterior and posterior arteries to form an arterial circle at the base of the brain known as the _____ _____ _____.

19. _____ are the ultimate extensions of capillaries.

20. When blood is in the capillaries of abdominal digestive organs, it must flow through the _____ _____ _____.

21. If either hepatic portal circulation or venous return from the liver is interfered with, a condition known as _____ may occur.

22. Many arteries have corresponding _____ _____ with the same name.

III—FETAL CIRCULATION

Multiple Choice—select the best answer.

23. The structure used to bypass the liver in the fetal circulation is the:
    a. foramen ovale.
    b. ductus venosus.
    c. ductus arteriosus.
    d. umbilical vein.

24. The foramen ovale serves the fetal circulation by:
    a. connecting the aorta and the pulmonary artery.
    b. shunting blood from the right atrium directly into the left atrium.
    c. bypassing the liver.
    d. bypassing the lungs.

25. The structure used to connect the aorta and pulmonary artery in the fetal circulation is the:
    a. ductus arteriosus.
    b. ductus venosus.
    c. aorta.
    d. foramen ovale.

Fill in the blanks.

26. Two _____ _____ carry circulation to the placenta, and one _____ _____ returns blood from the placenta.

27. The _____ _____ contracts as soon as respiration is established and eventually turns into a fibrous cord.

True or False

28. _____ The mixing of fetal and maternal blood occurs in the placenta.

29. _____ Almost all fetal blood is a mixture of oxygenated and deoxygenated blood.

Labeling—match each term with its corresponding number on the following illustration of the
principal veins of the body. Some numbers may be used more than once.

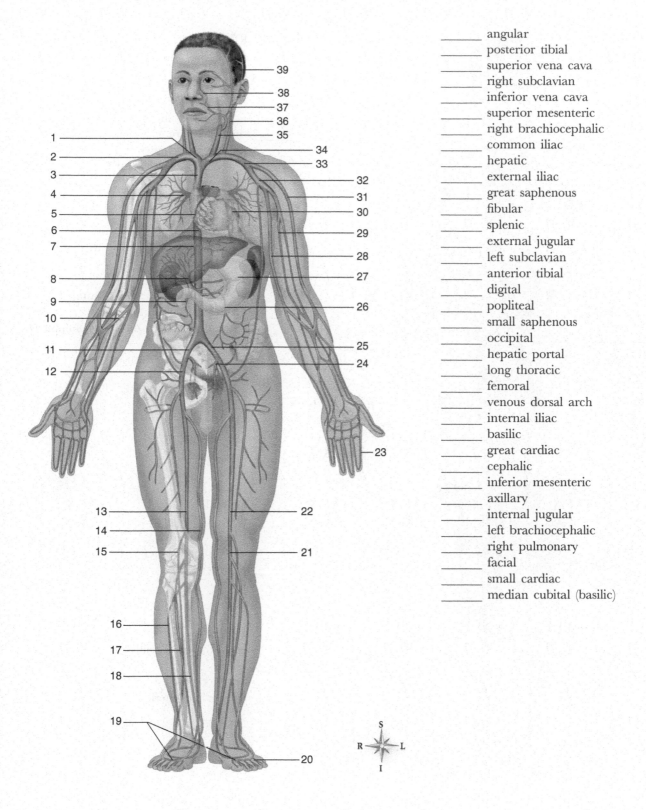

_____ angular
_____ posterior tibial
_____ superior vena cava
_____ right subclavian
_____ inferior vena cava
_____ superior mesenteric
_____ right brachiocephalic
_____ common iliac
_____ hepatic
_____ external iliac
_____ great saphenous
_____ fibular
_____ splenic
_____ external jugular
_____ left subclavian
_____ anterior tibial
_____ digital
_____ popliteal
_____ small saphenous
_____ occipital
_____ hepatic portal
_____ long thoracic
_____ femoral
_____ venous dorsal arch
_____ internal iliac
_____ basilic
_____ great cardiac
_____ cephalic
_____ inferior mesenteric
_____ axillary
_____ internal jugular
_____ left brachiocephalic
_____ right pulmonary
_____ facial
_____ small cardiac
_____ median cubital (basilic)

Labeling—match each term with its corresponding number on the following illustration of the principal arteries of the body. Some numbers may be used more than once.

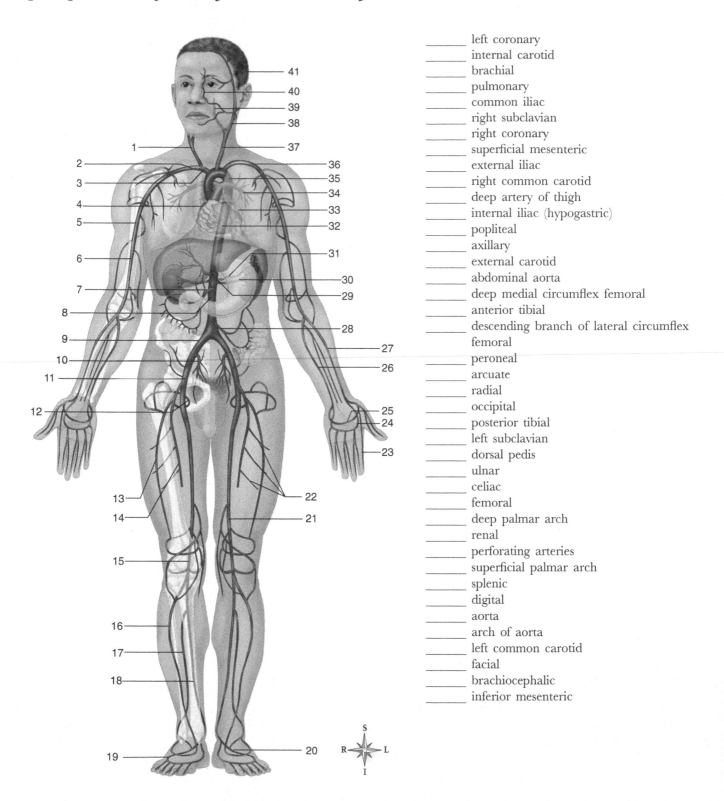

_____ left coronary
_____ internal carotid
_____ brachial
_____ pulmonary
_____ common iliac
_____ right subclavian
_____ right coronary
_____ superficial mesenteric
_____ external iliac
_____ right common carotid
_____ deep artery of thigh
_____ internal iliac (hypogastric)
_____ popliteal
_____ axillary
_____ external carotid
_____ abdominal aorta
_____ deep medial circumflex femoral
_____ anterior tibial
_____ descending branch of lateral circumflex femoral
_____ peroneal
_____ arcuate
_____ radial
_____ occipital
_____ posterior tibial
_____ left subclavian
_____ dorsal pedis
_____ ulnar
_____ celiac
_____ femoral
_____ deep palmar arch
_____ renal
_____ perforating arteries
_____ superficial palmar arch
_____ splenic
_____ digital
_____ aorta
_____ arch of aorta
_____ left common carotid
_____ facial
_____ brachiocephalic
_____ inferior mesenteric

Labeling—match each term with its corresponding number on the following depiction of fetal circulation.

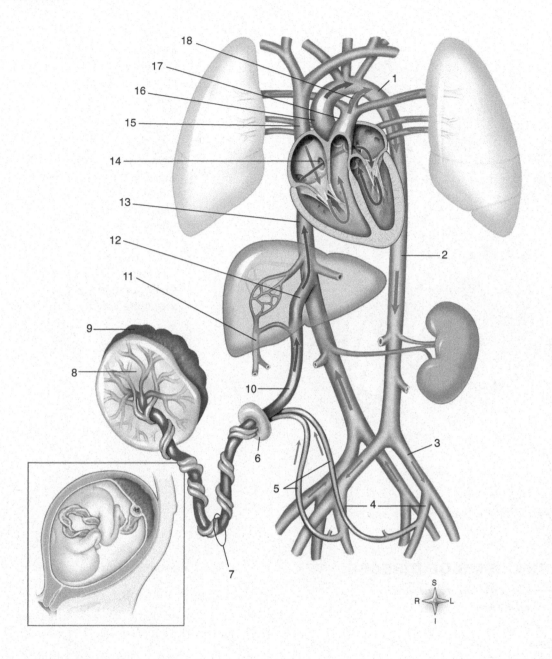

_____ ductus arteriosus	_____ abdominal aorta	_____ ductus venosus
_____ umbilical arteries	_____ foramen ovale	_____ umbilical vein
_____ pulmonary trunk	_____ hepatic portal vein	_____ common iliac arteries
_____ ascending aorta	_____ fetal umbilicus	_____ maternal side of placenta
_____ inferior vena cava	_____ internal iliac arteries	_____ umbilical cord
_____ aortic arch	_____ superior vena cava	_____ fetal side of placenta

Labeling—match each term with its corresponding number on this diagram of the hepatic portal circulation.

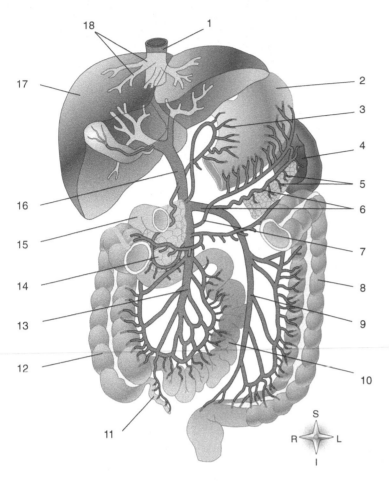

_____ liver
_____ gastric vein
_____ appendix
_____ pancreas
_____ hepatic veins
_____ inferior vena cava
_____ stomach
_____ spleen
_____ hepatic portal vein
_____ superior mesenteric vein
_____ duodenum
_____ pancreatic vein
_____ splenic vein
_____ gastroepiploic vein
_____ descending colon
_____ inferior mesenteric vein
_____ small intestine
_____ ascending colon

➔ *If you had difficulty with this section, review pages 670-691.*

IV—MECHANISMS OF DISEASE

Matching—identify the term with the proper selection.

a. arteriosclerosis
b. ischemia
c. aneurysm
d. necrosis
e. gangrene
f. hemorrhoids
g. phlebitis
h. stroke
i. myocardial infarction
j. thrombus
k. stents
l. atherectomies

30. _____ heart attack

31. _____ decreased blood supply to a tissue

32. _____ tissue death

33. _____ necrosis that has progressed to decay

34. _____ "hardening of the arteries"

35. _____ a section of an artery that has become abnormally widened

36. _____ varicose veins in the rectum

37. _____ vein inflammation

38. _____ clot formation

39. _____ cerebral vascular accident

40. _____ PCI that uses lasers, drills, or spinning loops of wire to clear the way for normal blood flow

41. _____ metal springs or mesh tubes inserted in narrowed arteries to hold them open

➔ *If you had difficulty with this section, review pages 692-694.*

CROSSWORD PUZZLE

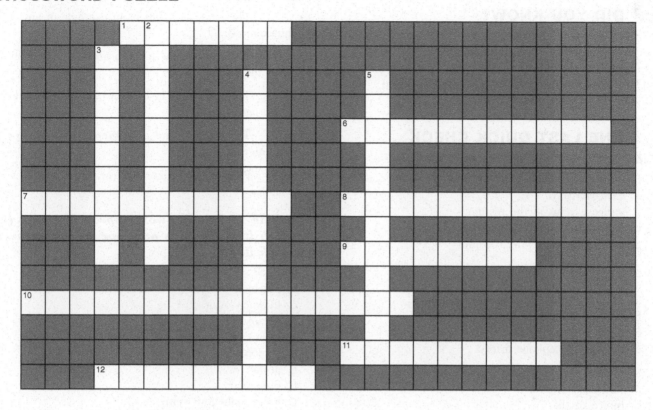

ACROSS
1. Belly; swelling
6. Within; nipple; thing
7. Vessel; widen; agent
8. Swollen vein; characterized by; blood vessel (2 words)
9. Widening
10. Vessel; hardening; condition
11. Hair; relating to
12. Vein; inflammation

DOWN
2. Below; key; relating to
3. Vessel; little
4. Against; curdle; agent
5. Tunic or coat; innermost (2 words)

 APPLYING WHAT YOU KNOW

42. Allison's friend just visited her with her new 6-month-old baby. She advised Allison that the pediatrician had detected a heart murmur and that there was a hole in the baby's heart. She further stated that if it didn't improve within the next few months that the baby would require surgery. What condition does the baby have and what are the possible outcomes?

43. Rochelle is a hairstylist who works long hours. Lately she has noticed that her feet are sore and edematous. What might be the cause of these symptoms? What advice could you offer Rochelle to provide some relief from these symptoms?

DID YOU KNOW?

- Capillaries are so small that it takes 10 of them to equal the thickness of a human hair.
- In one day, the blood travels a total of 12,000 miles. That's four times the distance across the United States from coast to coast!

ONE LAST QUICK CHECK

Multiple Choice—select the best answer.

44. Hemorrhoids can best be described as:
    a. varicose veins.
    b. varicose veins in the rectum.
    c. thrombophlebitis of the rectum.
    d. clot formation in the rectum.

45. All of the following are major branches of the aortic arch *except:*
    a. the left common carotid artery.
    b. the left subclavian artery.
    c. the coronary arteries.
    d. the brachiocephalic artery.

46. Smooth muscle in blood vessels is located in the:
    a. tunica adventitia.
    b. tunica media.
    c. tunica intima.
    d. all of the above.

47. Structures that control the direction of blood returning to the heart are:
    a. capillaries.
    b. valves.
    c. arterioles.
    d. venules.

48. The large veins of the cranial cavity, formed by the dura mater, are not usually called *veins* but are instead called:
    a. sinuses.
    b. venules.
    c. foramens.
    d. branches.

True or False

49. _____ The circle of Willis is an example of an anastomosis.

50. _____ The walls of the arteries are much thicker than the veins.

51. _____ The innermost layer of a blood vessel is the *tunica intima.*

52. _____ The thoracic and abdominal aorta compose the internal iliac.

53. _____ Precapillary sphincters are located within venules.

Matching—select the most appropriate answer for each item (there is only one correct answer for each item).

    a. FAS
    b. phlebitis
    c. foramen ovale
    d. aneurysm
    e. vena cava
    f. angioplasty
    g. aorta
    h. pulmonary
    i. great saphenous vein
    j. capillaries

54. _____ largest artery

55. _____ potential result of alcohol entering the fetal blood

56. _____ leg vein

57. _____ fetal circulation

58. _____ arterial procedure

59. _____ vein inflammation

60. _____ lung circulation

61. _____ weakened artery

62. _____ large vein that returns venous blood to the heart

63. _____ the eventual extension of arteries

CHAPTER 30
Circulation of Blood

This chapter reviews the circulation of the blood. A functional cardiovascular system is vital for survival because, without circulation, tissues would lack a supply of oxygen and nutrients. Waste products would also begin to accumulate and could become toxic.

The importance of blood pressure is also reviewed in this chapter. Blood pressure is the force of blood in the vessels. This force is highest in the arteries and lowest in the veins. Normal blood pressure varies among individuals and depends on the volume of blood in the arteries. The larger the volume of blood in the arteries, the more pressure is exerted on the walls of the arteries and the higher the arterial pressure. Conversely, the smaller volume of blood in the arteries, the lower the blood pressure. Your review of this system will provide you with an understanding of the complex transportation mechanism of the body necessary for survival.

I—HEMODYNAMICS AND ARTERIAL BLOOD PRESSURE

Multiple Choice—select the best answer.

1. The term used to describe a collection of mechanisms that influence the active and changing circulation of blood is:
   a. perfusion.
   b. cardiac output.
   c. stroke volume.
   d. hemodynamics.

2. Blood flows because of:
   a. a pressure gradient.
   b. Fick's formula.
   c. inotropic factors.
   d. the ejection fraction.

3. The greatest drop in pressure occurs as blood goes through the:
   a. arteries.
   b. arterioles.
   c. venules.
   d. veins.

4. Determining the cardiac output is usually accomplished by:
   a. using Fick's formula.
   b. using Starling's law.
   c. calculating: SV × CR = CO.
   d. using Poiseuille's law.

5. Which of the following has the ability to alter heart rate?
   a. chronotropic factors
   b. baroreceptors
   c. carotid sinus reflex
   d. all of the above

True or False

6. _____ A change in heart rate or stroke volume does not always change the heart's output, the amount of blood in the arteries, or the blood pressure.

7. _____ If blood pressure within the aorta or carotid sinus suddenly increases beyond the set point, the control center will increase vagal inhibition and return the blood pressure to normal.

8. _____ The amount that the CO can increase above the resting value is called the *inotropic factor*.

9. _____ The ejection fraction is related to the stroke volume.

10. _____ Peripheral resistance in arteries determines arterial blood pressure.

Matching—select the best answer from the list below.

a. vasoconstriction
b. cardiac output
c. viscosity
d. vasomotor pressure flex
e. hypoxia
f. hypercapnia
g. active hyperemia
h. ischemic
i. perfusion
j. contractility

11. _____ thickness of blood

12. _____ reduction in vessel diameter

13. _____ "flow through"

14. _____ amount of blood that flows out of a ventricle of the heart per unit of time

15. _____ deficiency of blood oxygen

16. _____ inadequate blood supply

17. _____ local vasodilation

18. _____ the ability of a muscle cell to shorten to produce movement

19. _____ excess carbon dioxide

20. _____ initiated by a change in arterial blood pressure

➡ *If you had difficulty with this section, review pages 699-711.*

II—VENOUS RETURN TO THE HEART

Fill in the blanks.

21. The ability of blood vessels to expand and adapt to higher pressure and maintain normal flow is called the _____ _____ _____.

22. Increased respirations and increased _____ tend to coincide.

23. _____ _____ is the exchange of materials between plasma in the capillaries and the surrounding interstitial fluid of the systemic tissues.

24. _____ _____ tends to promote diffusion of fluid into the plasma.

25. The more ADH that is secreted, the more water will be _____ into the blood from the urine and the greater the blood plasma volume will become.

26. _____ _____ _____ _____ of aldosterone secretion changes blood plasma volume.

27. _____ _____ is secreted by specialized cells in the atrial wall in response to overstretching.

28. _____ is high blood pressure.

➡ *If you had difficulty with this section, review pages 711-714.*

III—BLOOD PRESSURE

Multiple Choice—select the best answer.

29. The diastolic blood pressure is:
    a. the heart contracting.
    b. the heart relaxing.
    c. the pressure in the atria.
    d. the pressure in the ventricles.

30. With a blood pressure of 120/80, the number 80 indicates:
    a. the diastolic reading.
    b. the systolic reading.
    c. the Korotkoff sounds.
    d. the ejection phase.

31. The mean arterial pressure (MAP)* for a BP of 130/90 is:
    a. 90.
    b. 93.
    c. 100.
    d. 103.

Fill in the blanks.

32. _____ is the apparatus used to measure blood pressure.

33. If blood gushes forth in spurts with considerable force, you have most likely cut an _____.

34. The pressure points can be used to stop _____ bleeding.

➡ *If you had difficulty with this section, review pages 714-720.*

*MAP = [(2 × diastolic BP) + systolic BP] ÷ 3

Labeling—fill in the blank with the correct pulse point, as shown in the diagram.

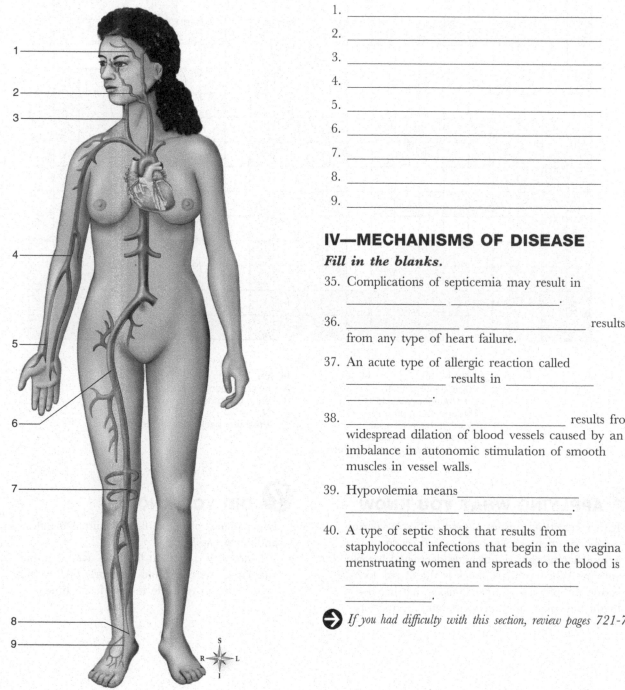

Pulse points.

1. _____
2. _____
3. _____
4. _____
5. _____
6. _____
7. _____
8. _____
9. _____

IV—MECHANISMS OF DISEASE

Fill in the blanks.

35. Complications of septicemia may result in
_____ _____.

36. _____ _____ results
from any type of heart failure.

37. An acute type of allergic reaction called
_____ results in _____
_____.

38. _____ _____ results from
widespread dilation of blood vessels caused by an
imbalance in autonomic stimulation of smooth
muscles in vessel walls.

39. Hypovolemia means_____
_____ _____.

40. A type of septic shock that results from
staphylococcal infections that begin in the vagina of
menstruating women and spreads to the blood is
_____ _____
_____.

➡ *If you had difficulty with this section, review pages 721-722.*

CROSSWORD PUZZLE

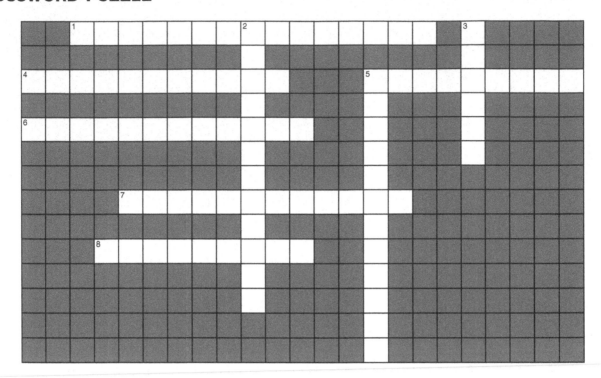

ACROSS
1. Pulse; thin; measure
4. Go around; relating to
5. Through; pour; process
6. Blood; force; relating to
7. Pressure; receive; agent
8. Apart or through; position; relating to

DOWN
2. Lifted; relating to; back or again; bend (2 words)
3. Noise
5. Pressure; back or again; bend

 APPLYING WHAT YOU KNOW

41. Kim received a gunshot wound to her leg during a robbery attempt. She experienced severe hemorrhaging that significantly decreased her blood volume. Which kind of shock is she at risk for? Name the physiologic mechanisms that her body might initiate to attempt to maintain circulatory homeostasis.

42. Students at Charlotte's high school were holding a car wash to collect money for an AED to be available at the school gymnasium. The coach had advised them that it could be used for emergencies such as VF. What is an AED and VF, and why is this so important?

 DID YOU KNOW?

• Every pound of excess fat contains 200 miles of additional capillaries.
• If laid out in a straight line, the average adult's circulatory system would be nearly 60,000 miles long—enough to circle the earth 2.5 times.

✓ ONE LAST QUICK CHECK

Multiple Choice—select the best answer.

43. Starling's law of the heart states that:
    a. blood flows from areas of high pressure to areas of low pressure.
    b. the volume of blood ejected from the ventricle is constant.
    c. the more stretched the heart fibers are at the beginning of a contraction, the stronger is their contraction.
    d. average heart rate is 72 beats per minute.

44. The vagus nerve is said to act as a(n) _____ on the heart.
    a. temperature monitor
    b. positive feedback loop
    c. ejection mechanism
    d. brake

45. Under normal conditions, blood viscosity changes:
    a. frequently.
    b. during hemorrhage only.
    c. under stress.
    d. very little.

46. The popliteal pulse point is found:
    a. at the bend of the elbow.
    b. on the dorsum of the foot.
    c. behind the knee.
    d. behind the medial malleolus.

47. Peripheral resistance is primarily affected by:
    a. the length of myocardial fibers.
    b. blood viscosity and the diameter of arterioles.
    c. the capacity of the blood reservoirs.
    d. the elasticity of the heart.

48. Septic shock is caused by:
    a. complications of toxins in the blood.
    b. a nerve condition.
    c. a drop in blood pressure.
    d. blood vessel dilation.

49. Hypovolemic shock is caused by:
    a. heart failure.
    b. dilated blood vessels.
    c. a loss in blood volume.
    d. a severe allergic reaction.

50. The shift of the blood reservoir to the veins in the legs when standing is called the:
    a. orthostatic effect.
    b. total peripheral resistance effect.
    c. vasomotor mechanism.
    d. medullary ischemic reflex.

51. Fick's formula is used for determining:
    a. stroke volume.
    b. cardiac output.
    c. cardiac reserve.
    d. ejection fraction.

52. The minute volume is equal to the:
    a. the pressure gradient divided by the resistance.
    b. mean arterial pressure divided by the cardiac output.
    c. cardiac output divided by the ejection fraction.
    d. cardiac output divided by the cardiac reserve.

Fill in the blanks.

53. The chief determinant of arterial blood pressure is the _____ of blood in the arteries.

54. Factors that affect the strength of myocardial contraction and, therefore, stroke volume are _____ factors.

55. Starling's law of the heart states that "within limits, the longer, or more stretched, the heart fibers at the beginning of contraction, the _____ is their contraction."

56. The _____ _____ is the ratio of the stroke volume (SV) to the end-diastolic volume (EDV).

57. The pumping work that the heart must do to push blood into the arteries is known as cardiac _____.

58. The hormone most known as a heart accelerator is _____.

59. During exercise blood from reservoirs is redistributed to more active structures such as _____ muscles and the heart.

60. The blood vessel commonly used to perform blood pressure readings is the _____ _____.

61. The sounds made during the measurement of a blood pressure are called _____ _____.

62. Blood flows most rapidly in the _____ and most slowly in the _____.

CHAPTER 31

Lymphatic System

The lymphatic system is similar to the circulatory system. Lymph, like blood, flows through an elaborate route of vessels. In addition to lymphatic vessels, the lymphatic system consists of lymph nodes, lymph, and the spleen. Unlike the circulatory system, the lymphatic vessels do not form a closed circuit. Lymph flows only once through the vessels before draining into the general blood circulation. This system is a filtering mechanism for microorganisms and a protective device against foreign invaders, such as cancer.

As your text suggests, this system can also be likened to the wastewater system of our communities. Lymph circulates to bring contaminants to the system that are harmful to the body. Toxins are filtered and the fluid is returned cleansed, just as our wastewater systems remove harmful substances from the water and return it cleansed for our eventual use. Your knowledge of this system is necessary to understand the function of the lymphatic system in maintaining fluid balance in the tissues and the role that plays in the body's immune system.

I—LYMPHATIC VESSELS, LYMPH, AND CIRCULATION OF LYMPH

Multiple Choice—select the best answer.

1. The most important function(s) of the lymphatic system is/are:
   a. fluid balance of the internal environment.
   b. immunity.
   c. both a and b.
   d. none of the above.

2. Lymphatic capillaries that operate in the villi of the small intestine are called:
   a. lymphatics.
   b. lacteals.
   c. Peyer patches.
   d. lymph nodes.

3. Lymph from the entire body drains into the thoracic duct, *except* lymph from the:
   a. upper right quadrant.
   b. upper left quadrant.
   c. lower limbs.
   d. entire head and neck.

4. Which of the following is *not* a difference between lymphatics and veins?
   a. Lymphatics have thinner walls.
   b. Lymphatics contain more valves.
   c. Lymphatics contain lymph nodes.
   d. Lymphatics endure greater pressure.

5. If lymphatic return is blocked, which of the following will *not* occur?
   a. Blood protein concentration will fall.
   b. Blood osmotic pressure will fall.
   c. CO_2 levels in the blood will rise.
   d. Fluid imbalance will occur.

6. Lymphatic circulation is maintained by all of the following *except*:
   a. breathing movements.
   b. heart.
   c. skeletal muscle contractions.
   d. valves.

7. Lymphatic circulation begins with lymphatic:
   a. capillaries.
   b. veins.
   c. venules.
   d. arterioles.

True or False

8. _____ The lymphatic system could be referred to as a specialized component of the circulatory system.

9. _____ Lymphatic vessels, like vessels in the blood vascular system, form a closed loop of circulation.

10. _____ Both lymph and interstitial fluid closely resemble blood plasma in composition.

11. _____ Lymphatics have one-way valves much like veins.

12. _____ The milky lymph found in lacteals after digestion is called *chyle*.

13. _____ A dilated structure on the thoracic duct that serves as a storage area for lymph moving toward its point of entry into the venous system is the *cisterna chyli*.

14. _____ Activities that result in central movement, or flow, of lymph are called *lymphokinetic actions*.

➡ *If you had difficulty with this section, review pages 729-733.*

201

II—LYMPH NODES

Multiple Choice—select the best answer.

15. The small depression of a lymph node from which the efferent lymph vessel arises is termed the:
    a. sinus.
    b. hilum.
    c. capsule.
    d. nodule.

16. The lymph nodes located in front of the ear are called the:
    a. submaxillary groups.
    b. inguinal lymph nodes.
    c. cervical lymph nodes.
    d. none of the above.

17. An infection of a lymph node is called:
    a. adenitis.
    b. noditis.
    c. lymphitis.
    d. lysis.

18. The lymphatic tissue of lymph nodes serves as the final maturation site for:
    a. monocytes.
    b. lymphocytes.
    c. both a and b.
    d. none of the above.

True or False

19. _____ Even though some lymph nodes occur in clusters, most occur as single nodes.

20. _____ Cortical nodules are composed of packed lymphocytes that surround an area called the *germinal center*.

Labeling—identify the principal organs of the lymphatic system by matching each term with its corresponding number on the following illustration.

_____ spleen
_____ tonsils
_____ right lymphatic duct
_____ aggregated lymphoid nodules (Peyer patches) in intestinal wall
_____ entrance of thoracic duct into subclavian vein
_____ superficial cubital (supratrochlear) lymph nodes
_____ axillary lymph node
_____ red bone marrow
_____ cisterna chyli
_____ cervical lymph node
_____ thoracic duct
_____ inguinal lymph node
_____ thymus gland

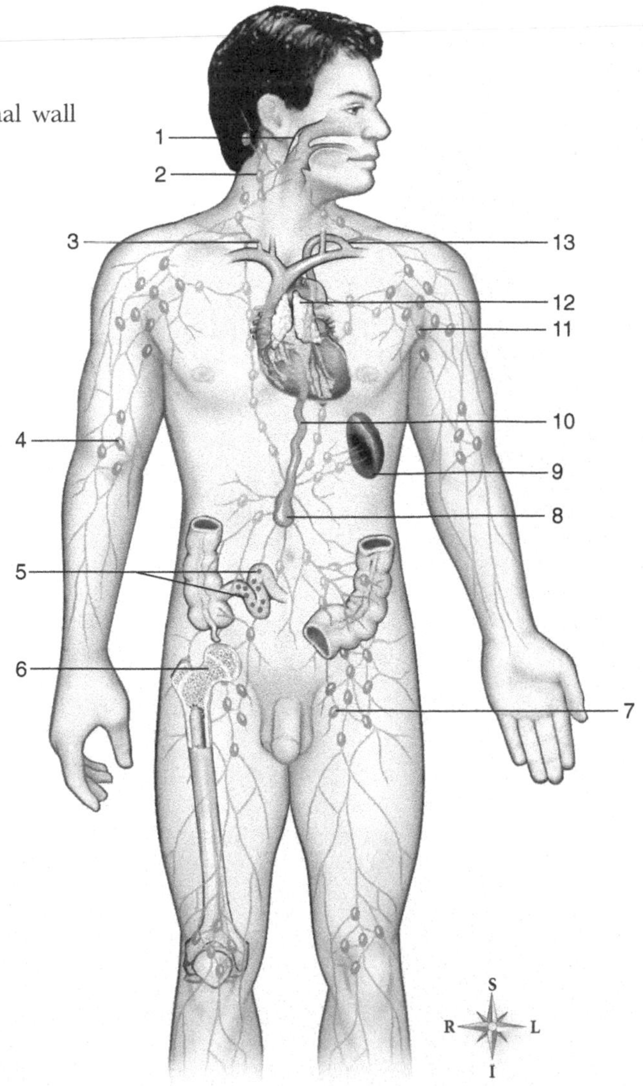

Labeling—using the terms provided, label the structure of a lymph node on the following diagram.

efferent lymph vessel　　　germinal center　　　　sinuses
medullary cords　　　　　　hilum　　　　　　　　　capsule
afferent lymph vessel　　　　cortical nodules

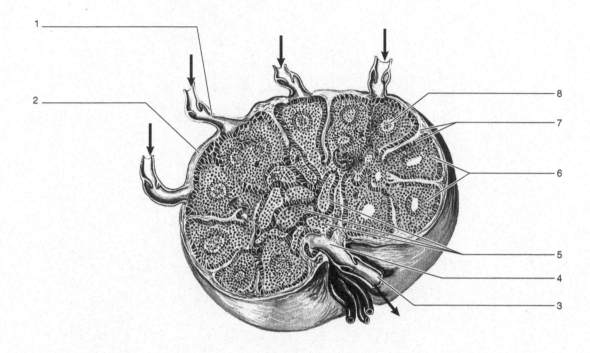

 If you had difficulty with this section, review pages 734-737.

III—LYMPHATIC DRAINAGE OF THE BREAST

Multiple Choice—select the best answer.

21. Over 85% of the lymph from the breast enters lymph nodes of the:
    a. axillary region.
    b. supraclavicular region.
    c. brachial region.
    d. subscapular region.

22. The breast—mammary gland and surrounding tissue—is drained by:
    a. lymphatics that originate in and drain the skin over the breast, with the exception of the areola and nipple.
    b. lymphatics that originate in and drain the substance of the breast itself, including the skin of the areola and nipple.
    c. both a and b.
    d. none of the above.

Labeling—label the lymphatic drainage of the breast on the following illustration.

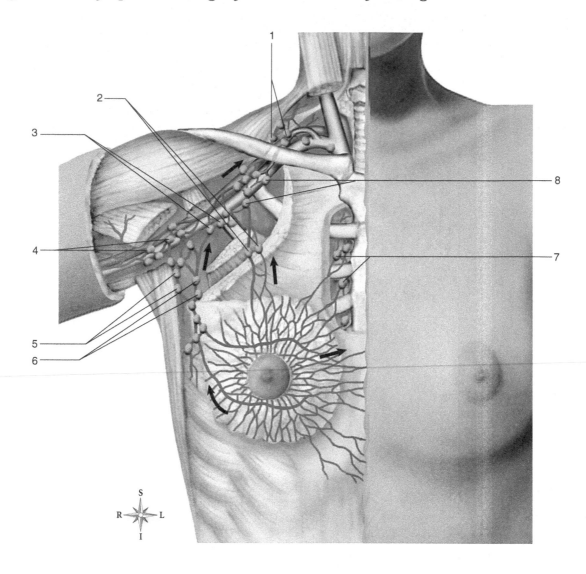

1. _____   5. _____

2. _____   6. _____

3. _____   7. _____

4. _____   8. _____

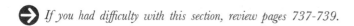 *If you had difficulty with this section, review pages 737-739.*

IV—TONSILS, THYMUS, AND SPLEEN

Multiple Choice—select the best answer.

23. Adenoids are swollen:
    a. pharyngeal tonsils.
    b. palatine tonsils.
    c. lingual tonsils.
    d. none of the above.

24. The thymus secretes:
    a. T_3.
    b. T_4.
    c. thymosin.
    d. both a and c.

25. The thymus is located:
    a. deep to the thyroid.
    b. in the axillary region.
    c. in the mediastinum.
    d. none of the above

True or False

26. _____ As a person ages, the thymus increases in size; this process is called *involution*.

27. _____ The spleen functions solely in defense from foreign microorganisms.

28. _____ The spleen removes imperfect platelets from the blood.

→ *If you had difficulty with this section, review pages 739-743.*

V—MECHANISMS OF DISEASE
Fill in the blanks.

29. _____ is a term that refers to a tumor of the cells of lymphoid tissue.

30. A middle ear infection is known as _____ _____ _____.

31. Septicemia is also known as _____ _____.

32. Lymphedema may be caused by small parasitic worms called _____ that infest the lymph nodes.

33. Two principal categories of lymphomas are _____ and _____ lymphoma.

→ *If you had difficulty with this section, review pages 743-745.*

CROSSWORD PUZZLE

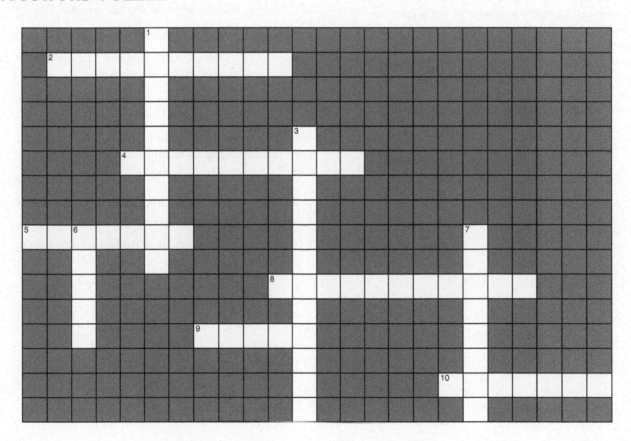

ACROSS
2. Water; swelling
4. In; roll; state
5. Milk; relating to
8. Anew; mouth; condition of
9. Water
10. Thread; like; things

DOWN
1. Throat; relating to
3. Vessel; of juice (2 words)
6. Juice
7. Breast; inflammation

APPLYING WHAT YOU KNOW

34. Ms. Langston was diagnosed with hemolytic anemia. Is a splenectomy a viable option? If so, why? Can she live without her spleen?

35. Baby Wilson was born without a thymus gland. Immediate plans were made for a transplant to be performed. In the meantime, baby Wilson was placed in strict isolation. For what reason was he placed in isolation?

 DID YOU KNOW?

- According to the Centers for Disease Control and Prevention, 18 million courses of antibiotics are prescribed for the common cold in the United States per year. Research shows that colds are caused by viruses. Fifty million unnecessary antibiotics are prescribed for viral respiratory infections every year.
- On average, at any time about 1 to 2 liters of lymph fluid circulate in the lymphatics and body tissues.

 ONE LAST QUICK CHECK

Matching—select the best response.

  a. thymus
  b. tonsils
  c. spleen

36. _____ palatine, pharyngeal, tubal, and lingual are examples

37. _____ hematopoiesis

38. _____ destroys worn-out red blood cells

39. _____ located in the mediastinum

40. _____ serves as a reservoir for blood

41. _____ T lymphocytes

42. _____ largest at puberty

True or False

43. _____ The cisterna chyli is a dilated structure on the thoracic duct that serves as a storage area for lymph moving into the venous system.

44. _____ Healthy capillaries "leak" proteins.

45. _____ Thoracic duct lymph is "pumped" into the venous system during inspiration.

46. _____ Lymph nodes have several afferent and efferent vessels.

47. _____ Lymphedema is swelling due to an accumulation of lymph.

48. _____ An anastomosis is the removal of a part.

49. _____ The spleen is located below the diaphragm, above the right kidney and descending colon.

50. _____ Splenomegaly is removal of the spleen.

CHAPTER 32
Innate Immunity

The immune system is the armed forces division of the body. Ready to attack at a moment's notice, the immune system defends us against the major enemies of the body: microorganisms, foreign transplanted tissue cells, and our own cells that have turned malignant.

We can further divide the immune system into innate immunity and adaptive immunity. Innate immunity may attack invading microorganisms and cells through species resistance, mechanical and chemical barriers, inflammation, fever, natural killer cells, and toll-like receptors.

Phagocytes, a large group of innate immunity cells, additionally assist with the destruction of foreign invaders by a process known as *phagocytosis*. Neutrophils and macrophages ingest and digest the invaders, rendering them harmless to the body.

Another weapon that innate immunity possesses is complement. Normally a group of inactive enzymes, called *complement*, is present in the blood and can be activated to kill invading cells by drilling holes in their cytoplasmic membranes, which allow fluid to enter the cell until it bursts. Your review of this chapter will give you an understanding of how the body defends itself from the daily invasion of destructive substances.

I—INNATE IMMUNITY

Multiple Choice—select the best answer.

1. Which of the following cells is *not* involved with innate immunity?
   a. natural killer cells
   b. neutrophils
   c. macrophages
   d. all of the above are involved with innate immunity

2. The "first line of defense" in innate immunity is:
   a. inflammation.
   b. phagocytosis.
   c. mechanical and chemical barriers.
   d. complement.

3. About 15% of the total number of lymphocyte cells are:
   a. natural killer (NK) cells.
   b. macrophages.
   c. neutrophils.
   d. interferon.

4. The most numerous type of phagocyte is the:
   a. neutrophil.
   b. macrophage.
   c. histocyte.
   d. Kupffer cell.

5. Which of the following is a phagocytic monocyte that migrates out of the bloodstream?
   a. neutrophil
   b. macrophage
   c. phagosome
   d. none of the above

True or False

6. _____ The immune mechanism that provides a general defense by acting against anything recognized as nonself is termed *adaptive immunity*.

7. _____ Species resistance is the genetic characteristics of the human species that protect the body from certain pathogens.

8. _____ Interferon has been proven effective as a treatment against most cancers.

9. _____ The complement cascade causes phagocytosis of the foreign cell that triggered it.

10. _____ Natural killer cells are a group of lymphocytes that kill many types of tumor cells and cells infected by different kinds of viruses.

Matching—select the best answer.

a. antigen
b. interferon
c. complement
d. innate immunity
e. toll-like receptors
f. non-specific
g. natural killer cells
h. immunocompetence
i. opsonization
j. phagocytosis

11. _____ molecular markers

12. _____ process used by complement to mark microbes for destruction by phagocytic cells

13. _____ cytokine

14. _____ pattern-recognition receptors in the membranes of host cells

15. _____ second line of defense

16. _____ ability to activate an effective response to an antigen

17. _____ must engage their target cells by direct contact to cause cell destruction

18. _____ another term for "innate" immunity

19. _____ major category of immune mechanisms

20. _____ name given to each of about 20 inactive enzymes in the plasma and on cell surfaces

➡ *If you had difficulty with this section, review pages 750-759.*

CROSSWORD PUZZLE

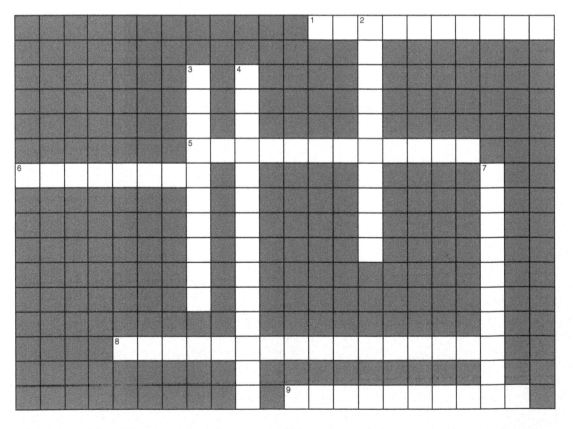

ACROSS
1. Large; eat
5. Eating; cell; condition
6. Cell; movement
8. Weird or amazing; receive; agent (3 words)
9. Complete; result of action

DOWN
2. Chemical; movement
3. Through; an oozing
4. Inborn; free; state (2 words)
7. Between; strike; substance

APPLYING WHAT YOU KNOW

21. Angela cut herself while cooking. She cleansed the area immediately with soap and water and put a band-aid on it. While checking it on the third day, she noticed a small area of pus in the center. She did not notice any redness or any other symptoms, and it appeared to be healing around the edges of the approximately ¾-inch cut. Should she be concerned about this sign? Explain your rationale for your decision.

❓ DID YOU KNOW?

• Approximately 5%-8% of the U.S. population has an autoimmune disease—about 78% of these people are women.
• Getting less than 5 hours of sleep a night has been shown to greatly depress immune function in your body.
• Dieting decreases natural killer (NK) cell functionality, therefore weakening the immune system.

✔ ONE LAST QUICK CHECK

Fill in the blanks.

22. Histamine, kinins, and interleukins are examples of _____ mediators.

23. A type of immune mechanism that provides a general defense by acting against anything recognized as "not-self" is called _____ _____.

24. Chemicals released from cells to trigger or regulate innate and adaptive responses are _____.

25. Natural killer (NK) cells are a group of _____ that kill many types of tumor cells and cells infected with different types of viruses.

26. The ability of our immune system to attack abnormal or foreign cells but spare our own normal cells is _____ _____.

True or False

27. _____ Phagocytosis is a specific defense mechanism.

28. _____ Diapedesis is the movement of neutrophils out of the bloodstream and around the tissue cells to the site of the injury.

29. _____ Innate immunity is also known as *adaptive immunity.*

30. _____ Sebum and mucus are part of the body's first line of defense.

31. _____ The primary cells involved in adaptive immunity are T cells and B cells.

CHAPTER 33

Adaptive Immunity

Adaptive immunity, in contrast to innate immunity, attacks specific enemies of the body that are considered abnormal. It is part of the third line of defense, and the primary cells are lymphocytes.

Lymphocytes are the most numerous cells of the immune system. They circulate in the body's fluids seeking invading organisms and destroying them with powerful lymphotoxins, lymphokines, or antibodies.

Two types of lymphocytes (B cells and T cells) attack specific antigens in different ways. B cells produce antibodies that either attack the pathogen or direct other cells to kill the invader. This is known as *antibody-mediated immunity* or *humoral immunity*. T cells attack abnormal cells more directly and are distinguished by the name *cell-mediated immunity* or *cellular immunity*.

Your review of this chapter will complete your knowledge of how the body protects itself from invading pathogens.

I—ADAPTIVE IMMUNITY

Multiple Choice—select the best answer.

1. B cells and T cells are examples of:
   a. monocytes.
   b. lymphocytes.
   c. neutrophils.
   d. macrophages.

2. Cell-mediated immunity involves:
   a. B cells.
   b. T cells.
   c. both a and b.
   d. neither a nor b.

3. The T cell subsets that are clinically important in diagnosing AIDS are:
   a. CD4.
   b. CD8.
   c. neither a nor b.
   d. both a and b.

4. An antibody consists of:
   a. two heavy and two light polypeptide chains.
   b. two heavy and one light polypeptide chains.
   c. one heavy and two light polypeptide chains.
   d. one heavy and one light polypeptide chain.

5. The amount of antibodies in a person's blood in response to exposure to a pathogen is called:
   a. toxoid.
   b. titer.
   c. both a and b.
   d. none of the above.

6. The most abundant circulating antibody is:
   a. IgM.
   b. IgG.
   c. IgA.
   d. IgE.

7. The specific cells that secrete antibodies are:
   a. B cells.
   b. T cells.
   c. plasma cells.
   d. none of the above.

8. T cells are sensitized by:
   a. direct exposure to an antigen.
   b. presentation of an antigen by an antigen-presenting cell.
   c. antibodies produced by B cells.
   d. lymphokines.

9. *Complement* can best be described as:
   a. an antibody.
   b. an enzyme in the blood plasma.
   c. a hormone.
   d. a lymphokine.

10. The chemical messengers that T cells release into inflamed tissues are called:
    a. pathogens.
    b. cytokines.
    c. lymphotoxins.
    d. suppressor cells.

Fill in the blanks.

11. Antibodies are proteins of the family called _____.

12. _____ is the predominant class of antibody produced after initial contact with an antigen.

13. The first vaccination was against the _____ _____.

14. Some vaccines use _____ (weakened) pathogens.

15. _____ _____
    generally lasts longer than passive immunity.

16. Abnormal antigens or _____
    _____ are present in the plasma
    membranes of some cancer cells in addition to
    self-antigens.

17. _____ is elevated in both benign
    and malignant prostate disease.

18. Helper T cells and suppressor T cells help regulate
    _____ _____
    function by regulating B cell and T cell function.

19. A fetus receives protection from the mother through
    _____ _____
    immunity.

20. A vaccination provides _____
    _____ immunity.

→ *If you had difficulty with this section, review pages 762-777.*

T Cell Development

Labeling—label the T cell as it progresses from the thymus through activation.

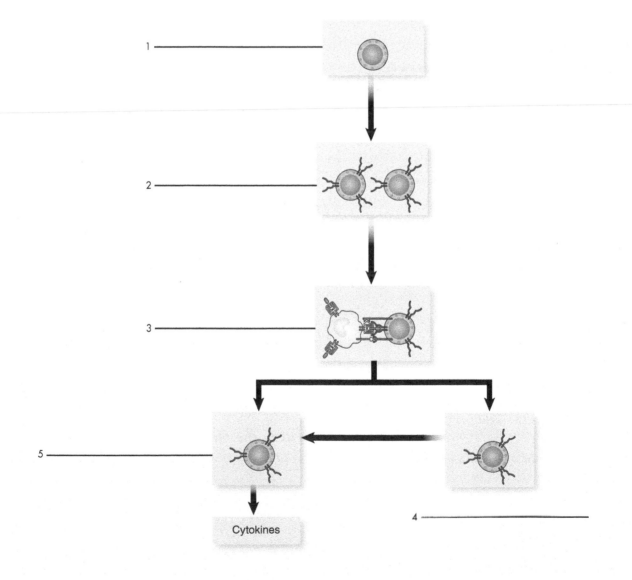

II—MECHANISMS OF DISEASE

Matching—match the term with the proper selection.

a. HIV
b. AZT
c. SCID
d. HLAs
e. SLE

21. _____ Stem cells are missing or unable to grow properly

22. _____ Retrovirus

23. _____ Inhibits symptoms of AIDS

24. _____ Chronic autoimmune inflammatory disease of the joints, blood vessels, skin, kidney, and nervous system

25. _____ Involved in transplant rejection

➜ *If you had difficulty with this section, review pages 778-782.*

CROSSWORD PUZZLE

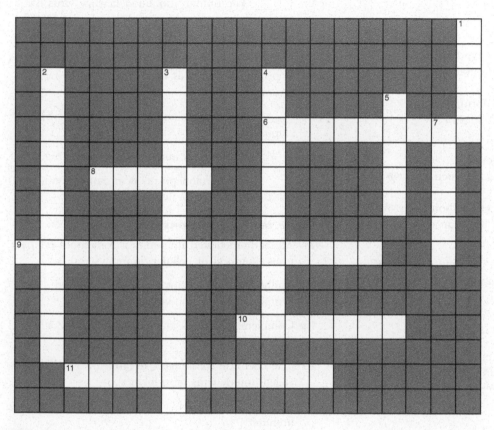

ACROSS
6. Thyme flower; cell
8. Plant cutting
9. Liquid; relating to; free; state (2 words)
10. Against; produce
11. Cow; process

DOWN
1. Natural
2. Self; free; state
3. Free; ball; small; substance
4. Between; white; substance
5. Thymus gland; storeroom (2 words)
7. Free (immunity)

 APPLYING WHAT YOU KNOW

26. Trent, a newborn, received immune protection from his mother through the placenta and breast milk. Which specific type of immunity is this? His older sister, Carrie, also recently received immune protection from a host of illnesses; however, hers was achieved deliberately via immunization by her pediatrician. What specific type of immunity is she experiencing? How do her types of immunity differ from her brother's?

27. Marcia is an intravenous drug user. She has developed a type of skin cancer known as Kaposi sarcoma. What, most likely, is Marcia's primary diagnosis? What are some of the medications that might be used to inhibit symptoms for a while?

DID YOU KNOW?

- The number one way to boost the immune system is to reduce stress.
- Although the body needs some sunshine to produce vitamin D, too much sunshine can suppress the immune system.

 ONE LAST QUICK CHECK

Multiple Choice—select the best answer.

28. T cells do which of the following?
    a. develop in the thymus
    b. form memory cells
    c. form plasma cells
    d. all of the above

29. Acquired immune deficiency syndrome is characterized by which of the following?
    a. caused by a retrovirus
    b. causes inadequate T cell formation
    c. can result in death from cancer
    d. all of the above

30. B cells do which of the following?
    a. develop into plasma cells and memory cells
    b. secrete antibodies
    c. develop from primitive cells in bone marrow called *stem cells* and then into naïve B cells
    d. all of the above

31. Which of the following kills invading cells by drilling a hole in their plasma membrane?
    a. interferon
    b. complement
    c. antibody
    d. memory cell

32. What is a rapidly growing population of identical cells that produce large quantities of specific antibodies called?
    a. complementary
    b. lymphotoxic
    c. chemotactic
    d. monoclonal

33. Which of the following is a form of passive natural immunity?
    a. A child develops measles and acquires immunity to subsequent exposure.
    b. Antibodies are injected into an infected individual.
    c. An infant receives protection through its mother's milk.
    d. Vaccinations are given against smallpox.

Fill in the blanks.

34. Hypersensitivity of the immune system to an environmental antigen is known as an _____.

35. Drugs used to relieve the symptoms of allergies are called _____.

36. Adaptive immunity is also known as _____ _____.

37. A _____ is a powerful poison that acts directly and quickly to kill any cell it attacks.

True or False

38. _____ The human immunodeficiency virus has a profound impact on a person's number of CD12 subset of T cells.

39. _____ Once inside a cell, HIV uses its viral RNA to produce DNA; this process is called *reverse transcription.*

40. _____ A common autoimmune disease is SLE or "lupus."

41. _____ SCID is an immunosuppressive drug.

42. _____ Glomerulonephritis is an autoimmune disease of the neuromuscular junction.

Circle the best response.

43. Antibody-mediated immunity is sometimes referred to as (humoral or cellular) immunity.

44. Antibodies are proteins of the family called (lymphotoxins or immunoglobulins).

45. Complement attacks antigens by (cytolysis or clonal deletion).

46. The chemical messengers released by T cells are called (interleukins or cytokines).

47. Vaccinations are (active or passive) forms of gaining immunity.

CHAPTER 34

Stress

Life without any stress would be very dull and boring. Often it is stress that stimulates us to achieve our dreams and experience success and happiness. However, too much stress becomes unpleasant and tiring and can seriously interfere with our ability to function effectively. The challenge is to keep stress at a level that is healthy and enjoyable.

Although we react differently and in various degrees to stressors, we must acknowledge that in most individuals, stress leads to a physiologic stress response. These responses may be as simple as an increase in heart rate or perspiration or as complex as a disease syndrome. And although we may not be aware of it on a day-to-day basis, stress can be cumulative and manifest itself long after apparent stressors have been resolved. Your study of this unit will alert you to the impact of stress on your body and the significant role it plays in homeostasis.

I—SELYE'S CONCEPT OF STRESS

Multiple Choice—select the best answer.

1. The stages of general adaptation syndrome in the correct order are:
   a. alarm reaction, stage of exhaustion, stage of resistance.
   b. alarm reaction, stage of resistance, stage of exhaustion.
   c. stage of exhaustion, alarm reaction, stage of resistance.
   d. stage of exhaustion, stage of resistance, stage of alarm.

2. The "stress triad" refers to:
   a. alarm, exhaustion, resistance.
   b. hypertrophied adrenals, atrophied thymus and lymph nodes, and bleeding ulcers.
   c. stressor, stress, and response.
   d. health, stress, and disease.

3. Which of the following is *not* an alarm reaction response resulting from hypertrophy of the adrenal cortex?
   a. hyperglycemia
   b. hypertrophy of thymus
   c. decreased immunity
   d. decreased allergic responses

4. All of the following are true statements *except:*
   a. stressors are extreme stimuli.
   b. stressors are always unpleasant, injurious, or painful.
   c. the emotions of fear, anxiety, and grief can act as stressors.
   d. stressors differ in individuals.

5. What determines which stimuli are stressors for each individual?
   a. past experience
   b. diet
   c. heredity
   d. all of the above

True or False

6. _____ Selye's stage of exhaustion is reached in each exposure to stressors.

7. _____ High-stress, hard-driving, competitive individuals who may be at greater risk of coronary heart disease are classified as "Type B."

8. _____ The stage of resistance can also be described as *adaptation.*

9. _____ Stressors are "bad" stimuli that should always be avoided.

10. _____ The stress response commonly referred to as "fight or flight" is evoked by increased sympathetic activity.

Matching—identify the best answer from the choices given and insert the letter in the answer blank.

a. FAS
b. resistance stage
c. general adaptation syndrome
d. alarm stage
e. exhaustion state
f. stressor

11. _____ group of changes that make the presence of stress in the body known

12. _____ occurs when stress is extremely severe or continues over long periods

13. _____ increased activity of the sympathetic nervous system

14. _____ agent that produces stress

15. _____ "fight or flight" reaction disappears

16. _____ can occur as the result of stress in a developing fetus

➡ *If you had difficulty with this section, review pages 785-795.*

II—SOME CURRENT CONCEPTS ABOUT STRESS

Multiple Choice—select the best answer.

17. Corticotropin-releasing hormone (CRH) stimulates the anterior pituitary gland to secrete increased amounts of:
a. glucocorticoids.
b. aldosterone.
c. ACTH.
d. ADH.

18. All of the following are effects of cortisol *except:*
a. increased protein catabolism.
b. decreased immune responses.
c. decreased allergic responses.
d. "fight or flight" responses.

19. The dominant subjective reaction that occurs with psychological stress is:
a. guilt.
b. anxiety.
c. depression.
d. fear.

True or False

20. _____ The current definition of stress is "any stimulus that directly or indirectly stimulates neurons of the hypothalamus to release corticotropin-releasing hormone (CRH)."

21. _____ It is accepted among physiologists that a higher-than-normal blood level of corticoids results in a greater ability to resist stress.

22. _____ Physiologic stress and psychological stress are clearly different phenomena.

23. _____ Hypervolemia and antidiuresis are common responses to stress.

24. _____ Stress is an issue only among adolescents and adults.

25. _____ The brain's limbic system is often called the "emotional brain."

➡ *If you had difficulty with this section, review pages 788 and 790-796.*

CROSSWORD PUZZLE

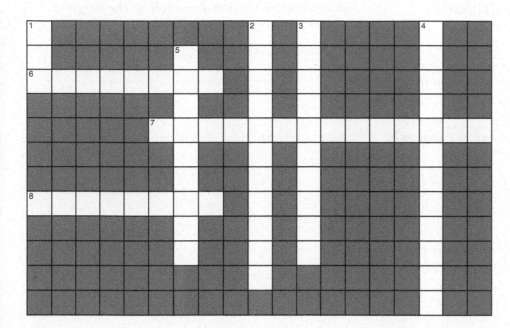

ACROSS
6. Tighten; agent
7. Tighten; together; running or (race) course (2 words)
8. Adjust; process

DOWN
1. Adjust; process; together; running or (race) course (3 words; abbreviation)
2. Tighten; group of three (2 words)
3. Different; standing still
4. Nerve; digest; chemical
5. Cortex or bark; like

 APPLYING WHAT YOU KNOW

26. Merrilee has an adolescent crush on John. Whenever she is near him, she feels anxious, her pupils dilate, heart rate elevates, systolic blood pressure rises, blood glucose levels are above normal, and blood and urine levels of epinephrine and norepinephrine are elevated. What is the physiologic term used to describe this syndrome? Beginning in the hypothalamus, trace the mechanisms that are causing this response. If this physiologic scenario were extended and intense, what illnesses might Merrilee be at risk for?

27. Bill is going to his boss for his annual evaluation. He is planning to ask for a raise and hopes the evaluation will be good. Which subdivision of the autonomic nervous system will be active during this stressful conference? Should he have a large meal before his appointment? Support your answer with facts.

 DID YOU KNOW?

• Laughing lowers levels of stress hormones and strengthens the immune system. Six-year-olds laugh an average of 300 times a day. Adults only laugh 15-100 times a day.
• A survey conducted at Iowa State College in 1969 suggests that a parent's stress at the time of conception plays a major role in determining a baby's sex. The child tends to be of the same sex as the parent who is under less stress.
• Cocoa and chocolate, which are rich in antioxidants, have been known to reduce stress.

✓ ONE LAST QUICK CHECK

Fill in the blanks.

28. _____ _____
_____ is the term for the group of
changes that make the presence of stress in the body
known.

29. The stage of _____ develops
only when stress is extremely severe or continues
over a long period.

30. The hypothalamus releases _____
_____ _____, which
acts as a trigger that initiates many diverse changes
in the body.

31. The term that describes the stress responses that
occur as a result of stimulation of the sympathetic
centers is known as the _____
_____ _____
_____.

32. _____ investigates
physiologic responses made by individuals to
psychological stressors.

True or False

33. _____ Type B personalities are at greater risk of
coronary disease than Type A personalities.

34. _____ Stress causes disruption in homeostasis.

35. _____ Smoking increases plasma adrenocorticoids
by as much as 77%.

36. _____ Identical psychological stressors induce
identical physiologic responses in different
individuals.

37. _____ Hans Selye identified a group of changes
classic to stress and called them the *stress triad*.

38. _____ Prolonged stress is thought to produce the
hormone neuropeptide Y.

Fill in the blanks—provide an example of a disease or condition for each of the target organs or systems.

39. Cardiovascular system _____

_____

40. Muscles _____

_____

41. Connective tissue _____

_____

42. Pulmonary system _____

_____

43. Immune system _____

_____

44. Gastrointestinal system _____

_____

45. Genitourinary system _____

_____

46. Skin _____

_____

47. Endocrine system _____

_____

48. Central nervous system _____

_____

CHAPTER 35
Respiratory Tract

As you sit reviewing this system, your body needs 16 quarts of air per minute. Walking requires 24 quarts of air and running requires 50 quarts per minute. The respiratory system provides the air necessary for you to perform your daily activities and eliminates the waste gases from the air that you breathe. Take a deep breath and think of the air as it enters some 250 million tiny air sacs similar in appearance to clusters of grapes. These microscopic air sacs expand to let air in and contract to force it out. These tiny sacs, or *alveoli*, are the functioning units of the respiratory system. They provide the necessary volume of oxygen and eliminate carbon dioxide 24 hours a day.

Air enters either through the mouth or the nasal cavity. Next it passes through the pharynx and past the epiglottis, through the glottis and the rest of the larynx. It then continues down the trachea, into the bronchi to the bronchioles, and finally through the alveoli. The reverse occurs for expelled air. Your review of this system is necessary to provide you with an understanding of this essential homeostatic mechanism—the breath of life.

I—UPPER RESPIRATORY TRACT

Multiple Choice—select the best answer.

1. Which of the following structures is *not* part of the upper respiratory tract?
   a. trachea
   b. larynx
   c. oropharynx
   d. nose

2. Which part of the respiratory system does *not* function as an air distributor?
   a. trachea
   b. bronchioles
   c. alveoli
   d. bronchi

3. Which sequence is the correct pathway for air movement through the nose and into the pharynx?
   a. anterior nares, posterior nares, vestibule, nasal cavity meatuses
   b. anterior nares, vestibule, posterior nares, nasal cavity meatuses
   c. nasal cavity meatuses, anterior nares, vestibule, posterior nares
   d. anterior nares, vestibule, nasal cavity meatuses, posterior nares

4. Which of the following is *not* a paranasal sinus?
   a. frontal
   b. maxillary
   c. mandibular
   d. sphenoid

5. The true vocal cords and the rima glottidis are called the:
   a. glottis.
   b. epiglottis.
   c. vestibular fold.
   d. both a and b.

True or False

6. _____ Failure of the palatine bones to unite is called *cribriform palate*.

7. _____ The pharynx is a tubelike structure that opens only into the mouth and larynx.

8. _____ Enlarged pharyngeal tonsils are called *adenoids*.

9. _____ The more common name for the thyroid cartilage is the *voice box*.

10. _____ The epiglottis moves up and down during swallowing to prevent food or liquids from entering the trachea.

Labeling—match each term with its corresponding number on the following illustration of the respiratory system.

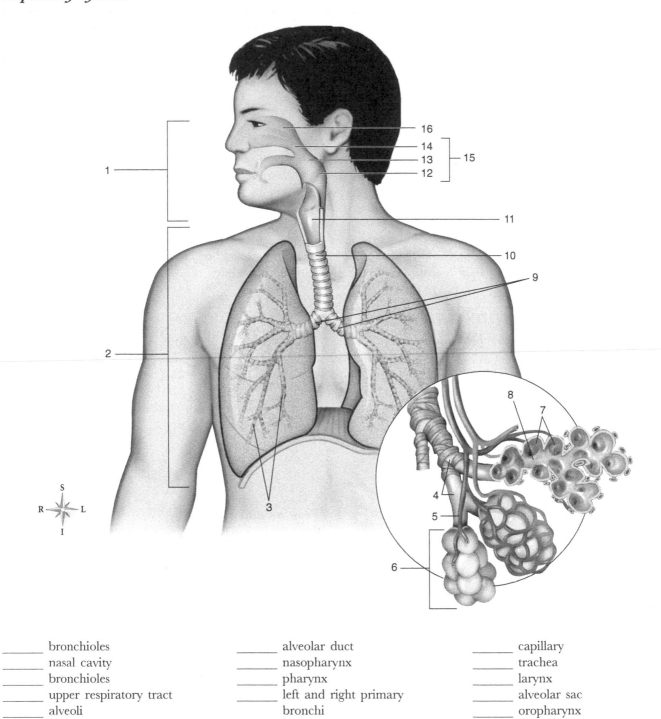

_____ bronchioles	_____ alveolar duct	_____ capillary
_____ nasal cavity	_____ nasopharynx	_____ trachea
_____ bronchioles	_____ pharynx	_____ larynx
_____ upper respiratory tract	_____ left and right primary	_____ alveolar sac
_____ alveoli	bronchi	_____ oropharynx
_____ lower respiratory tract	_____ laryngopharynx	

Labeling—using the terms provided, label the three divisions of the pharynx and nearby structures on the following illustration.

_____ opening of the auditory
(eustachian) tube
_____ laryngopharynx
_____ esophagus
_____ oropharynx
_____ vocal cords
_____ pharyngeal tonsil
(adenoids)
_____ epiglottis
_____ uvula
_____ lingual tonsil
_____ hyoid bone
_____ trachea
_____ nasopharynx
_____ soft palate
_____ palatine tonsil

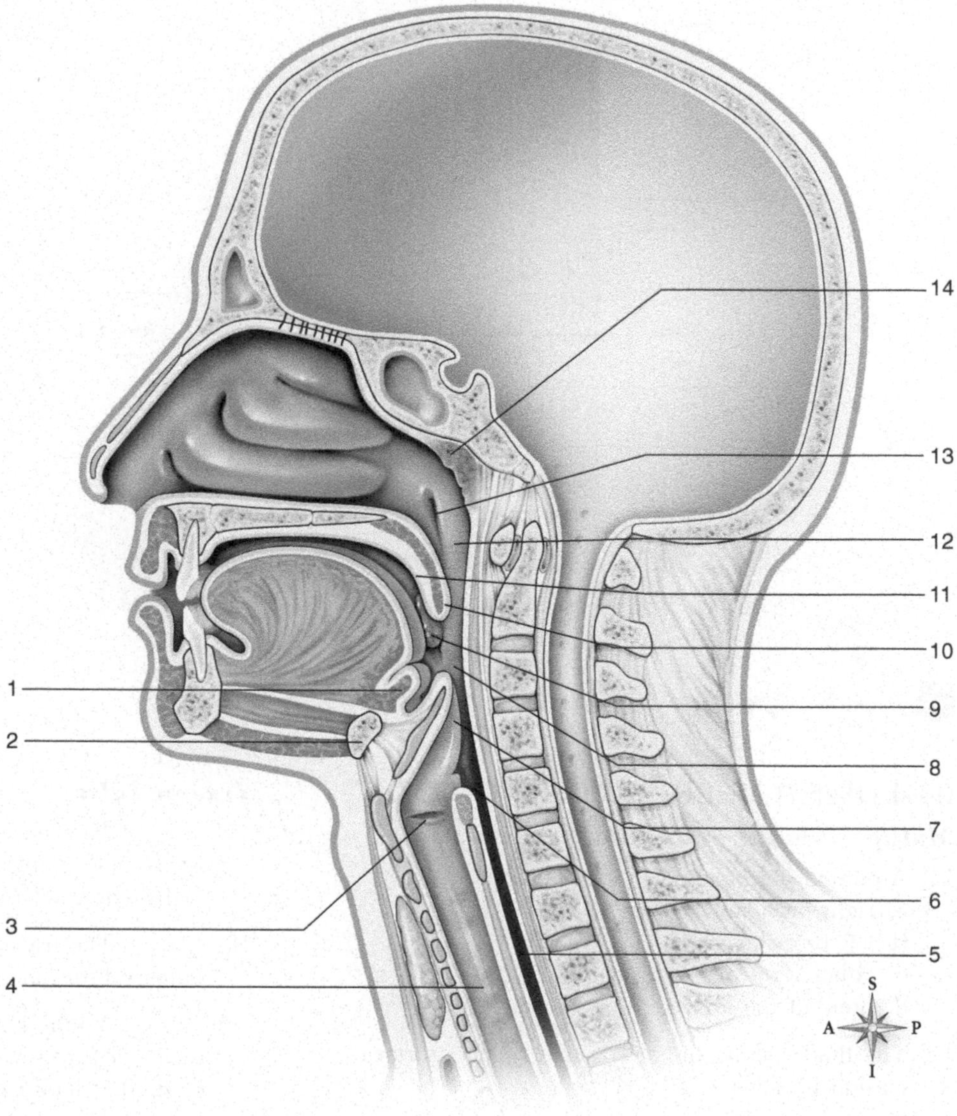

Labeling—label the structures related to the paranasal sinuses on the following illustration. Some terms may be used more than once.

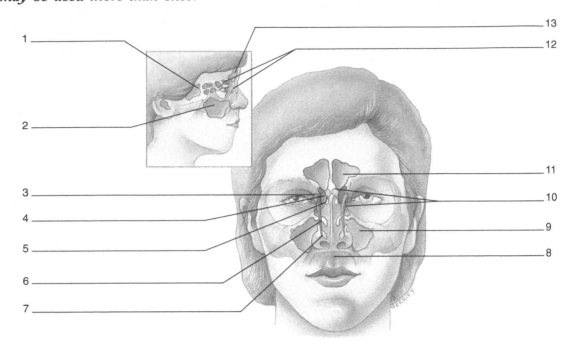

1 _____

2 _____

3 _____

4 _____

5 _____

6 _____

7 _____

13 _____

12 _____

11 _____

10 _____

9 _____

8 _____

 If you had difficulty with this section, review pages 800-807.

II—LOWER RESPIRATORY TRACT

Multiple Choice—select the best answer.

11. Aspirated objects tend to lodge in the:
    a. right bronchus.
    b. left bronchus.
    c. either right or left bronchus.
    d. none of the above.

12. The fluid coating the alveoli that reduces surface tension is called:
    a. bronchus.
    b. surfactant.
    c. alveolus.
    d. none of the above.

13. Which of the following is *not* an area of the lungs?
    a. oblique fissure
    b. horizontal fissure
    c. superior fissure
    d. hilum

14. Which of the following is *false*?
    a. When the diaphragm relaxes, it returns to a domelike shape.
    b. When the diaphragm contracts, it pulls the floor of the thoracic cavity downward.
    c. Changes in thorax size bring about inspiration and expiration.
    d. Raising the ribs decreases the depth and width of the thorax.

True or False

15. _____ The rings of cartilage that form the trachea are complete rings that prevent it from collapsing and shutting off the vital airway.

16. _____ The trachea divides into symmetrical primary bronchi.

17. _____ A tube is often placed in the trachea before a patient leaves the operating room, especially if he or she has had a muscle relaxant.

18. _____ The left lung is divided into three lobes by horizontal and oblique fissures.

19. _____ The apex of each lung is lateral and inferior.

20. _____ The exchange of gases between air and blood occurs in the alveoli.

21. _____ LVRS is the treatment of choice for emphysema.

22. _____ The barrier across which gases are exchanged between alveolar air and blood is called the *respiratory membrane*.

23. _____ Prolonged exposure to cigarette smoke can paralyze respiratory cilia.

24. _____ The visceral pleura lines the entire thoracic cavity.

Labeling—identify the lobes and fissures of the lungs by matching each term with its corresponding number on the following illustration (anterior view).

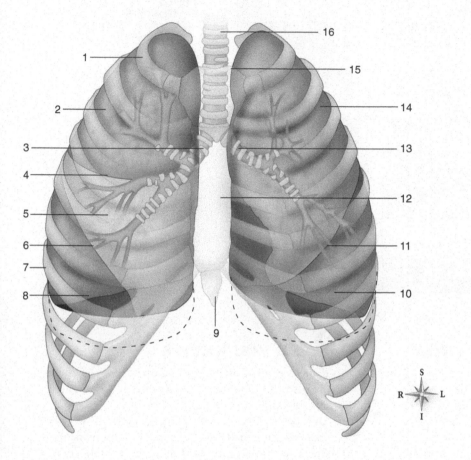

_____ right primary bronchus
_____ oblique fissure
_____ trachea
_____ right superior lobe
_____ sternum (manubrium)
_____ horizontal fissure
_____ seventh rib
_____ left primary bronchus
_____ right inferior lobe
_____ right middle lobe
_____ oblique fissure
_____ sternum (xiphoid process)
_____ body of sternum
_____ first rib
_____ left superior lobe
_____ left inferior lobe

➜ *If you had difficulty with this section, review pages 807-816.*

III—MECHANISMS OF DISEASE

Matching—identify each disorder with its corresponding description.

a. acute bronchitis
b. deviated septum
c. epistaxis
d. lung cancer
e. pharyngitis
f. rhinitis
g. tuberculosis
h. croup

25. _____ malignancy of pulmonary tissue

26. _____ very serious, chronic, and highly contagious infection

27. _____ displacement of the nasal septum

28. _____ a common infection of the lower respiratory tract characterized by acute inflammation of the bronchial tree

29. _____ nosebleed

30. _____ an inflammation of the mucosa of the nasal cavity

31. _____ sore throat

32. _____ difficulty breathing with a harsh, vibrating cough

➜ *If you had difficulty with this section, review pages 817-819.*

CROSSWORD PUZZLE

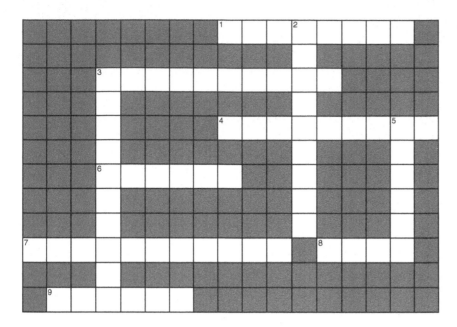

ACROSS
1. Hollow; little
3. Windpipe; inflammation
4. Entrance hall
6. Sea shell
7. Nose; throat
8. Tip
9. Side of body

DOWN
2. Upon; drip
3. Windpipe; little
5. Voice box

 APPLYING WHAT YOU KNOW

33. Mrs. Metheny's 6-year-old child had trouble swallowing. She had a high fever, appeared very anxious, and was drooling from her mouth. Mrs. Metheny called the EMS personnel, who assessed the child, inserted an airway, and transported her immediately to the emergency department. What is a possible explanation for why the child is experiencing these symptoms? What is the causative agent for these symptoms? Is this a serious threat to the child?

34. Mr. Gorski is a heavy smoker. Recently, he has noticed that when he gets up in the morning, he has a bothersome cough that brings up a large accumulation of mucus. This cough persists for several minutes and then leaves until the next morning. What is a possible explanation for this problem?

? DID YOU KNOW?

- If the roof of your mouth is narrow, you are more likely to snore because you are not getting enough oxygen through your nose.
- Only about 10% of the air in the lungs is actually changed with each cycle of inhaling and exhaling when an at-rest person is breathing, but up to 80% can be exchanged during deep breathing or strenuous exercise.

ONE LAST QUICK CHECK

Matching—choose the correct response.

    a. nose
    b. pharynx
    c. larynx

35. _____ warms and humidifies air

36. _____ air and food pass through here

37. _____ sinuses

38. _____ conchae

39. _____ septum

40. _____ tonsils

41. _____ middle ear infections

42. _____ epiglottis

43. _____ rhinitis

44. _____ sore throat

45. _____ epistaxis

Fill in the blanks.

The organs of the respiratory system are designed to perform two basic functions. They serve as an (46) _____ _____ and as a (47) _____ _____ . In addition to the above, the respiratory system (48) _____ , (49) _____ , and (50) _____ the air we breathe. Respiratory organs include the (51) _____ , (52) _____ , (53) _____ , (54) _____ , (55) _____ , and the (56) _____ . The respiratory system ends in millions of tiny, thin-walled sacs called (57) _____ .

(58)_____ of gases takes place in these sacs. Two aspects of the structure of these sacs assist them in the exchange of gases. First, an extremely thin membrane, the (59) _____ _____ , allows for easy exchange and second, the large number of air sacs makes an enormous (60)_____ area.

CHAPTER 36
Ventilation

The respiratory system functions to diffuse gases into and out of the blood so that the organs of our body receive blood that is rich in oxygen and low in carbon dioxide. The exchange of gases that occurs within the body is a complex operation, and each component of the pulmonary system contributes to successful ventilation. Air must enter the lungs (inspiration) from the external environment, an exchange must occur between the blood and the cells, and then air high in CO_2 is returned to the environment (expiration). The proper exchange of gases is necessary for survival and if disturbed can cause death within minutes.

I—RESPIRATORY PHYSIOLOGY/ VENTILATION

Multiple Choice—select the best answer.

1. Boyle's law states that:
   a. fluids move from areas of high pressure to low.
   b. the volume of a gas is inversely proportional to its pressure.
   c. the atmosphere exerts a pressure of 760 mm Hg.
   d. volume is directly proportional to temperature.

2. When the diaphragm contracts, the volume of the thorax increases, thoracic pressure:
   a. increases, and air is forced from the lungs.
   b. decreases, and air is forced from the lungs.
   c. decreases, and air rushes into the lungs.
   d. increases, and air rushes into the lungs.

3. Quiet inspiration is the function of:
   a. the diaphragm and the internal intercostal muscles.
   b. the diaphragm and the external intercostal muscles.
   c. the internal intercostal and external intercostal muscles.
   d. none of the above.

4. During normal, quiet respiration, the amount of air exchanged between the lungs and atmosphere is called _____ and has a volume of _____ mL.
   a. tidal volume; 1200
   b. vital capacity; 4500
   c. tidal volume; 500
   d. residual volume; 1200

5. Functional residual capacity (FRC) equals:
   a. TV + IRV.
   b. TV + IRV + ERV + RV.
   c. TV + IRV + ERV.
   d. ERV + RV.

6. *Eupnea* is a term used to describe:
   a. rapid, deep respiration.
   b. cessation of respiration.
   c. slow, shallow respiration.
   d. normal breathing.

7. Under normal conditions, air in the atmosphere exerts a pressure of:
   a. 500 mm Hg.
   b. 560 mm Hg.
   c. 660 mm Hg.
   d. 760 mm Hg.

8. Areas where gas exchange cannot take place are:
   a. anatomical dead spaces.
   b. nose, pharynx, larynx.
   c. trachea and bronchi.
   d. all of the above.

9. All of the following are regulated processes associated with the functioning of the respiratory system *except*:
   a. control of cell reproduction.
   b. gas exchange in lungs and tissue.
   c. pulmonary ventilation.
   d. transport of gases.

10. Dalton's law is also known as:
    a. Henry's law.
    b. Boyle's law.
    c. Charles' law.
    d. the law of partial pressures.

True or False

11. _____ Temperature is the measurement of the motion of molecules.

12. _____ The largest amount of air that can enter and leave the lungs during respiration is termed total lung capacity (TLC).

13. _____ Residual volume (RV) is the volume remaining in the respiratory tract after maximum expiration.

14. _____ The temporary cessation of breathing is termed *apnea*.

15. _____ It is not possible to exhale all of the air from your lungs.

Fill in the blanks.

16. The ability of the lungs and thorax to stretch, referred to as _____, is essential to normal respiration.

17. Intrapleural pressure is always less, or "negative," with respect to alveolar pressure. The difference is called the _____ _____.

18. Tidal volume multiplied by the respiratory rate yields the _____ _____ _____.

19. The constant alternation between inspiration and expiration is called the _____ _____.

20. The basic rhythm of the respiratory cycle of inspiration and expiration seems to be generated by the _____ _____ _____.

Labeling—label the following diagram with the correct terminology for the lung volumes displayed.

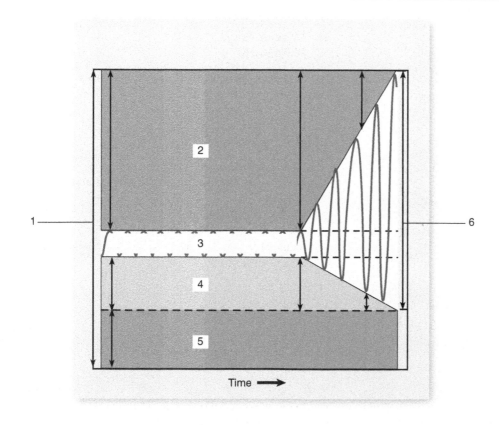

1. _____
2. _____
3. _____
4. _____
5. _____
6. _____

Labeling—identify the respiratory centers of the brain stem by matching each term to its corresponding number on the following illustration.

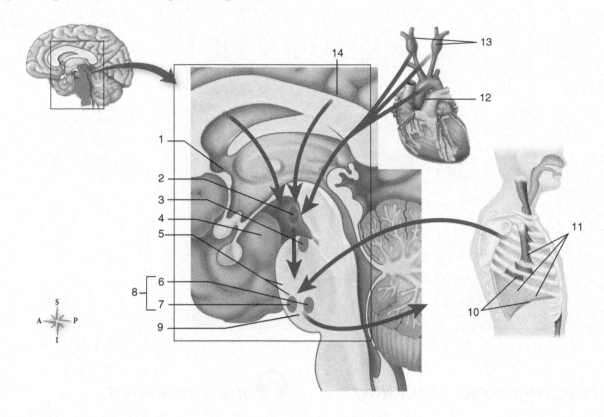

_____ carotid chemoreceptors and
      baroreceptors
_____ respiratory muscles
_____ apneustic center
_____ DRG
_____ limbic system (emotional
      responses)

_____ aortic chemoreceptors and
      baroreceptors
_____ PRG
_____ pons
_____ VRG
_____ medulla

_____ stretch receptors in lungs
      and thorax
_____ cortex (voluntary control)
_____ medullary rhythmicity area
_____ central chemoreceptors

➔ *If you had difficulty with this section, review pages 824-841.*

II—MECHANISMS OF DISEASE

Fill in the blanks.

21. _____ or _____
_____ _____
_____ is a broad term used to describe
conditions of progressive, irreversible obstruction of
expiratory air flow.

22. _____ results from excessive
tracheobronchial secretions that obstruct air flow.

23. _____ may result from the
progression of chronic bronchitis or other conditions
as air becomes trapped within alveoli, causing them
to enlarge and eventually rupture.

24. _____ is an obstructive disorder
characterized by recurring spasms of the smooth
muscle in the walls of the bronchial air passages.

25. _____ _____ _____
_____ is sometimes called "crib death"
because it occurs most frequently in babies with no
obvious medical problems who are younger than
3 months of age.

➔ *If you had difficulty with this section, review pages 842-843.*

CROSSWORD PUZZLE

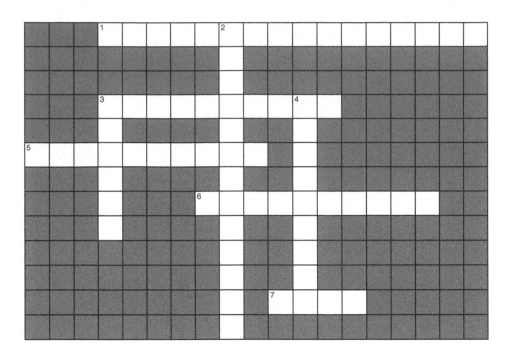

ACROSS
1. Excessive; fan or create wind; process
3. Out; breathe; process
5. Complete; act of
6. Breathe; measure
7. Gape

DOWN
2. Life; relating to; hold; state (2 words)
3. Easily; breathe; condition
4. Straight or upright; breathe; condition

 APPLYING WHAT YOU KNOW

26. Mr. Gaines has smoked a considerable number of cigars and cigarettes during the last 2 decades. He is beginning to have difficulty breathing—especially on exhalation. Which broad category of diseases may he be exhibiting symptoms of? What other diseases is he at risk for? What are the physiologic mechanisms of these diseases?

 DID YOU KNOW?

- Sinusitis affects 37 million Americans, causing difficulty in breathing and chronic headaches.
- A person's nose and ears continue to grow throughout his or her life.

27. While sledding on a frozen creek, Heather, a 12-year-old girl, fell through the ice. Her situation wasn't discovered for about half an hour. Upon rescue, she displayed fixed, dilated pupils; cyanosis; and no pulse. Miraculously, she recovered. Identify and explain the physiologic phenomena that resulted in this astonishing recovery.

ONE LAST QUICK CHECK

Multiple Choice—select the best answer.

28. The term that means the same thing as *breathing* is:
    a. gas exchange.
    b. respiration.
    c. inspiration.
    d. pulmonary ventilation.

29. Which of the following does *not* occur during inspiration?
    a. elevation of the ribs
    b. the diaphragm relaxes
    c. alveolar pressure decreases
    d. chest cavity becomes longer from top to bottom

30. A young adult male would have a vital capacity of about _____ mL.
    a. 500
    b. 1200
    c. 3300
    d. 4800

31. The amount of air that can be forcibly exhaled after expiring the tidal volume is known as the:
    a. total lung capacity.
    b. vital capacity.
    c. inspiratory reserve volume.
    d. expiratory reserve volume.

32. Which one of the following is correct?
    a. VC = TV − IRV + ERV
    b. VC = TV + IRV − ERV
    c. VC = TV + IRV x ERV
    d. VC = TV + IRV + ERV

33. The diving reflex:
    a. explains why some people can hold their breath for extended periods while under water.
    b. is responsible for the astonishing recovery of near-drowning victims in cold water.
    c. forces a submerged individual to exhale prior to surfacing.
    d. both a and c.

True or False

34. _____ Air in the pleural space of the thoracic cavity is called a *pneumothorax*.

35. _____ A deficiency of surfactant in premature infants is called *SIDS*.

36. _____ Cheyne-Stokes is characterized by repeated sequences of deep gasps and apnea.

37. _____ Exercise physiologists use maximum oxygen consumption as a predictor of a person's capacity to do aerobic exercise.

Matching—identify the term with the proper selection.

a. collapsed lung
b. reduces surface tension in lungs
c. approximately 3300 mL
d. P_{O_2}
e. normal exhalation volume
f. increased in emphysema
g. helps control respirations
h. respiratory stimulant
i. cessation of breathing
j. sensitive to changes in arterial CO_2 and pH

38. _____ tidal volume
39. _____ inspiratory reserve volume
40. _____ pneumothorax
41. _____ physiologic dead space
42. _____ oxygen pressure
43. _____ surfactant
44. _____ apneusis
45. _____ chemoreceptors
46. _____ Hering-Breuer reflexes
47. _____ CO_2

CHAPTER 37
Gas Exchange and Transport

Numerous anatomic and physiologic mechanisms influence the successful exchange of gases throughout the process of breathing. The rate, depth, and pressure of pulmonary ventilation are determined by how adequately these mechanisms are functioning.

The actual exchange of gases in the lungs takes place between the alveolar air and blood flowing through lung capillaries surrounding the alveoli. Oxygen and carbon dioxide are transported as solutes and as parts of molecules of certain chemical compounds. The exchange of gases in tissues takes place between arterial blood flowing through tissue capillaries and cells. Carbon dioxide exchange between tissues and blood occurs in the opposite direction from oxygen exchange.

Gas exchange and the transport of gases are critical elements to successful respiration. A lung full of air is of no value if the essential gases cannot be distributed to all body cells. Your study of the exchange and transportation of these gases throughout the body gives you an immediate appreciation for their importance to survival.

I—PULMONARY GAS EXCHANGE

Multiple Choice—select the best answer.

1. If oxygen is 21% of the atmosphere, it will contribute _____ of the total atmospheric pressure.
   a. 21%
   b. 79%
   c. 0.21%
   d. 0.79%

2. The amount of oxygen that diffuses into blood each minute depends on the:
   a. total functional surface area of the respiratory membrane.
   b. respiratory minute volume.
   c. alveolar ventilation.
   d. all of the above.

3. P_{O_2} at standard atmospheric pressure is approximately:
   a. 21 mm Hg.
   b. 0.2 mm Hg.
   c. 160 mm Hg.
   d. 760 mm Hg.

4. Anything that decreases the total functional surface area of the respiratory membrane:
   a. tends to decrease oxygen diffusion into the blood.
   b. tends to increase oxygen diffusion into the blood.
   c. has little effect on oxygen diffusion.
   d. increases the humidity of oxygen as it diffuses.

True or False

5. _____ *Partial pressure* and *tension* can be used interchangeably.

6. _____ The diameter of the pulmonary capillaries allows red blood cells to travel through at 10 abreast.

7. _____ Nitrogen is the gas of greatest concentration in atmospheric air.

→ *If you had difficulty with this section, review pages 848-852.*

II—BLOOD TRANSPORTATION OF GASES / SYSTEMIC GAS EXCHANGE

Multiple Choice—select the best answer.

8. Oxygen is carried in blood:
   a. as oxyhemoglobin.
   b. dissolved in plasma.
   c. molecularly as HbO_2.
   d. all of the above.

9. Which of the following is *not* a manner in which CO_2 is transported in the blood?
   a. dissolved in plasma
   b. bound to the heme group of the hemoglobin molecule
   c. as bicarbonate ions
   d. bound to the polypeptide chains of hemoglobin

10. Increasing the carbon dioxide content of blood results in:
    a. increased H^+ concentration of plasma.
    b. decreased blood pH.
    c. increased blood pH.
    d. both a and b.
    e. both a and c.

11. Approximately 97% of oxygen is transported as
_____, whereas the remaining 3% is
transported dissolved in _____.
a. plasma; hemoglobin
b. oxyhemoglobin; bicarbonate ion
c. oxyhemoglobin; plasma
d. bicarbonate ion; carbonic acid

True or False

12. _____ The exact amount of oxygen in blood
depends mainly upon the amount of hemoglobin
present.

13. _____ As plasma P_{CO_2} increases, the CO_2 carrying
capacity of blood decreases.

14. _____ Interstitial fluid P_{O_2} and intracellular fluid
P_{O_2} are essentially the same.

15. _____ A right shift of the oxygen-hemoglobin
dissociation curve due to increased P_{CO_2} is known as
the Bohr effect.

➔ *If you had difficulty with this section, review pages 852-858.*

CROSSWORD PUZZLE

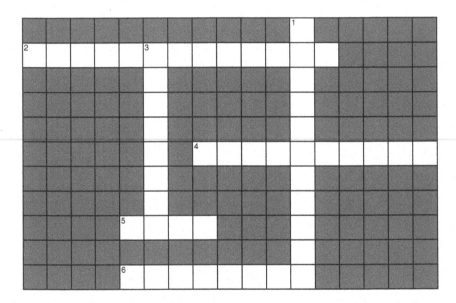

ACROSS
2. Sharp; blood; ball; substance
4. Able to dissolve; state
5. Blood
6. Green; chemical

DOWN
1. Two; coal; oxygen compound
3. Single; sharp; chemical

APPLYING WHAT YOU KNOW

16. Alex's father has emphysema. He has been advised
that this disease causes a problem with gas
exchange. Describe to Alex what emphysema is and
what structures in the lung are directly affected.
Name the resultant gas exchange issue that occurs.
(Refer to Chapter 36 if necessary.)

17. Carbon monoxide poisoning can cause death quickly
if not addressed within minutes after exposure. Why
is this gas is so deadly and why isn't it detected
early during exposure?

DID YOU KNOW?

- Each red blood cell contains about 250 million hemoglobin molecules. Each hemoglobin molecule can carry four oxygen molecules.
- When the Earth was first formed, about 4.6 billion years ago, there was almost no oxygen in the atmosphere.

ONE LAST QUICK CHECK

Multiple Choice—select the best answer.

18. Carbaminohemoglobin is formed when _____ bind(s) to hemoglobin.
    a. oxygen
    b. amino acids
    c. carbon dioxide
    d. nitrogen

19. Most of the oxygen transported by the blood is:
    a. dissolved to white blood cells.
    b. bound to white blood cells.
    c. bound to hemoglobin.
    d. bound to carbaminohemoglobin.

20. The increased total CO_2 loading caused by a decrease in P_{O_2} is a phenomenon known as the:
    a. Haldane effect.
    b. Bohr effect.
    c. Boyle effect.
    d. Dalton effect.

21. Fick's law
    a. describes the formation of oxyhemoglobin.
    b. describes the diffusion of carbon dioxide and oxygen across the respiratory membrane.
    c. describes the principle that states that a gas's volume is inversely proportional to its pressure.
    d. states that volume is directly proportional to temperature when pressure is held constant.

22. Which of the following is true regarding the diffusion of oxygen from the alveolar air into the blood in lung capillaries?
    a. The walls of the alveoli and the capillaries together form a very thin barrier for the gases to cross.
    b. Alveolar and capillary surfaces are both extremely large.
    c. Lung capillaries accommodate a large amount of blood at one time.
    d. All of the above are true.

23. Gases:
    a. move in both directions through the respiratory membrane.
    b. cause a decrease in acidity or an increase in pH in the blood when there is an increase in carbon dioxide.
    c. enter and leave the internal environment by osmosis.
    d. none of the above.

Fill in the blanks.

24. Oxygen travels in two forms: (1) as dissolved O_2 in the _____ and (2) as O_2 associated with _____.

25. The compound formed when carbon dioxide combines with hemoglobin is _____.

26. According to the rate law of chemistry, as more CO_2 is added to the plasma, more will be converted to _____ _____.

27. _____ _____ binds to hemoglobin (Hb) more than 200 times more strongly than oxygen.

CHAPTER 38
Upper Digestive Tract

Think of the last meal you ate, with the different shapes, sizes, tastes, and textures that you so recently enjoyed. Now think of those items circulating in your bloodstream in those same original shapes and sizes. Impossible? Of course. Because of this impossibility you can begin to understand and marvel at the close relationship of the digestive system to the circulatory system. It is the digestive system that changes our food, both mechanically and chemically, into a form that is acceptable to the blood and the body.

This change begins the moment you take the very first bite. Digestion starts in the mouth, where food is chewed and mixed with saliva. It then moves down the pharynx and esophagus by deglutition and peristalsis and enters the stomach. In the stomach it is churned and mixed with gastric juices to continue the digestive process. These gastric secretions help prepare the food for absorption along the course of the small intestine. Your review of the upper digestive system will help you to understand the various organs and mechanisms that prepare your food for proper nourishment and absorption in your body.

I—OVERVIEW OF THE DIGESTIVE SYSTEM

Multiple Choice—select the best answer.

1. Starting from the deepest layer and moving toward the most superficial, the layers of the wall of the GI tract are:
   a. mucosa, submucosa, serosa, muscularis.
   b. submucosa, mucosa, muscularis, serosa.
   c. mucosa, submucosa, muscularis, serosa.
   d. submucosa, serosa, muscularis, mucosa.

2. The serosa is actually:
   a. parietal peritoneum.
   b. visceral peritoneum.
   c. mesentery.
   d. none of the above.

True or False

3. _____ *Gastrointestinal tract* and *alimentary canal* are often used synonymously.

4. _____ The tissue layers of the GI tract are constant, with no variation in the different organs.

Matching—identify each digestive organ with its correct classification.

a. GI tract segment
b. accessory organ

5. _____ mouth

6. _____ jejunum

7. _____ cecum

8. _____ pancreas

9. _____ teeth

10. _____ liver

11. _____ salivary glands

12. _____ vermiform appendix

13. _____ oropharynx

14. _____ sigmoid colon

Labeling—identify the principal organs of the digestive system by matching each term with its corresponding number on the following illustration.

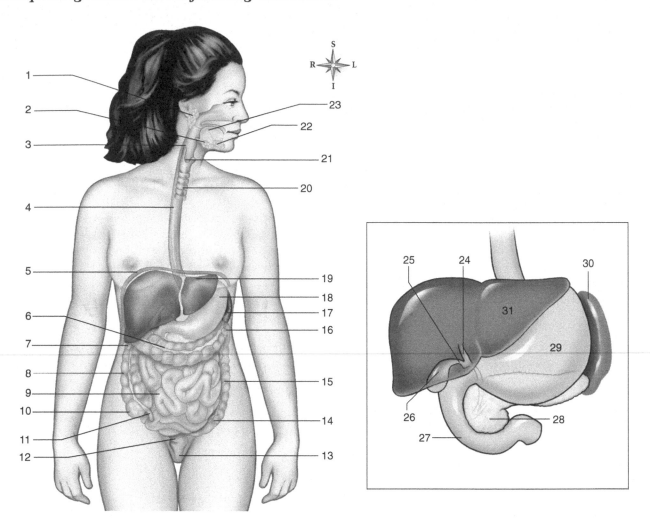

_____ submandibular salivary
gland
_____ ascending colon
_____ liver
_____ esophagus
_____ transverse colon
_____ parotid gland
_____ spleen
_____ cystic duct
_____ ileum
_____ gallbladder

_____ vermiform appendix
_____ splenic flexure of colon
_____ cecum
_____ diaphragm
_____ duodenum
_____ common hepatic duct
_____ rectum
_____ descending colon
_____ anal canal
_____ spleen
_____ pancreas

_____ liver
_____ hepatic flexure of colon
_____ sigmoid colon
_____ tongue
_____ stomach
_____ trachea
_____ larynx
_____ sublingual salivary gland
_____ stomach
_____ pharynx

➡ *If you had difficulty with this section, review pages 860-863.*

II—MOUTH AND PHARYNX

Multiple Choice—select the best answer.

15. The hard palate consists of portions of:
    a. three bones: two maxillae and one palatine.
    b. two bones: one maxillae and one palatine.
    c. three bones: one maxillae and two palatine.
    d. four bones: two maxillae and two palatine.

16. Which of the following is an accurate description of salivary glands?
    a. There are four pairs of salivary glands.
    b. They secrete about 1 liter of saliva per day.
    c. They are associated with buccal glands, which secrete about 50% of the saliva.
    d. Both b and c are true.

17. The crown of a tooth is covered with:
    a. dentin.
    b. cementum.
    c. enamel.
    d. alveolar bone.

18. Teeth that do *not* appear as deciduous teeth are:
    a. incisors.
    b. canines.
    c. second molars.
    d. premolars.

19. The act of swallowing moves a mass of food called a _____ from the mouth to the stomach.
    a. dentin
    b. bolus
    c. fauces
    d. philtrum

True or False

20. _____ A typical tooth can be divided into three main parts: crown, neck, and root.

21. _____ The philtrum is a fold of mucous membrane that helps anchor the tongue to the floor of the mouth.

22. _____ There are 20 deciduous teeth and 30 permanent teeth.

23. _____ The act of swallowing is termed *deglutition*.

24. _____ The soft palate forms a partition between the mouth and oropharynx.

Labeling—label the structures of the tooth on the following illustration.

1. _____
2. _____
3. _____
4. _____
5. _____
6. _____
7. _____
8. _____
9. _____
10. _____
11. _____
12. _____
13. _____

➜ *If you had difficulty with this section, review pages 863-869.*

III—ESOPHAGUS AND STOMACH

Multiple Choice—select the best answer.

25. Which of the following statements is *not* true of the esophagus?
    a. It extends from the pharynx to the stomach.
    b. It lies anterior to the trachea and posterior to the heart.
    c. It resides in both the thoracic and abdominal cavities.
    d. It pierces the diaphragm.

26. Which of the following controls the opening of the stomach into the small intestine?
    a. pylorus
    b. cardiac sphincter
    c. duodenal bulb
    d. pyloric sphincter

27. Which of the layers of the muscularis is present only in the stomach?
    a. longitudinal muscle layer
    b. circular muscle layer
    c. oblique muscle layer
    d. horizontal muscle layer

True or False

28. _____ The folds in the lining of the stomach are called *rugae*.

29. _____ The cardiac sphincter controls the opening of the esophagus into the stomach.

30. _____ Parietal cells secrete hydrochloric acid and are thought to produce intrinsic factor.

Labeling—match each term with its corresponding number on the following illustration of the stomach.

_____ rugae	_____ pylorus	_____ submucosa
_____ fundus	_____ esophagus	_____ lesser curvature
_____ mucosa	_____ oblique muscle layer	_____ circular muscle layer
_____ lower esophageal sphincter (LES)	_____ duodenum	_____ pyloric sphincter
_____ cardia	_____ serosa	_____ muscularis
_____ longitudinal muscle layer	_____ duodenal bulb	_____ gastroesophageal opening
	_____ greater curvature	_____ body of stomach

➡ *If you had difficulty with this section, review pages 869-874.*

IV—MECHANISMS OF DISEASE

Fill in the blanks.

31. An autoimmune disease in which the body's immune system targets the salivary and tear glands is _____ _____.

32. Tooth decay is also referred to as _____ _____.

33. _____ is the general term for inflammation or infection of the gums.

34. A precancerous change in the mucous membrane characterized by thickened, white, and slightly raised patches of tissue is known as _____.

35. The most common congenital defects affecting the mouth are _____ _____ and _____ _____.

36. The lay term for acid indigestion is _____.

37. A loss of appetite is known as _____.

38. The primary cause of ulcers is _____ _____.

→ *If you had difficulty with this section, review pages 874-878.*

CROSSWORD PUZZLE

ACROSS
1. Under; slime; relating to; thing
5. Groin or flank
6. Will carry; food
8. Around; stretched; thing
9. Chew; process
10. Gate; to guard; relating to; bind tight; agent (2 words)

DOWN
2. Sore
3. Bad; close up; state
4. Swallow; process
7. Beside; ear; relating to

APPLYING WHAT YOU KNOW

39. Jack is 30 and was recently diagnosed with parotitis. He had fever, inflammation, pain, and a loss of appetite. The doctor advised him that he should follow his instructions specifically so that he would avoid orchitis. What is the common name for Jack's diagnosis? What is orchitis, and why should Jack be concerned about it?

40. Baby Billy has been regurgitating his bottle-feeding at every meal. The milk is curdled, but does not appear to be digested. He has become dehydrated, so his mother, Amanda, is taking him to the pediatrician. What is a possible diagnosis from your textbook reading?

DID YOU KNOW?

- The human stomach lining replaces itself every 3 days.
- Every 2 weeks the human stomach produces a new layer of mucous lining to protect itself; otherwise, the stomach would digest itself.

✓ ONE LAST QUICK CHECK

Multiple Choice—select the best answer.

41. The first baby tooth, on average, appears at age:
    a. 2 months.
    b. 1 year.
    c. 1 month.
    d. 6 months.

42. The dentin of the tooth contains the _____, which consists of connective tissue, blood and lymphatic vessels, and nerves.
    a. pulp cavity
    b. neck
    c. root
    d. crown

43. Which of the following teeth is missing from the deciduous arch?
    a. central incisor
    b. canine
    c. second premolar
    d. first molar

44. The third molars generally erupt around the age of _____.
    a. 9
    b. 10
    c. 12
    d. 17

45. A general term for infection of the gums is:
    a. dental caries.
    b. leukoplakia.
    c. Vincent's angina.
    d. gingivitis.

46. The ducts of the _____ glands open into the floor of the mouth.
    a. sublingual
    b. submandibular
    c. parotid
    d. carotid

47. The stomach:
    a. is lined with villi.
    b. lies in a vertical position of the left side of the abdomen.
    c. secretes intrinsic factor.
    d. serves as a breeding ground for nonpathogenic bacteria.

48. Another name for the third molar is:
    a. central incisor.
    b. wisdom tooth.
    c. canine.
    d. lateral incisor.

49. After food has been chewed, it is formed into a small rounded mass called a:
    a. moat.
    b. chyme.
    c. bolus.
    d. protease.

True or False

50. _____ Following mastication, deglutition occurs.

51. _____ The oral cavity is also known as the *buccal cavity.*

52. _____ The esophagus is voluntary in the upper third, mixed in the middle, and involuntary in the lower third.

53. _____ The upper lip is marked near the midline by a shallow vertical groove called the *philtrum.*

54. _____ The complete process of altering the physical and chemical composition of ingested food material so that it can be absorbed and used by the body is called *digestion.*

55. _____ The fundus, pylorus, and plicae are the three main divisions of the stomach.

CHAPTER 39

Lower Digestive Tract

Digestion and absorption continue throughout the small intestine (duodenum, jejunum, and ileum). Food products that are not absorbed throughout the small intestine continue on and enter the cecum, ascending colon, transverse colon, descending colon, sigmoid colon, the rectum, and out the anus.

Products that are used in the cells must undergo absorption. Absorption allows newly processed nutrients to pass through the walls of the digestive tract and into the bloodstream to be distributed to the cells. Your review of this portion of the digestive tract will help you understand an important segment of the alimentary canal, which provides the mechanical and chemical processes necessary to convert food into energy sources and compounds necessary for survival.

I—SMALL INTESTINE, LARGE INTESTINE, APPENDIX, AND PERITIONEUM

Multiple Choice—select the best answer.

1. The correct order of small intestine divisions, starting proximal to the stomach, is:
   a. ileum, duodenum, jejunum.
   b. duodenum, ileum, jejunum.
   c. duodenum, jejunum, ileum.
   d. ileum, jejunum, duodenum.

2. Beginning with the largest structures, which of the following is a correct description of the small intestine's adaptation for absorption?
   a. villi, microvilli, plicae
   b. plicae, villi, microvilli
   c. microvilli, villi, plicae
   d. microvilli, plicae, villi

3. The terminal inch of the rectum is called the:
   a. anal canal.
   b. fistula.
   c. anus.
   d. sigmoid.

4. The lesser omentum attaches the:
   a. transverse colon to the posterior abdominal wall.
   b. liver to the lesser curvature of the stomach.
   c. ileum and jejunum to the posterior abdominal wall.
   d. greater omentum to the posterior abdominal wall.

True or False

5. _____ The hepatic flexure of the large intestine is also called the *left colic flexure.*

6. _____ The nonpathogenic bacteria of the colon are thought to be produced in the sigmoid colon.

7. _____ The pouchlike structures of the large intestine are called *haustra.*

8. _____ The kidneys, adrenal glands, and descending colon are examples of retroperitoneal organs.

9. _____ Villi are important modifications of the mucosal layer of the small intestine.

10. _____ Paneth cells produce enzymes and other molecules that inhibit bacterial growth in the small intestine.

Labeling—using the terms provided, label the wall of the small intestine on the following illustration.

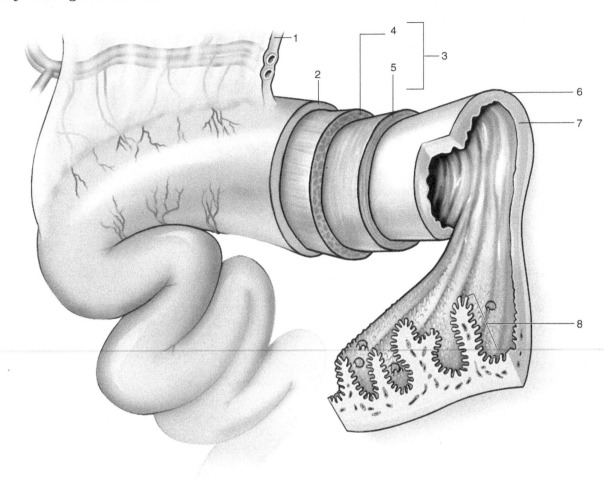

_____ circular muscle   _____ longitudinal muscle   _____ submucosa
_____ plica (fold)   _____ mesentery   _____ mucosa
_____ serosa   _____ muscularis

Labeling—using the terms provided, label the divisions of the large intestine on the following illustration.

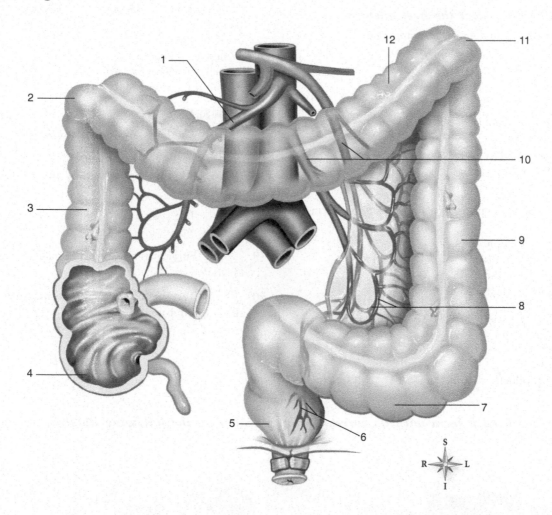

_____ hepatic (right colic) flexure	_____ ascending colon	_____ transverse colon
_____ splenic (left colic) flexure	_____ superior mesenteric artery	_____ sigmoid artery and vein
_____ superior rectal artery and vein	_____ cecum	_____ rectum
_____ inferior mesenteric artery and vein	_____ sigmoid colon	_____ descending colon

➜ *If you had difficulty with this section, review pages 882-889.*

II—LIVER, GALLBLADDER, AND PANCREAS

Multiple Choice—select the best answer.

11. The anatomic units of the liver are called:
    a. lobes.
    b. lobules.
    c. sinusoids.
    d. none of the above.

12. Blood flows to hepatic lobules via branches of the:
    a. hepatic artery.
    b. hepatic portal vein.
    c. hepatic vein.
    d. both a and b.

13. A merger of the hepatic duct and cystic duct form the:
    a. common hepatic duct.
    b. common bile duct.
    c. right hepatic duct.
    d. left hepatic duct.

14. Bile salts aid in the absorption of:
    a. fat.
    b. carbohydrates.
    c. proteins.
    d. waste products.

15. Within the sinusoids of the liver are many cells that remove bacteria, worn red blood cells, and other products from the bloodstream. These cells are known as:
    a. alpha cells.
    b. hepatic leukocells.
    c. stellate macrophages.
    d. haustra.

True or False

16. _____ The liver consists of two lobes separated by the falciform ligament.

17. _____ Bile is manufactured by the Kupffer cells of the liver.

18. _____ The pancreas is both an endocrine and exocrine gland.

19. _____ Surgical removal of the gallbladder is called *cholecystectomy.*

20. _____ The small intestine is the main site of digestion and absorption.

Labeling—match each term with its corresponding number on the following illustration of the liver.

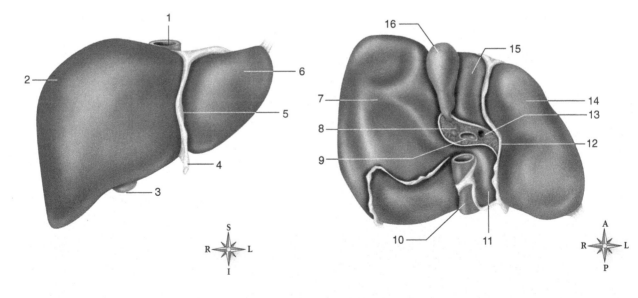

_____ hepatic artery	_____ falciform ligament	_____ inferior vena cava
_____ right lobe	_____ right lobe proper	_____ inferior vena cava
_____ caudate lobe	_____ gallbladder	_____ falciform ligament
_____ gallbladder	_____ left lobe	_____ left lobe
_____ round ligament	_____ common hepatic duct	
_____ quadrate lobe	_____ hepatic portal vein	

Labeling—match each term with its corresponding number on the following illustration of the common bile duct and its tributaries.

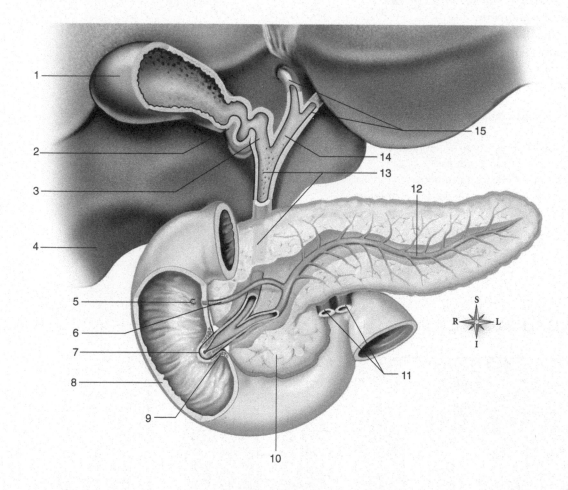

_____ neck of gallbladder

_____ superior mesenteric artery
         and vein

_____ common bile duct

_____ cystic duct

_____ duodenum

_____ pancreas

_____ minor duodenal papilla

_____ accessory pancreatic duct

_____ major duodenal papilla

_____ corpus (body) of gallbladder

_____ common hepatic duct

_____ liver

_____ sphincter muscles

_____ right and left hepatic ducts

_____ pancreatic duct

➡ *If you had difficulty with this section, review pages 884 and 889-895.*

III—MECHANISMS OF DISEASE

Matching—Identify the term with the appropriate description.

a. irritable bowel syndrome
b. passageway between the rectal wall and the skin around the anus
c. degenerative liver condition
d. dilated veins
e. abnormal saclike outpouchings of the intestinal wall
f. elimination of feces often accompanied by cramps
g. low incidence in older adults
h. inflammation of the rectal mucosa
i. inflammatory condition of the large intestine
j. gallstone formation

21. _____ hemorrhoids
22. _____ appendicitis
23. _____ diarrhea
24. _____ diverticula
25. _____ colitis
26. _____ spastic colon
27. _____ proctitis
28. _____ anal fistula
29. _____ cirrhosis
30. _____ cholelithiasis

➡ *If you had difficulty with this section, review pages 895-897 and page 893.*

CROSSWORD PUZZLE

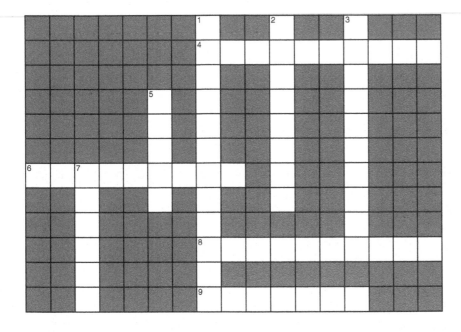

ACROSS
4. Around; stretched; thing
6. Yellow-orange; condition
8. Across; turn
9. Letter of Greek alphabet; like

DOWN
1. Hang upon; inflammation
2. Through; flow
3. Intestine; cell
5. Large intestine
7. Straight; thing

APPLYING WHAT YOU KNOW

31. Brian is experiencing difficulty digesting fatty foods and is displaying a yellow discoloration of his skin. What may be causing his condition? What is the clinical term used to describe the yellow appearance of his skin and what is the physiology? How could doctors treat his condition and what are the names of the procedures?

32. Billy is 17. He was admitted to the emergency department complaining of pain in the lower right abdominal quadrant. What is the probable diagnosis? Why is this diagnosis more likely than in a 60-year-old patient?

DID YOU KNOW?

- If one were to unravel the entire human alimentary canal (esophagus, stomach, small and large intestines), it would reach the height of a three-story building.
- Borborygmi, or stomach rumblings, are the result of peristalsis in the stomach and small intestines. When the tract is empty, however, borborygmi are louder because there's nothing to muffle the sound.

ONE LAST QUICK CHECK

Multiple Choice—select the best answer.

33. Which one is *not* part of the small intestine?
    a. jejunum
    b. ileum
    c. cecum
    d. duodenum

34. The union of the cystic duct and the _____ forms the common bile duct.
    a. hepatic duct
    b. major duodenal papilla
    c. minor duodenal papilla
    d. pancreatic duct

35. Each villus in the intestine contains a lymphatic vessel or _____ that serves to absorb lipid or fat materials from the chyme.
    a. plica
    b. lacteal
    c. villa
    d. microvilli

36. *Cholelithiasis* is the term used to describe:
    a. biliary colic.
    b. jaundice.
    c. portal hypertension.
    d. gallstones.

37. The largest gland in the body is the:
    a. pituitary.
    b. thyroid.
    c. liver.
    d. thymus.

True or False

38. _____ The splenic flexure is the bend between the ascending colon and the transverse colon.

39. _____ The splenic colon is the S-shaped segment that terminates in the rectum.

40. _____ The mesentery is a fan-shaped projection of the parietal peritoneum.

41. _____ The normal microbiome of the colon produces essential molecules such as vitamin K and biotin.

42. _____ The last 7 to 8 inches of the intestinal tube is called the *sigmoid colon.*

CHAPTER 40
Digestion and Absorption

Digestion is the process of breaking down complex nutrients into simpler units suitable for absorption. It involves two major processes: mechanical and chemical. Mechanical digestion occurs during mastication and the churning and propelling mechanisms that take place along the alimentary canal. Chemical digestion occurs with the help of the many digestive enzymes and various substances that are added to the nutrients as they progress the length of the digestive tube. These substances include saliva and gastric, pancreatic, and intestinal enzymes. Delicate nervous and hormonal reflex mechanisms control the flow of these juices so that the proper amount is released at the appropriate time.

Absorption is the passage of substances (digested foods, water, salts, and vitamins) through the intestinal mucosa and into the blood or lymph. After the body has determined the nutrients necessary for absorption, it sends the residue of digestion to the final segment of the GI tract to be eliminated as feces.

Your review of this system will help you understand the mechanical and chemical processes necessary to convert food into energy sources and compounds necessary for survival.

I—DIGESTION

Multiple Choice—select the best answer.

1. Which of the following describes the pharyngeal stage of deglutition?
   a. mouth to oropharynx
   b. oropharynx to esophagus
   c. esophagus to stomach
   d. none of the above

2. Which step of deglutition is under voluntary control?
   a. oral
   b. pharyngeal
   c. esophageal
   d. all of the above

3. The final product of carbohydrate digestion is a:
   a. disaccharide.
   b. monosaccharide.
   c. polysaccharide.
   d. fatty acid.

4. Enzymes that catalyze the hydrolysis of proteins are:
   a. proteases.
   b. amylases.
   c. lactases.
   d. lipases.

5. A micelle is:
   a. a disaccharide attached to the brush border of the small intestine.
   b. a tiny sphere of lipid and water.
   c. a thick, milky material comprised of food and digestive enzymes.
   d. synonymous with *bolus*.

6. Which of the following is *not* true concerning the gastric emptying of water?
   a. Large volumes of water leave the stomach more rapidly than small volumes.
   b. Warm fluids empty more quickly than cool fluids.
   c. High-solute concentration fluids empty more slowly than dilute concentrations.
   d. All of the above are true.

7. The process of fat emulsification consists of:
   a. chemically breaking down fat molecules.
   b. absorption of fats.
   c. breaking down fats into small droplets.
   d. the secretion of digestive juices for fat digestion.

True or False

8. _____ Peristalsis can be described as a mixing movement.

9. _____ The volumes of the stomach and the duodenum are approximately equal.

10. _____ Enzymes are organic catalysts.

11. _____ Digestive enzymes catalyze chemical reactions with great efficiency within a wide range of pH.

12. _____ Cellulose resists digestion and is eliminated in feces.

13. _____ Water is readily absorbed in the stomach.

14. _____ Amino acids are the end product of protein digestion.

➜ *If you had difficulty with this section, review pages 901-913.*

II—SECRETION AND CONTROL OF DIGESTIVE GLAND SECRETION

Multiple Choice—select the best answer.

15. The principal enzyme of saliva is:
    a. protease.
    b. amylase.
    c. lipase.
    d. salivase.

16. Which of the following is true?
    a. Saliva contains large amounts of lipase.
    b. Pepsinogen is converted into pepsin by hydrochloric acid.
    c. Chief cells secrete pepsin.
    d. Zymogenic cells produce intrinsic factor.

17. Which of the following is present in bile?
    a. lecithin
    b. gastrin
    c. bile salts
    d. both a and c

18. The hormone that stimulates the gallbladder to release bile is:
    a. enterogastrone.
    b. insulin.
    c. gastrin.
    d. cholecystokinin.

True or False

19. _____ Pancreatic juice is secreted by exocrine acinar cells of the pancreas.

20. _____ Olfactory and visual stimuli are factors concerning the control of digestive gland secretion.

21. _____ The cephalic phase is initiated by the presence of food in the stomach.

22. _____ Chyme is liquefied food found in the stomach.

→ *If you had difficulty with this section, review pages 906 and 913-920.*

CHEMICAL DIGESTION

Fill in the blank areas on the chart below.

Digestive Juices and Enzymes	Substance Digested (or Hydrolyzed)	Resulting Product
Saliva		
1. Amylase	1.	1. Maltose
Gastric Juice		
2. Protease (pepsin) plus hydrochloric acid	2. Proteins	2.
Pancreatic Juice		
3. Protease (trypsin)	3. Proteins (intact or partially digested)	3.
4. Lipase	4.	4. Fatty acids, monoglycerides, and glycerol
5. Amylase	5.	5. Maltose
Intestinal Juice		
6. Peptidases	6.	6. Amino acids
7.	7. Sucrose	7. Glucose and fructose
8. Lactase	8.	8. Glucose and galactose (simple sugars)
9. Maltase	9. Maltose	9.
10. Nucleotidases and phosphatases		10. Nucleosides

III—ABSORPTION AND ELIMINATION

Multiple Choice—select the best answer.

23. Fats are absorbed primarily into which of the following structures?
    a. blood in intestinal capillaries
    b. lymph in intestinal lacteals
    c. villi in large intestine
    d. none of the above

24. Movement of lower colon and rectum contents at a rate slower than normal can cause:
    a. defecation.
    b. constipation.
    c. diarrhea.
    d. both b and c.

25. Which blood vessel carries absorbed nutrients from the GI tract to the liver?
    a. hepatic artery
    b. hepatic vein
    c. portal vein
    d. inferior vena cava

True or False

26. _____ Both water and sodium are absorbed via simple diffusion.

27. _____ The majority of substances are absorbed in the small intestine.

28. _____ Cholera is an intestinal infection that kills more than 600,000 infants and children worldwide each year.

29. _____ Vitamins A, C, D, and E are known as "fat-soluble" vitamins.

30. _____ Impaired fat absorption produces large, greasy, foul-smelling stools known as *steatorrhea*.

Labeling—fill in the functions of each organ of digestion in the boxes provided below.

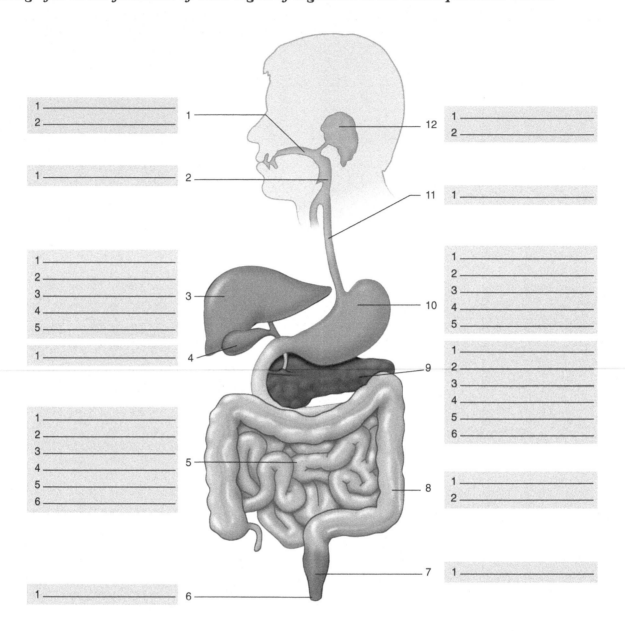

1 _____
2 _____

1 _____

1 _____
2 _____
3 _____
4 _____
5 _____

1 _____

1 _____
2 _____
3 _____
4 _____
5 _____
6 _____

1 _____

1 _____
2 _____

1 _____

1 _____
2 _____
3 _____
4 _____
5 _____

1 _____
2 _____
3 _____
4 _____
5 _____
6 _____

1 _____
2 _____

1 _____

➡ *If you had difficulty with this section, review pages 912 and 920-925.*

CROSSWORD PUZZLE

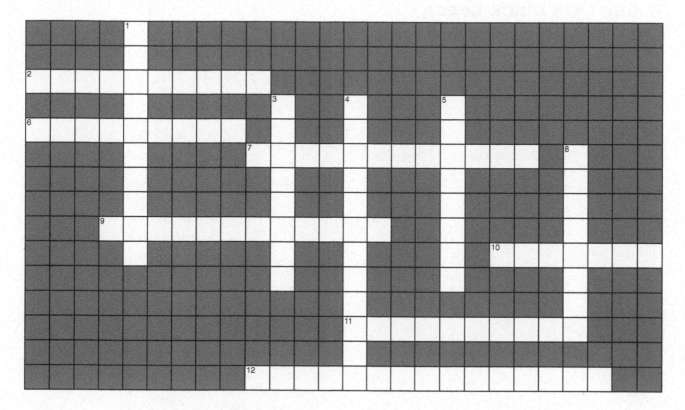

ACROSS
2. In front; drive; process
6. Break apart; process
7. Crowd together; process
9. Cut section; process
10. Stomach; substance
11. From; suck; process
12. Bile; bladder; move; substance

DOWN
1. Out; milk; combining form; process
3. Protein enzyme
4. Intestine; movement; enzyme
5. Move; relating to; state
8. Yolk; substance

 APPLYING WHAT YOU KNOW

31. Janice complained of cramping and diarrhea. When the doctor told her that she had "colitis," or inflammation of the bowel, she asked what the diagnosis meant. He responded that the end products of digestion were moving through the digestive tract too rapidly. Why does the speed of food going through the digestive tract have anything to do with Janice's diarrhea?

32. Cliff and Pete like to play soccer vigorously in the heat of the day. What kind of recommendations should they observe concerning the replacement of fluids? Be sure to consider parameters such as fluid temperature, volume, and solute concentration.

 DID YOU KNOW?

- Even if the stomach, the spleen, 75% of the liver, 80% of the intestines, one kidney, one lung, and virtually every organ from the pelvic and groin area are removed, the human body can still survive!
- The human body takes 6 hours to digest a high-fat meal and 2 hours to digest a carbohydrate meal.

ONE LAST QUICK CHECK

Multiple Choice—select the best answer.

33. During the process of digestion, stored bile is poured into the duodenum by which of the following?
    a. gallbladder
    b. liver
    c. pancreas
    d. spleen

34. The portion of the alimentary canal that mixes food with gastric juice and breaks it down into a mixture called *chyme* is the:
    a. gallbladder.
    b. small intestine.
    c. stomach.
    d. large intestine.

35. Polysaccharides are hydrolyzed to disaccharides by enzymes known as:
    a. amylases.
    b. peptides.
    c. micelles.
    d. colipases.

36. Which of the following is *not* a stage of deglutition?
    a. oral
    b. pharyngeal
    c. esophageal
    d. gastric

37. Protein digestion begins in the:
    a. esophagus.
    b. small intestine.
    c. stomach.
    d. large intestine.

38. The enzyme pepsin is concerned primarily with the digestion of which of the following?
    a. sugars
    b. starches
    c. proteins
    d. fats

39. The enzyme amylase converts which of the following?
    a. starches to sugars
    b. sugars to starches
    c. proteins to amino acids
    d. fatty acids and glycerols to fats

40. Which of the following substances does *not* contain any enzymes?
    a. saliva
    b. bile
    c. gastric juice
    d. intestinal juice

41. Which of the following is a simple sugar?
    a. maltose
    b. sucrose
    c. lactose
    d. glucose

42. Fats are broken down into:
    a. amino acids.
    b. simple sugars.
    c. fatty acids.
    d. disaccharides.

43. Which hormone decreases peristalsis and slows the passage of food from the stomach to the duodenum?
    a. CCK
    b. GIP
    c. secretin
    d. gastrin

44. The union of the cystic duct and hepatic duct form the:
    a. common bile duct.
    b. major duodenal papilla.
    c. minor duodenal papilla.
    d. pancreatic duct.

45. The process of swallowing is known as:
    a. mastication.
    b. segmentation.
    c. peristalsis.
    d. deglutition.

46. Peristalsis begins in the:
    a. mouth.
    b. pharynx.
    c. esophagus.
    d. stomach.

True or False

47. _____ The mechanical process that occurs in the rectum is churning.

48. _____ Mechanical digestion begins in the mouth.

49. _____ The hormones secretin and CCK stimulate ejection of bile.

50. _____ Segmentation is a mixing movement.

51. _____ Bilirubin is the result of hemolysis by the liver.

52. _____ Most digestive enzymes are synthesized and secreted as inactive kinases.

CHAPTER 41
Nutrition and Metabolism

Most of us love to eat, but do the foods we enjoy provide us with the basic food types necessary for good nutrition? The body, a finely tuned machine, requires a balance of carbohydrates, fats, proteins, vitamins, and minerals to function properly. These nutrients must be digested, absorbed, and circulated to cells constantly to accommodate the numerous activities that occur throughout the body. The use the body makes of foods once these processes are completed is called *metabolism*.

Although the body relies on many organs to prepare nutrients, the liver plays a major role in the metabolism of food. It helps maintain a normal blood glucose level, removes toxins from the blood, processes blood immediately after it leaves the gastrointestinal tract, and initiates the first steps of protein and fat metabolism.

The study of metabolism is not complete without a discussion of the basal metabolic rate (BMR). The BMR is the rate at which food is catabolized under basal conditions. The total metabolic rate (TMR) is the amount of energy, expressed in calories, used by the body each day. This chapter also demonstrates the use of metabolic testing to measure thyroid functioning.

Finally, the hypothalamus appears to be a critical component in determining appetite and satiety. While many theories suggest various ways that the hypothalamus might perform these functions, it is imperative that we acknowledge its importance in nutrition and metabolism. Review of this chapter is necessary to provide you with an understanding of the *fuel*, or nutrition, necessary to maintain that complex homeostatic machine—the body.

I—OVERVIEW OF NUTRITION AND METABOLISM

Multiple Choice—select the best answer.

1. The universal biological currency is:
   a. ATP.
   b. ADP.
   c. carbohydrates.
   d. NADH.

2. *Nutrition* refers to the:
   a. complex set of chemical processes that make life possible.
   b. breaking down of food into small molecular compounds.
   c. release of energy in two main forms.
   d. food we eat and the nutrients they contain.

True or False

3. _____ Catabolism is a process that breaks down molecules into smaller molecular compounds.

4. _____ Metabolism is identical in all cells.

➡ *If you had difficulty with this section, review pages 930-933.*

II—CARBOHYDRATES

Multiple Choice—select the best answer.

5. Glucose, fructose, and galactose are important:
   a. monosaccharides.
   b. disaccharides.
   c. polysaccharides.
   d. starches.

6. The carbohydrate most useful to the human cell is:
   a. cellulose.
   b. glucose.
   c. fructose.
   d. galactose.

7. The process of glucose phosphorylation forms the molecule:
   a. ATP.
   b. ADP.
   c. glucose-6-phosphate.
   d. glycogen.

8. The breakdown of one glucose molecule into two pyruvic acid molecules is called:
   a. glycolysis.
   b. glycogenesis.
   c. glycogenolysis.
   d. glycogen.

9. The amount of heat necessary to raise the temperature of 1 g of water by 1°C is a:
   a. calorie.
   b. Celsius.
   c. kilocalorie.
   d. none of the above.

10. To enter the citric acid cycle, glucose must be transformed into:
    a. pyruvic acid.
    b. acetyl-CoA.
    c. ATP.
    d. NADH.

11. Which of the following defines *glycogenesis?*
    a. process of glycogen formation
    b. joining of glucose molecules
    c. catabolism of glycogen
    d. both a and b

12. Which of the following hormones helps glucose enter cells and therefore decreases blood glucose?
    a. glucagon
    b. insulin
    c. epinephrine
    d. growth hormone

True or False

13. _____ Glycolysis is an anaerobic process.

14. _____ Glycolysis prepares glucose for the citric acid cycle.

15. _____ Glycolysis occurs in the mitochondria, whereas the citric acid cycle occurs in the cytoplasm.

16. _____ Erythrocytes rely on aerobic respiration.

17. _____ The process of gluconeogenesis synthesizes new glucose molecules.

18. _____ Glycogenesis is a homeostatic mechanism that functions when blood glucose levels increase above normal.

19. _____ Hyperglycemia occurs when the blood glucose dips below the normal set point level.

20. _____ The conversion of proteins to glucose is an example of gluconeogenesis.

21. _____ Glucagon stimulates glycogenolysis in the liver.

22. _____ ACTH decreases blood glucose concentration.

23. _____ Disaccharides do not need to be chemically digested before they can be absorbed.

24. _____ The *citric acid cycle*, the *TCA cycle*, and the *Krebs cycle* are all synonymous.

25. _____ Oxidative phosphorylation refers to the joining of a phosphate group to ADP to form ATP.

26. _____ The breakdown of ATP molecules provides 50% of all of the energy needed for cellular work.

27. _____ Glycogenolysis is consistent in all cells.

→ *If you had difficulty with this section, review pages 933-943.*

III—LIPIDS

Multiple Choice—select the best answer.

28. _____ contains fatty acid chains in which all available bonds of its hydrocarbon chain are filled with hydrogen atoms.
    a. Saturated fat
    b. Unsaturated fat
    c. Cholesterol
    d. Both a and b

29. The most common lipids in the diet are:
    a. phospholipids.
    b. cholesterol.
    c. triglycerides.
    d. prostaglandins.

30. A high risk for atherosclerosis is associated with a high blood concentration of:
    a. LDL.
    b. HDL.
    c. CVA.
    d. both a and b.

31. All of the following hormones control lipid metabolism *except:*
    a. ACTH.
    b. glucocorticoids.
    c. epinephrine.
    d. insulin.

32. Which of the following lab results would indicate high risk for atherosclerosis?
    a. 100 mg LDL/100 mL of blood
    b. 180 mg HDL/100 mL of blood
    c. 60 mg HDL/100 mL of blood
    d. 200 mg LDL/100 mL of blood

True or False

33. _____ A diet high in saturated fats and cholesterol tends to increase blood concentration of high-density lipoproteins.

34. _____ Lipid catabolism yields 9 kcal/g.

35. _____ Essential fatty acids are not synthesized by the body and must be obtained through the diet.

36. _____ Lipids are transported in the blood as chylomicrons, lipoproteins, and free fatty acids.

37. _____ The liver is the chief site of ketogenesis.

→ *If you had difficulty with this section, review pages 944-946.*

IV—PROTEINS

Multiple Choice—select the best answer.

38. Which of the following is a nonessential amino acid?
    a. lysine
    b. alanine
    c. tryptophan
    d. valine

39. The process by which proteins are synthesized by the ribosomes in all cells is called:
    a. protein catabolism.
    b. protein anabolism.
    c. protein metabolism.
    d. both a and b.

40. Which of the following hormones tends to promote protein anabolism?
    a. testosterone
    b. growth hormone
    c. thyroid hormone
    d. all of the above

True or False

41. _____ In protein metabolism, catabolism is primary and anabolism is secondary.

42. _____ Foods from animal sources high in proteins contain the essential amino acids.

43. _____ Glucocorticoids are protein catabolic hormones.

44. _____ Growth and pregnancy usually result in a negative nitrogen balance.

45. _____ The first step in protein catabolism takes place in the liver and is called *deamination*.

→ *If you had difficulty with this section, review pages 946-948.*

V—VITAMINS AND MINERALS

Multiple Choice—select the best answer.

46. Which of the following plays an important role in detecting light in the sensory cells of the eye?
    a. vitamin D
    b. retinal
    c. biotin
    d. pantothenic acid

47. Which of the following vitamins is fat soluble?
    a. vitamin A
    b. vitamin B
    c. vitamin C
    d. none of the above

48. Which of the following illnesses can result from an iodine deficiency?
    a. anemia
    b. bone degeneration
    c. goiter
    d. acid-base imbalance

True or False

49. _____ Athletic performance can be enhanced by vitamin supplementation.

50. _____ Vitamin E is thought to neutralize free radicals.

51. _____ Vitamin C deficiency could result in scurvy.

52. _____ Coenzymes are inorganic catalysts.

→ *If you had difficulty with this section, review pages 948-952 and page 959.*

VI—METABOLIC RATE AND MECHANISMS FOR REGULATING FOOD INTAKE

Multiple Choice—select the best answer.

53. Which of the following is *not* a condition required for the BMR?
    a. The individual is lying down and not moving.
    b. The individual is sleeping.
    c. It has been 12 to 18 hours since the individual's last meal.
    d. The individual is in a comfortable, warm environment.

54. Which of the following does *not* influence BMR?
    a. age
    b. gender
    c. ethnicity
    d. size

55. One pound of adipose tissue equals:
    a. 1000 kcal.
    b. 350 kcal.
    c. 3500 kcal.
    d. 10,000 kcal.

56. The appetite center is most likely located in the:
    a. cerebrum.
    b. hypothalamus.
    c. small intestine.
    d. stomach.

True or False

57. _____ Males have a BMR approximately 15%-20% higher than females.

58. _____ Increases in blood temperature and glucose concentration may be linked to satiety.

59. _____ Body weight is linked to both energy input and energy output.

60. _____ When body temperature decreases, metabolism increases.

61. _____ Metabolic rate is the amount of energy released in the body in a given time by anabolism.

→ *If you had difficulty with this section, review pages 952-956.*

CROSSWORD PUZZLE

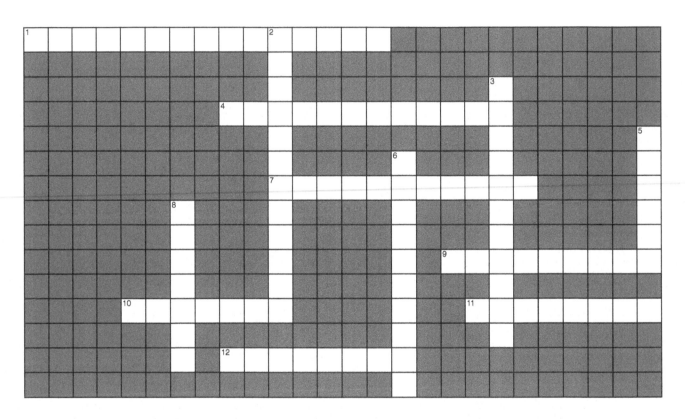

ACROSS
1. Light; carry; chemical; process
4. Three; sweet; chemical
7. Fat; produce; process
9. Nourish; process
10. Island; substance
11. Together; in; ferment
12. Life; ammonia compound

DOWN
2. Make alike; process
3. Undo; ammonia compound; process
5. Thin; substance
6. Over; throw; action
8. Acetone; process

VII—MECHANISMS OF DISEASE

Matching—choose the correct response.

    a. phenylketonuria
    b. anorexia nervosa
    c. bulimia
    d. obesity
    e. protein-calorie malnutrition
    f. marasmus
    g. ascites

62. _____ characterized by a refusal to eat

63. _____ results from a deficiency of calories in general and protein in particular

64. _____ inborn error of metabolism

65. _____ advanced form of PCM

66. _____ not a disorder, but may be a symptom of abnormal behavior

67. _____ binge-purge syndrome

68. _____ abdominal bloating

→ *If you had difficulty with this section, review pages 957-960.*

 APPLYING WHAT YOU KNOW

69. Dr. Reeder was concerned about Myrna. Her daily food intake provided fewer calories than her TMR. If this trend continues, what will be the result? If it continues over a long period of time, what eating disorder might Myrna develop?

70. Tom was experiencing fatigue, and a blood test revealed that he was slightly anemic. What mineral(s) will his doctor most likely prescribe? What dietary sources might you suggest that he emphasize in his daily diet?

? DID YOU KNOW?

- The body's daily requirement of vitamins and minerals is less than a thimbleful.
- The average person consumes 2000 to 2500 calories a day, but if you had the metabolism of a shrew you would need to consume approximately 200,000 calories a day! Smaller animals have higher metabolic rates because they have to work harder to keep their bodies warm.

ONE LAST QUICK CHECK

Multiple Choice—select the best answer.

71. What is the process by which pyruvic acid is broken down into carbon dioxide and high-energy electrons called?
    a. glycogenesis
    b. citric acid cycle
    c. glycolysis
    d. pyruvic acid cycle

72. The anabolism of glucose produces which of the following?
    a. glycogen
    b. amino acid
    c. rennin
    d. starch

73. Which of the following is a major hormone in the body that aids carbohydrate metabolism?
    a. oxytocin
    b. prolactin
    c. insulin
    d. ADH

74. The total metabolic rate is which of the following?
    a. the amount of fats we consume in a 24-hour period
    b. the same as the BMR
    c. the amount of energy expressed in calories used by the body per day
    d. cannot be calculated

75. When your consumption of calories equals your TMR, your weight will do which of the following?
    a. increase
    b. remain the same
    c. fluctuate
    d. decrease

76. What is the primary molecule the body usually breaks down as an energy source?
    a. amino acids
    b. pepsin
    c. maltose
    d. glucose

77. When glucose is *not* available, the body will next catabolize which of the following energy sources?
    a. fats
    b. hormones
    c. minerals
    d. vitamins

Circle the word or phrase that does not belong.

78. glycolysis	citric acid cycle	ATP	bile
79. adipose	amino acids	triglycerides	lipid
80. A	D	M	K
81. iron	protein	amino acids	essential
82. ACTH	insulin	growth hormone	epinephrine
83. sodium	calcium	zinc	folic acid
84. thiamine	niacin	ascorbic acid	riboflavin

Matching—identify the term that best matches the definition.

a. carbohydrate
b. fat
c. protein
d. vitamins
e. minerals

85. _____ preferred energy food

86. _____ amino acids

87. _____ fat-soluble

88. _____ required for nerve conduction

89. _____ glycolysis

90. _____ inorganic elements found naturally in the earth

91. _____ pyruvic acid

92. _____ chylomicrons

93. _____ triglycerides

CHAPTER 42
Urinary System

Living produces wastes. Wherever people live or work or play, wastes accumulate. To keep these areas healthy, there must be a method of disposing of these wastes such as a sanitation department.

Wastes also accumulate in your body. The conversion of food and gases into substances and energy necessary for survival results in waste products. A large percentage of these wastes is removed by the urinary system.

Two vital organs, the kidneys, cleanse the blood of the many waste products that are continually produced as a result of the metabolism of food in the body cells. They eliminate these wastes in the form of urine.

Urine formation is the result of three processes: filtration, reabsorption, and secretion. These processes occur in successive portions of the microscopic units of the kidneys known as *nephrons*. The amount of urine produced by the nephrons is controlled primarily by the hormones antidiuretic hormone (ADH) and aldosterone. After the urine is produced, it is drained from the renal pelvis by the ureters to flow into the bladder. The bladder then stores the urine until it is voided through the urethra.

If waste products are allowed to accumulate in the body, they soon become poisonous, a condition called *uremia*. A knowledge of the urinary system is necessary to understand how the body rids itself of waste and avoids toxicity.

I—ANATOMY OF THE URINARY SYSTEM

Multiple Choice—select the best answer.

1. Which of the following is regulated by the kidneys?
   a. water content of the blood
   b. blood pH level
   c. blood ion concentration
   d. all of the above

2. The medial surface of each kidney has a notch called the:
   a. medulla.
   b. cortex.
   c. hilum.
   d. pelvis.

3. At the beginning of the "plumbing system" of the urinary system, urine leaving the renal papilla is collected in the cuplike structures called:
   a. renal columns.
   b. renal pyramids.
   c. calyces.
   d. ureters.

4. The functional unit of the kidney is the:
   a. renal corpuscle.
   b. nephron.
   c. juxtaglomerular apparatus.
   d. Bowman's capsule.

5. Which of the following is a component of the renal corpuscle?
   a. glomerulus
   b. Bowman's capsule
   c. afferent arteriole
   d. both a and b

6. Which of the following structures secretes renin when blood pressure in the afferent arteriole drops?
   a. renal tubule
   b. proximal convoluted tubule
   c. juxtaglomerular apparatus
   d. both a and b

7. Substances pass from the glomerulus and into the Bowman's capsule by:
   a. diffusion.
   b. active transport.
   c. filtration.
   d. osmosis.

8. The juxtaglomerular cells reside in the:
   a. afferent arteriole.
   b. efferent arteriole.
   c. proximal convoluted tubule.
   d. distal convoluted tubule.

True or False

9. _____ The left kidney is often slightly larger and positioned slightly lower than the right kidney.

10. _____ Blood is brought to the kidneys by the renal vein.

11. _____ *Micturition* and *urination* are synonymous terms.

12. _____ The glomerulus is one of the most important capillary networks for survival.

13. _____ Once urine enters the renal pelvis, it travels to the renal calyces.

14. _____ As the basic functional unit of the kidney, the nephron's function is blood processing and urine formation.

15. _____ The kidneys are covered with visceral peritoneum.

Labeling—match each term with its corresponding number on the following illustration of the kidney.

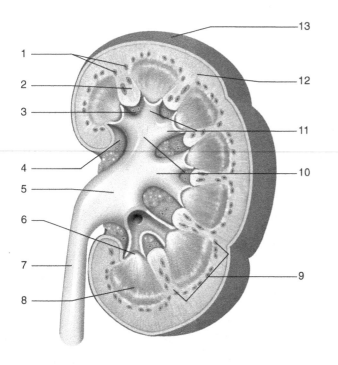

_____ renal pelvis
_____ renal papilla of pyramid
_____ minor calyces
_____ renal column
_____ cortex
_____ hilum
_____ ureter
_____ renal sinus
_____ interlobular arteries
_____ capsule (fibrous)
_____ medulla
_____ major calyces
_____ medullary pyramid

Labeling—match each term with its corresponding number on the following illustration of the nephron.

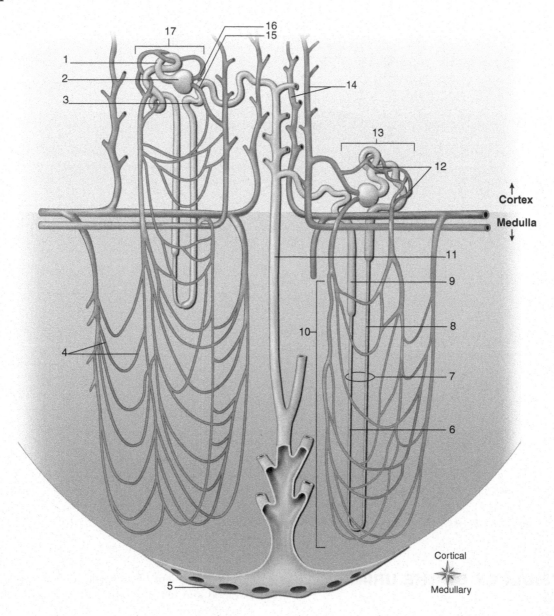

_____ renal corpuscle

_____ thick ascending limb of Henle loop (TAL)

_____ peritubular capillaries

_____ arcuate artery and vein

_____ proximal convoluted tubule (PCT)

_____ efferent arteriole

_____ thin ascending limb of Henle loop (tALH)

_____ cortical nephron

_____ Henle loop

_____ vasa recta

_____ papilla of renal pyramid

_____ afferent arteriole

_____ descending limb of Henle loop

_____ collecting duct (CD)

_____ juxtamedullary nephron

_____ distal convoluted tubule (DCT)

_____ interlobular artery and vein

Labeling—label the following structure of the male urinary bladder.

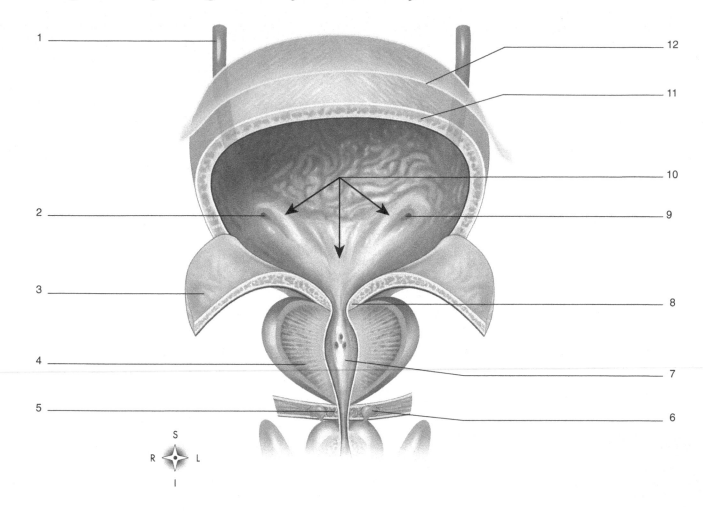

→ *If you had difficulty with this section, review pages 966-976 and page 978.*

II—PHYSIOLOGY OF THE URINARY SYSTEM

Multiple Choice—select the best answer.

16. Which of the following is *not* one of the processes of urine formation?
    a. filtration
    b. diffusion
    c. reabsorption
    d. secretion

17. The movement of water and solutes from the plasma in the glomerulus, across the glomerular-capsular membrane, and into the capsular space of the Bowman's capsule is termed:
    a. filtration.
    b. diffusion.
    c. reabsorption.
    d. secretion.

18. The movement of molecules out of the peritubular blood and into the tubule for excretion is:
    a. filtration.
    b. diffusion.
    c. reabsorption.
    d. secretion.

19. Under normal conditions, most water, electrolytes, and nutrients are reabsorbed in the:
    a. proximal convoluted tubule.
    b. distal convoluted tubule.
    c. Henle loop.
    d. collecting duct.

20. Which of the following is considered a countercurrent structure?
    a. glomerulus
    b. proximal convoluted tubule
    c. Henle loop
    d. distal convoluted tubule

21. Water loss from the blood is reduced by:
    a. ADH.
    b. atrial natriuretic hormone (ANH).
    c. aldosterone.
    d. both a and c.

22. *Dysuria* is a term describing:
    a. blood in the urine.
    b. pus in the urine.
    c. painful urination.
    d. absence of urine.

23. All of the following are normal contents of urine *except*:
    a. nitrogenous wastes.
    b. hormones.
    c. pigments.
    d. plasma proteins.

24. Which of the following is *not* symptomatic of diabetes mellitus?
    a. copious urination
    b. glycosuria
    c. anuria
    d. diuresis

True or False

25. _____ Proximal convoluted tubules reabsorb nutrients from the tubule fluid, notably glucose and amino acids, into peritubular blood by a special type of active transport mechanism called *sodium cotransport*.

26. _____ Postexercise proteinuria is considered serious and often indicative of kidney disease.

27. _____ Fluid exiting the Henle loop becomes less concentrated with Na^+ and Cl^- ions.

28. _____ A hydrostatic pressure gradient drives the filtration out of the plasma and into the nephron.

29. _____ The efferent arteriole has a larger diameter than the afferent arteriole.

30. _____ Stress causes an increase in glomerular hydrostatic pressure.

31. _____ In the renal tubule, Na^+ is reabsorbed via active transport.

32. _____ Glomerular filtration separates only harmful substances from the blood.

33. _____ Urine consists of approximately 75% water.

34. _____ Urine has a pH of 4.6 to 8.0 and is generally alkaline.

35. _____ More than 99% of filtrates must be reabsorbed from the tubular segments of the nephron.

➡ *If you had difficulty with this section, review pages 976-990.*

III—MECHANISMS OF DISEASE

Matching—select the correct disorder from the choices provided.

   a. pyelonephritis
   b. renal colic
   c. renal calculi
   d. acute glomerulonephritis
   e. proteinuria
   f. uremia
   g. neurogenic bladder
   h. acute renal failure
   i. hydronephrosis
   j. chronic renal failure
   k. cystitis
   l. urethritis

36. _____ urine backs up into the kidneys, causing swelling of the renal pelvis and calyces

37. _____ kidney stones

38. _____ final stage of chronic renal failure

39. _____ involuntary retention of urine with subsequent distention of the bladder

40. _____ inflammation of the bladder

41. _____ inflammation of the renal pelvis and connective tissues of the kidney

42. _____ an abrupt reduction in kidney function characterized by oliguria and a sharp rise in nitrogenous compounds in the blood

43. _____ progressive condition resulting from gradual loss of nephrons

44. _____ intense kidney pain caused by destruction of the ureters by large kidney stones

45. _____ most common form of kidney disease caused by a delayed immune response to streptococcal infection

46. _____ albumin in the urine

47. _____ inflammation of the urethra that commonly results from bacterial infection

➡ *If you had difficulty with this section, review pages 989-993.*

CROSSWORD PUZZLE

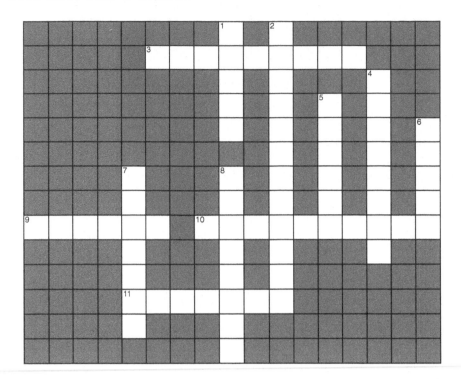

ACROSS
3. Vessel; straight or upright (2 words)
9. Urine; blood; condition
10. Strain; process
11. Kidney; unit

DOWN
1. Cup-like
2. Back again; from; suck; process
4. Bag; inflammation
5. Pus; urine; condition
6. Kidney; substance
7. Three; corner
8. Few or little; urine; condition

 APPLYING WHAT YOU KNOW

48. Mr. Dietz, an accident victim, was admitted to the hospital several hours ago. His chart indicates that he had been hemorrhaging at the scene of the accident. Nurse Petersen has been closely monitoring his urinary output and has noted that it has dropped to 10 mL/hr (the normal urine output for a healthy adult is approximately 30 to 60 mL/hr). What might explain this drop in urine output?

49. Madison developed chronic renal failure. Describe the progression of each of the three phases of chronic renal failure.

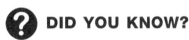 **DID YOU KNOW?**

- If the tubules in a kidney were stretched and untangled, there would be 70 miles of them.
- While examining urine, German chemist Hennig Brand discovered phosphorus.

ONE LAST QUICK CHECK

Multiple Choice—select the best answer.

50. Which of the following processes is used by the artificial kidney to remove waste materials from the blood?
    a. pinocytosis
    b. dialysis
    c. catheterization
    d. active transport

51. Failure of the kidneys to remove wastes from the blood will result in which of the following?
    a. retention
    b. anuria
    c. incontinence
    d. uremia

52. Hydrogen ions are transferred from blood into the urine during which of the following processes?
    a. secretion
    b. filtration
    c. reabsorption
    d. all of the above

53. Which of the following conditions would be considered normal in an infant younger than 2 years of age?
    a. retention
    b. cystitis
    c. incontinence
    d. anuria

54. Which of the following steps involved in urine formation allows the blood to retain most body nutrients?
    a. secretion
    b. filtration
    c. reabsorption
    d. all of the above

55. Voluntary control of micturition is achieved by the action of which of the following?
    a. internal urethral sphincter
    b. external urethral sphincter
    c. trigone
    d. bladder muscles

56. What is the structure that carries urine from the kidney to the bladder called?
    a. urethra
    b. Bowman's capsule
    c. ureter
    d. renal pelvis

57. What are the capillary loops contained within Bowman's capsule called?
    a. convoluted tubules
    b. glomeruli
    c. limbs of Henle
    d. collecting ducts

58. The triangular divisions of the medulla of the kidney are known as:
    a. pyramids.
    b. papillae.
    c. calyces.
    d. nephrons.

59. The trigone is located in the:
    a. kidney.
    b. bladder.
    c. ureter.
    d. urethra.

Matching—select the best answer to describe the terms.

    a. involuntary voiding
    b. passes through prostate gland
    c. absence of urine
    d. urination
    e. blood in the urine
    f. inflammation of the kidney
    g. large amount of protein in urine
    h. large amount of urine
    i. folds that line the bladder
    j. scanty amount of urine
    k. test for renal dysfunction

60. _____ hematuria

61. _____ anuria

62. _____ nephritis

63. _____ micturition

64. _____ oliguria

65. _____ polyuria

66. _____ incontinence

67. _____ proteinuria

68. _____ rugae

69. _____ urethra

70. _____ BUN

CHAPTER 43

Fluid and Electrolyte Balance

Referring to the very first chapter in your text, you will recall that survival depends on the body's ability to maintain or restore homeostasis. Specifically, *homeostasis* means that the body fluids remain constant within very narrow limits. These fluids are classified as either intracellular fluid (ICF) or extracellular fluid (ECF). As their names imply, intracellular fluid lies within the cells and extracellular fluid is located outside the cells. A balance between these two fluids is maintained by several body mechanisms. Among them are: 1) the adjustment of fluid output to fluid intake under normal circumstances, 2) the concentration of electrolytes, 3) the capillary blood pressure, and 4) the concentration of proteins in the blood. Knowledge of how these mechanisms maintain and restore fluid balance is necessary for an understanding of the complexities of homeostasis and its relationship to the survival of the individual.

I—OVERVIEW OF FLUID AND ELECTROLYTE BALANCE

Multiple Choice—select the best answer.

1. The majority of total body water is found in the:
   a. plasma.
   b. interstitial fluid.
   c. ICF.
   d. ECF.

2. The most abundant intracellular cation is:
   a. Na^+.
   b. Cl^-.
   c. K^+.
   d. Mg^{++}.

3. The most abundant extracellular cation is:
   a. Na^+.
   b. Cl^-.
   c. K^+.
   d. Mg^{++}.

4. The most abundant anion in ECF is:
   a. Na^+.
   b. Cl^-.
   c. K^+.
   d. Mg^{++}.

5. Electrolyte reactivity is measured in:
   a. mg/100 L.
   b. milliequivalents.
   c. mEq/L.
   d. both b and c.

6. Which of the following mechanisms varies fluid output so that it equals input?
   a. antidiuretic device
   b. aldosterone mechanism
   c. renin-angiotensin-aldosterone mechanism
   d. both b and c

7. Which of the following statements is true?
   a. Total body water as a percentage of total body weight does *not* differ due to age.
   b. Total body water as a percentage of total body weight is approximately 30% in a healthy nonobese female.
   c. Males that are healthy and nonobese will have 60% of their body weight as water.
   d. Adipose tissue contains less water than bone tissue.

True or False

8. _____ Obese people have a higher water content per kilogram of body weight than slender people.

9. _____ When compared chemically, plasma and interstitial fluid are nearly identical.

10. _____ Fluid intake usually equals fluid output.

11. _____ Electrolytes are substances that bind in water.

12. _____ Thirst is associated with any condition that decreases total volume of body water.

13. _____ Water exits the body only through the urinary and digestive systems.

14. _____ *Hypervolemia* refers to excess blood volume.

→ *If you had difficulty with this section, review pages 1000-1004.*

II—MECHANISMS THAT MAINTAIN HOMEOSTASIS OF TOTAL FLUID VOLUME

Multiple Choice—select the best answer.

15. The two factors that determine urine volume are:
    a. the amount of antidiuretic hormone (ADH) and aldosterone secretion.
    b. the amount of adrenocorticotropic hormone (ACTH) and ADH secretion.
    c. fluid intake and ADH secretion.
    d. the glomerular filtration rate and the rate of water reabsorption by the renal tubules.

16. Which of the following is an example of obligatory fluid output?
    a. water vapor in expired air
    b. water diffusion through the skin
    c. both a and b
    d. none of the above

True or False

17. _____ If a person takes nothing by mouth for several days, fluid output decreases to zero to compensate and maintain homeostasis.

18. _____ Dehydration is often detected by loss of skin elasticity.

➡ *If you had difficulty with this section, review pages 1004-1007.*

III—REGULATION OF WATER AND ELECTROLYTE LEVELS IN PLASMA, INTERSTITIAL FLUID, AND INTRACELLULAR FLUID

Multiple Choice—select the best answer.

19. Blood hydrostatic pressure:
    a. tends to force fluid out of capillaries and into interstitial fluid.
    b. tends to force fluid out of interstitial fluid and into capillaries.
    c. allows for an equilibrium across the capillary membrane.
    d. none of the above.

20. Which of the following is *not* a correct statement regarding severe dehydration?
    a. Loss of skin turgor is a symptom of severe dehydration.
    b. The relative loss of water in sweat is greater than the loss of electrolytes.
    c. Sweating serves the body by increasing body heat.
    d. Treatment of dehydration requires appropriate electrolyte replacement therapy.

21. The formula representing Starling's law of the capillaries is:
    a. (BHP + BCOP) − (IFCOP + IFHP) = EFP.
    b. (BHP + IFHP) − (IFCOP + BCOP) = EFP.
    c. (BHP + IFCOP) − (IFHP + BCOP) = EFP.

22. Which large molecules are retained by the selectively permeable cell membrane?
    a. sodium ions
    b. potassium ions
    c. proteins
    d. water

True or False

23. _____ Edema can be defined as "the presence of abnormally large amounts of fluid in the intercellular spaces of the body."

24. _____ The most common cause of edema is glomerulonephritis.

25. _____ The most significant player regulating ICF composition is the plasma membrane.

26. _____ Osmotic pressure is influenced by large protein molecules in the intracellular fluid.

➡ *If you had difficulty with this section, review pages 1007-1011.*

IV—REGULATION OF SODIUM AND POTASSIUM LEVELS IN BODY FLUIDS

True or False

27. _____ The release of ADH causes an increase in the reabsorption of sodium and water by the renal tubules.

28. _____ Over 8 liters of various internal secretions are produced daily.

29. _____ Potassium deficit is termed *hypokalemia*.

30. _____ ECF depletion is said to be the "last line of defense" against dehydration.

31. _____ By volume, intestinal secretions are the largest sodium-containing internal secretions.

➡ *If you had difficulty with this section, review page 1008 and pages 1011-1013.*

V—MECHANISMS OF DISEASE

Matching—identify the best answer for the terms.

a. dehydration
b. excessive perspiration
c. excess fluid volume
d. increased serum potassium
e. decreased serum sodium

32. _____ hypovolemia

33. _____ hyperkalemia

34. _____ hyponatremia

35. _____ diaphoresis

36. _____ hypervolemia

True or False

37. _____ Skin turgor is an important indicator of fluid volume stability.

38. _____ Cushing syndrome can cause hypokalemia.

39. _____ Overuse of diuretics can result in hyponatremia.

40. _____ Hyperkalemia is not a serious threat to the body.

➔ *If you had difficulty with this section, review pages 1014-1015.*

CROSSWORD PUZZLE

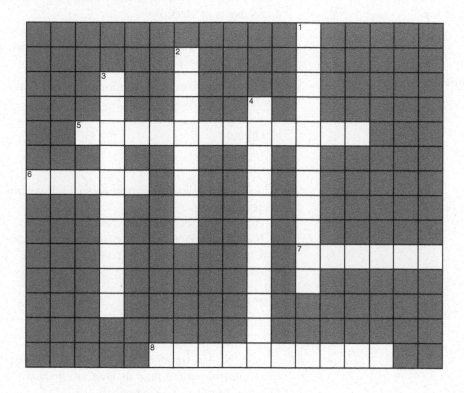

ACROSS
5. Push; receive; agent
6. Up; to go
7. Swollen; condition
8. Beside; intestine; relating to

DOWN
1. Electricity; loosening
2. Through; urine; relating to
3. Apart; unite; action
4. Remove; water; process

APPLYING WHAT YOU KNOW

41. Ms. Titus was asked to keep an accurate record of her fluid intake and output. She was concerned because the two did not balance, even though the physician assured her that she had no kidney pathology. What is a possible explanation for this?

42. Jack Sprat was 6' 5" and weighed 185 lbs. His wife was 5' 6" and weighed 185 lbs. Whose body contained more water?

DID YOU KNOW?

- The best fluid replacement drink is to add ½ tsp of table salt to 1 quart of water.
- If all of the water were drained from the body of an average 160-lb. man, the body would weigh 64 lbs.

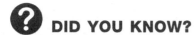 **ONE LAST QUICK CHECK**

Circle the correct answer.

43. The largest volume of water by far lies (inside or outside) cells.

44. Interstitial fluid is (intracellular or extracellular).

45. Plasma is (intracellular or extracellular).

46. Obese people have a (lower or higher) water content per pound of body weight than thin people.

47. Infants have (more or less) water in comparison to body weight than adults of either sex.

48. In general, as age increases, the amount of water per pound of body weight (increases or decreases).

Multiple Choice—select the best answer.

49. Which one of the following is *not* a positively charged ion?
    a. chloride
    b. calcium
    c. sodium
    d. potassium

50. Which one of the following is *not* a negatively charged ion?
    a. chloride
    b. bicarbonate
    c. phosphate
    d. sodium

51. The smallest amount of water comes from:
    a. water in foods that are eaten.
    b. ingested food.
    c. water formed from catabolism.
    d. none of the above.

52. The greatest amount of water lost from the body is from the:
    a. lungs.
    b. skin by diffusion.
    c. skin by sweat.
    d. feces.
    e. kidneys.

53. Excessive water loss and fluid imbalance can result from which of the following?
    a. diarrhea
    b. vomiting
    c. severe burns
    d. all of the above

54. Signals generated by osmoreceptors in the subfornical organ and hypothalamus stimulate the secretion of:
    a. aldosterone.
    b. insulin.
    c. ADH.
    d. ANH.

55. If blood sodium concentration decreases, what does blood volume do?
    a. increases
    b. decreases
    c. remains the same

56. Which of the following is true of body water?
    a. It is obtained from the liquids we drink.
    b. It is obtained from the foods we eat.
    c. It is formed by the catabolism of food.
    d. All of the above are true.

57. Edema may result from which of the following?
    a. retention of electrolytes
    b. decreased blood pressure
    c. increased concentration of blood plasma proteins
    d. all of the above

58. The most abundant and important positive plasma ion is which of the following?
    a. sodium
    b. chloride
    c. calcium
    d. oxygen

59. Which of the following is true when ECF volume decreases?
    a. Aldosterone secretion increases.
    b. Kidney tubule reabsorption of sodium increases.
    c. Urine volume decreases.
    d. All of the above are true.

True or False

60. _____ Interstitial fluid contains hardly any protein anions.

61. _____ No net transfer of water occurs between blood and interstitial fluid as long as effective filtration pressure (EFP) equals 0.

62. _____ Any change in the solute concentration of ECF will have a direct effect on water movement across the cell.

CHAPTER 44
Acid-Base Balance

It has been established in previous chapters that an equilibrium between intracellular and extracellular fluid volume must exist for homeostasis. Equally important to homeostasis is the chemical acid-base balance of the body fluids. The degree of acidity or alkalinity of a body fluid is expressed as pH value. The neutral point, where a fluid would be neither acid nor alkaline, is pH 7. Increasing acidity is expressed as less than 7, and increasing alkalinity as greater than 7. Examples of body fluids that are acidic are gastric juice (pH 1.6) and urine (pH 6.0). Blood, on the other hand, is considered alkaline with a pH of 7.4.

Buffers are substances that prevent a sharp change in the pH of a fluid when an acid or base is added to it. They are one of several mechanisms that are constantly monitoring the pH of fluids in the body. If for any reason these mechanisms do not function properly, a pH imbalance occurs. These two kinds of imbalances are known as *alkalosis* and *acidosis*.

Maintaining the acid-base balance of body fluids is a matter of vital importance. If this balance varies even slightly, necessary chemical and cellular reactions cannot occur. Your review of this chapter is necessary to understand the delicate fluid balance necessary for survival.

I—MECHANISMS THAT CONTROL pH OF BODY FLUIDS

Multiple Choice—select the best answer.

1. As pH goes down, a:
   a. solution becomes more basic.
   b. solution's hydrogen ion concentration decreases.
   c. solution becomes more acidic.
   d. solution thickens.

2. The most acidic body substance of the following is:
   a. gastric juice.
   b. pancreatic juice.
   c. bile.
   d. urine.

3. Which of the following is an acid-forming food?
   a. grapefruit
   b. meat
   c. orange juice
   d. coffee

4. Which of the following is a base-forming food?
   a. fruit
   b. vegetable
   c. egg
   d. both a and b

5. Which of the following describes the narrow pH range of blood?
   a. 7.21 to 7.49
   b. 7.00 to 7.20
   c. 7.36 to 7.41
   d. 7.50 to 7.77

6. An acid-forming element is:
   a. sulfur.
   b. calcium.
   c. potassium.
   d. sodium.

7. Acidic ketone bodies are associated with cellular metabolism of:
   a. proteins.
   b. carbohydrates.
   c. fats.
   d. minerals.

True or False

8. _____ Blood is slightly alkaline.

9. _____ Citrus fruits, such as oranges and grapefruit, have a significant effect on acid-base balance.

10. _____ Chemical buffer systems are fast acting.

11. _____ The carbon dioxide present in venous blood causes it to become slightly more basic than arterial blood.

12. _____ A vegetarian diet would tend to produce an alkaline state in body fluids.

13. _____ The respiratory and urinary systems can serve as physiologic buffer systems.

➔ *If you had difficulty with this section, review pages 1020-1025.*

II—BUFFER MECHANISMS FOR CONTROLLING pH OF BODY FLUIDS

Multiple Choice—select the best answer.

14. Potassium salts of hemoglobin inside the red blood cell primarily buffer:
    a. carbonic acid.
    b. lactic acid.
    c. phosphoric acid.
    d. sulfuric acid.

15. A serious complication of vomiting is:
    a. carbonic acid.
    b. bicarbonate deficit.
    c. metabolic alkalosis.
    d. metabolic acidosis.

True or False

16. _____ The process of exchanging a bicarbonate ion formed in the red blood cell with a chloride ion from the plasma is called *chloride shift*.

17. _____ Buffers control pH in a manner that requires no other mechanism of pH control to maintain homeostasis.

18. _____ The blood buffer system normally converts a strong acid to a weak acid.

19. _____ Bicarbonate loading by athletes has proven to be mildly successful in diminishing the muscle soreness and fatigue associated with strenuous exercise.

20. _____ Elevated CO_2 levels result in increased formation of carbonic acid in red blood cells.

→ *If you had difficulty with this section, review pages 1022-1025.*

III—RESPIRATORY AND URINARY MECHANISMS OF pH CONTROL

Multiple Choice—select the best answer.

21. With each expiration, which substances leave the body?
    a. CO_2
    b. H_2O
    c. O_2
    d. both a and b

22. All of the following would increase the respiration rate *except*:
    a. decreased blood pH.
    b. decreased carbon dioxide.
    c. increased arterial blood CO_2.
    d. all increase respirations.

23. The kidney tubules secrete hydrogen ions in exchange of:
    a. K^+.
    b. Na^+.
    c. Ca^{++}.
    d. Cl^-.

24. Acidosis causes:
    a. hyperventilation.
    b. hypoventilation.
    c. an increase in blood pH.
    d. increase in potassium ion excretion.

25. A decrease in blood pH accelerates tubule excretion of:
    a. hydrogen.
    b. ammonia.
    c. both a and b.
    d. none of the above.

True or False

26. _____ Prolonged hyperventilation may increase blood pH enough to cause alkalosis.

27. _____ Respiratory mechanisms are much more effective in expelling hydrogen ions than are urinary mechanisms.

28. _____ The more hydrogen ions secreted by the renal tubule, the fewer potassium ions secreted.

29. _____ Intravenous administration of normal saline is used for metabolic acidosis.

30. _____ An increase in blood pH above normal (alkalosis) causes hypoventilation.

→ *If you had difficulty with this section, review pages 1024-1029.*

IV—MECHANISMS OF DISEASE

Matching—write the letter of the correct term on the blank next to the appropriate definition.

    a. metabolic acidosis
    b. metabolic alkalosis
    c. respiratory acidosis
    d. respiratory alkalosis
    e. treatment for metabolic and respiratory acidosis
    f. uncompensated metabolic acidosis
    g. hyperventilation

31. _____ result of untreated diabetes

32. _____ sodium lactate

33. _____ bicarbonate deficit

34. _____ bicarbonate excess

35. _____ rapid breathing

36. _____ carbonic acid excess

37. _____ carbonic acid deficit

→ *If you had difficulty with this section, review page 1026 and pages 1030-1034.*

CROSSWORD PUZZLE

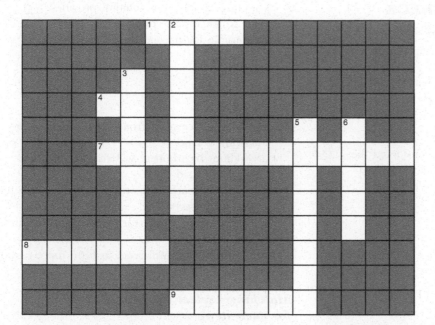

ACROSS
1. Foundation
4. Abbreviation for power; hydrogen
7. Soda; thing or substance; milk; chemical (2 words)
8. Cushion; agent
9. To vomit

DOWN
2. Ashes; relating to
3. Green; chemical
5. Sour; condition
6. A reckoning

APPLYING WHAT YOU KNOW

38. Desi was pregnant and was experiencing repeated vomiting episodes for several days. Her doctor became concerned, admitted her to the hospital, and began intravenous administrations of normal saline. How will this help Desi?

DID YOU KNOW?

• English ships carried limes to protect the sailors from scurvy. American ships carried cranberries.

39. Ginny had a minor bladder infection. She had heard that this is often the result of the urine being less acidic than necessary and that she should drink cranberry juice to correct the acid problem. She had no cranberry juice, so she decided to substitute orange juice. What was wrong with this substitution?

ONE LAST QUICK CHECK

Multiple Choice—select the best answer.

40. What happens as blood flows through lung capillaries?
    a. Carbonic acid in blood decreases.
    b. Hydrogen ions in blood decrease.
    c. Blood pH increases from venous to arterial blood.
    d. All of the above are true.

41. Which of the following organs is considered the most effective regulator of blood carbonic acid levels?
    a. kidneys
    b. intestines
    c. lungs
    d. stomach

42. Which of the following organs is/are considered the most effective regulator(s) of blood pH?
    a. kidneys
    b. intestines
    c. lungs
    d. stomach

43. What is the pH of the blood?
    a. 7.0 to 8.0
    b. 7.6 to 7.8
    c. 6.2 to 7.4
    d. 7.3 to 7.4

44. If the ratio of sodium bicarbonate to carbonate ions is lowered (perhaps 10 to 1) and blood pH is also lowered, what is the condition called?
    a. uncompensated metabolic acidosis
    b. uncompensated metabolic alkalosis
    c. compensated metabolic acidosis
    d. compensated metabolic alkalosis

45. If a person hyperventilates for a sufficient time period, which of the following will probably develop?
    a. metabolic acidosis
    b. metabolic alkalosis
    c. respiratory acidosis
    d. respiratory alkalosis

46. Normal saline is a therapy option for severe vomiting because this solution provides _____ ions, which replace bicarbonate ions that are responsible for the metabolic imbalance.
    a. hydrogen
    b. sodium
    c. potassium
    d. chloride

47. In the presence of a strong acid, which of the following is true?
    a. Sodium bicarbonate will react to produce carbonic acid.
    b. Sodium bicarbonate will react to produce more sodium bicarbonate.
    c. Carbonic acid will react to produce sodium bicarbonate.
    d. Carbonic acid will react to form more carbonic acid.

Matching—select the best answer for each item.

a. untreated diabetes mellitus
b. excessive vomiting
c. lab analysis of blood as related to acid-base imbalance
d. "fixed" acid
e. barbiturate overdose
f. fever
g. acidic solution
h. prevent sharp pH changes

48. _____ pH lower than 7.0

49. _____ ABG

50. _____ buffers

51. _____ decrease in respirations

52. _____ increase in respirations

53. _____ metabolic acidosis

54. _____ metabolic alkalosis

55. _____ lactic acid

CHAPTER 45

Male Reproductive System

The reproductive system consists of those organs that participate in propagating the species. It is a unique body system in that its organs differ between the two sexes, and yet the goal of creating a new being is the same. Of interest also is the fact that this system is the only one not necessary to the survival of the individual, and yet survival of the species depends on the proper functioning of the reproductive organs. The male reproductive system is divided into the external genitals, testes, duct system, and accessory glands. The testes, or gonads, are considered essential organs because they produce the sex cells—sperm—which join with the female sex cells—ova—to form a new human being. They also secrete testosterone, the male sex hormone, which is responsible for the physical transformation of a boy to a man.

Sperm are formed in the testes by the seminiferous tubules. From there they enter a long narrow duct, the epididymis. They continue onward through the vas deferens into the ejaculatory duct, down the urethra, and out of the body. Throughout this journey, various glands secrete substances that add motility to the sperm and create a chemical environment conducive to reproduction.

Knowledge of the male reproductive system is necessary to understand the role of the male and the phenomena necessary to produce an offspring.

I—MALE REPRODUCTIVE ORGANS

Multiple Choice—select the best answer.

1. The male gonads are known as the:
   a. testes.
   b. prostate.
   c. epididymis.
   d. perineum.

2. The region within a "triangle" created by the ischial tuberosities and the symphysis is the:
   a. anal triangle.
   b. urogenital triangle.
   c. perineal triangle.
   d. testicular triangle.

3. Which of the following is *not* a supporting structure?
   a. penis
   b. scrotum
   c. prostate
   d. spermatic cord

4. Each testicular lobule contains:
   a. seminiferous tubules.
   b. interstitial cells.
   c. Leydig cells.
   d. all of the above.

5. The blood-testis barrier is formed by tight junctions between which cells?
   a. Leydig cells
   b. interstitial cells
   c. sustentacular cells
   d. all of the above

6. Sperm production occurs in the:
   a. seminiferous tubules.
   b. interstitial cells.
   c. Sertoli cells.
   d. prostate.

7. Which hormone is responsible for the stimulation of sperm production?
   a. follicle-stimulating hormone (FSH)
   b. luteinizing hormone (LH)
   c. testosterone
   d. both b and c

8. Which of the following is *not* a specific region of a spermatozoon?
   a. head
   b. middle piece
   c. body
   d. tail

True or False

9. _____ The testes perform two primary functions: spermatogenesis and secretion of hormones.

10. _____ Testosterone is secreted by the anterior pituitary.

11. _____ The urogenital triangle surrounds the anus.

12. _____ *Capacitation* refers to the release of enzymes contained within the acrosome.

13. _____ *Sustentacular cells* and *efferent ductules* are synonymous.

14. _____ The bulbourethral glands are a supporting structure of the male reproductive system.

15. _____ Testosterone is sometimes referred to as "the anabolic hormone."

Labeling—match each term with its corresponding number on the following sagittal section of the pelvis depicting placement of male reproductive organs.

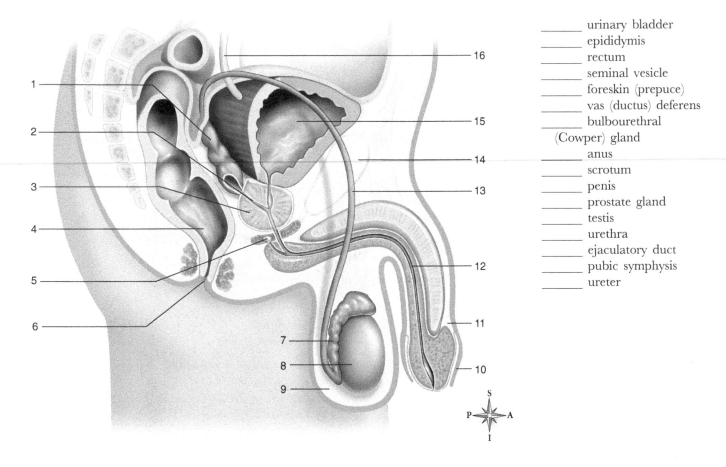

_____ urinary bladder
_____ epididymis
_____ rectum
_____ seminal vesicle
_____ foreskin (prepuce)
_____ vas (ductus) deferens
_____ bulbourethral (Cowper) gland
_____ anus
_____ scrotum
_____ penis
_____ prostate gland
_____ testis
_____ urethra
_____ ejaculatory duct
_____ pubic symphysis
_____ ureter

Labeling—using the terms provided, label the following tubules of the testis and epididymis.

seminiferous tubules
tunica albuginea
epididymis
lobule

septum
nerves and blood vessels in the
    spermatic cord

vas (ductus) deferens
testis

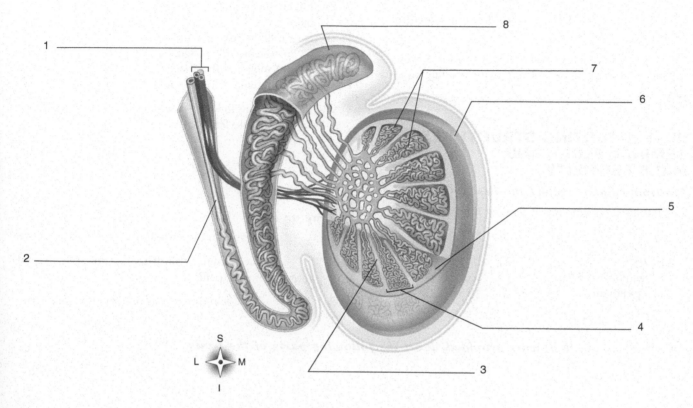

→ *If you had difficulty with this section, review pages 1039-1045.*

II—REPRODUCTIVE DUCTS AND ACCESSORY REPRODUCTIVE GLANDS

Multiple Choice—select the best answer.

16. Which of the following is *not* a function of the epididymis?
    a. a duct through which sperm travel on their journey to the exterior of the body
    b. production of spermatozoa
    c. maturation of spermatozoa
    d. secretion of a portion of seminal fluid

17. The ejaculatory ducts are formed by the union of the:
    a. seminal vesicles and ampulla.
    b. vas deferens and urethra.
    c. seminal vesicles and vas deferens.
    d. seminal vesicles and urethra.

18. Which of the following accessory reproductive glands produce(s) a secretion rich in fructose?
    a. seminal vesicles
    b. prostate
    c. bulbourethral gland
    d. Cowper glands

19. Which of the following accessory glands secrete(s) an alkaline substance?
    a. seminal vesicles
    b. bulbourethral gland
    c. all of the above
    d. none of the above

20. The most common cancer in American men is cancer of the:
    a. testes.
    b. prostate.
    c. penis.
    d. bladder.

True or False

21. _____ The duct of the vas deferens is an extension of the tail of the epididymis.

22. _____ Sperm may be stored in the vas deferens for up to a month with no loss of fertility.

23. _____ A vasectomy is a procedure intended to render a man sterile.

24. _____ Prostate-specific antigen (PSA) is always elevated in the blood of men with prostate cancer.

→ *If you had difficulty with this section, review pages 1045-1048.*

III—SUPPORTING STRUCTURES, SEMINAL FLUID, AND MALE FERTILITY

Multiple Choice—select the best answer.

25. The greatest amount of seminal fluid is secreted by the:
    a. prostate.
    b. testes.
    c. seminal vesicles.
    d. epididymis.

26. Elevation of the testes is caused by contraction of the:
    a. dartos fascia and muscle.
    b. cremaster muscle.
    c. corpora cavernosa.
    d. corpus spongiosum.

27. Functional sterility results when sperm count falls below:
    a. 5 million/mL of semen.
    b. 25 million/mL of semen.
    c. 100 million/mL of semen.
    d. 500 million/mL of semen.

28. Which of the following factors related to sperm does *not* affect male fertility?
    a. size
    b. shape
    c. texture
    d. motility

True or False

29. _____ The urethra lies within the corpora cavernosa.

30. _____ The terminal end of the corpus spongiosum forms the glans penis.

31. _____ *Emission* and *ejaculation* are synonymous terms.

Labeling—using the terms provided, label the following parts of the penis.

corpus cavernosum
bulb
glans penis
bulbourethral gland
deep artery
openings of ejaculatory ducts
prostate
urethra
crus penis
corpus spongiosum
foreskin (prepuce)
external urinary meatus
bladder
opening of bulbourethral gland

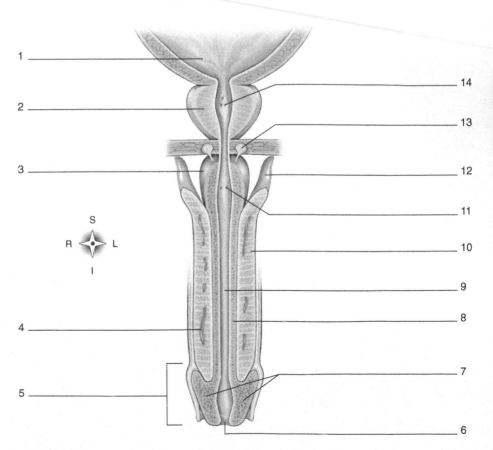

If you had difficulty with this section, review pages 1048-1051.

IV—MECHANISMS OF DISEASE

Fill in the blanks.

32. Decreased sperm production is called
    _____.

33. Testes normally descend into the scrotum about
    _____ before birth.

34. If a baby is born with undescended testes, a
    condition called _____ results.

35. A common noncancerous condition of the prostate
    in older men is known as _____
    _____ _____.

36. _____ is a condition in which the
    foreskin fits so tightly over the glans that it cannot
    retract.

37. Failure to achieve an erection of the penis is called
    _____ or _____
    _____.

38. An accumulation of fluid in the scrotum is known as
    a _____.

39. An _____
    _____ results when the
    intestines push through the weak area of the
    abdominal wall that separates the abdominopelvic
    cavity from the scrotum.

→ *If you had difficulty with this section, review pages 1051-1052.*

CROSSWORD PUZZLE

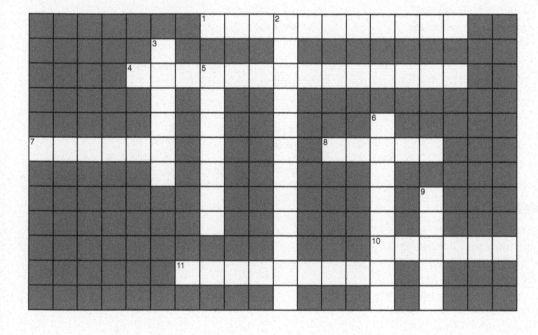

ACROSS
1. Out or away; throw; process
4. Hidden; testis; condition
7. Witness
8. Offspring; relating to
10. Marriage partner
11. Water; tumor

DOWN
2. Around; cut; process
3. Excitement
5. Before; penis
6. Male; produce
9. Seed

APPLYING WHAT YOU KNOW

40. Trent is an infant who was born with undescended testes. What is the clinical term for his condition? How easily is this diagnosed? What can Trent's doctor do to treat his condition? How serious is his condition if left untreated? What are his chances of normal testicular and sexual development?

41. John noticed an unusual swelling of his scrotum. What possible conditions may he be experiencing? Also, he noticed that the swelling occurred after a day of heavy lifting while moving out of his apartment. Based on this detail, which condition is he more likely to be experiencing? Describe the anatomy of this condition. How will the doctor treat John?

DID YOU KNOW?

- The testes produce approximately 50 million sperm per day. Every 2 to 3 months they produce enough cells to populate the entire earth.
- Men reach the peak of their sexual powers in their late teens or early twenties, and then begin to slowly decline. Women, however, do not reach their sexual peak until their late twenties or early thirties, and then remain at this level through their late fifties or early sixties.

ONE LAST QUICK CHECK

Multiple Choice—select the best answer.

42. The testes are suspended outside the body cavity to do which of the following?
    a. protect them from trauma
    b. keep them cooler
    c. keep them supplied with a greater number of blood vessels
    d. protect them from infection

43. What is the removal of the foreskin from the glans penis called?
    a. vasectomy
    b. sterilization
    c. circumcision
    d. ligation

44. The testes are surrounded by a tough membrane called the:
    a. ductus deferens.
    b. tunica albuginea.
    c. septum.
    d. seminiferous membrane.

45. The _____ lie(s) near the septa that separate the lobules.
    a. ductus deferens
    b. sperm
    c. interstitial cells
    d. nerves

46. Sperm are found in the walls of the:
    a. seminiferous tubule.
    b. interstitial cells.
    c. septum.
    d. blood vessels.

47. The scrotum provides an environment that is approximately _____ for the testes.
    a. the same as the body temperature
    b. 5° C warmer than the body temperature
    c. 3° C warmer than the body temperature
    d. 3° C cooler than the body temperature

48. The _____ produce(s) testosterone.
    a. seminiferous tubules
    b. prostate gland
    c. bulbourethral glands
    d. interstitial cells

49. The part of the sperm that contains genetic information that will be inherited is the:
    a. tail.
    b. acrosome.
    c. middle piece.
    d. head.

50. Which one of the following is *not* a function of testosterone?
    a. It causes deepening of the voice.
    b. It promotes development of the male accessory organs.
    c. It has a stimulatory effect on protein catabolism.
    d. It causes greater muscular development and strength.

51. Sperm production is called:
    a. spermatogonia.
    b. spermatids.
    c. spermatogenesis.
    d. spermatocyte.

52. The section of the sperm that contains enzymes that enable it to break down the covering of the ovum and permit entry should contact occur is the:
    a. acrosome.
    b. middle piece.
    c. tail.
    d. stem.

Matching—insert the letter in the space next to the appropriate description.

a. epididymis
b. vas deferens
c. ejaculatory duct
d. prepuce
e. seminal vesicles
f. prostate gland
g. Cowper glands
h. corpus spongiosum
i. semen
j. spermatic cord

53. _____ continuation of ducts that start in the epididymis

54. _____ erectile tissue

55. _____ also known as *bulbourethral*

56. _____ narrow tube that lies along the top of and behind the testes

57. _____ doughnut-shaped gland beneath the bladder

58. _____ union of the vas deferens with the ducts from the seminal vesicles

59. _____ mixture of sperm and secretions of accessory sex glands

60. _____ contributes 60% of the seminal fluid volume

61. _____ removed during circumcision

62. _____ enclose the vas deferens, blood vessels, lymphatics, and nerves

CHAPTER 46

Female Reproductive System

The female reproductive system is truly extraordinary and diverse. It produces ova, receives the penis and sperm during intercourse, is the site of conception, houses and nourishes the embryo during the prenatal development, and nourishes the infant after birth.

Because of its diversity, the physiology of the female is generally considered to be more complex than that of the male. Much of the activity of this system revolves around the menstrual cycle and the monthly preparation that the female undergoes for a possible pregnancy.

The organs of this system are divided into essential organs and accessory organs of reproduction. The essential organs of the female are the ovaries. Just as with the male, the essential organs of the female are referred to as the *gonads*. The gonads of the female produce ova and are responsible for producing hormones necessary for the appearance of the secondary sex characteristics.

The menstrual cycle of the female typically covers a period of 28 days. Each cycle consists of three phases: menstrual period, postmenstrual phase, and premenstrual phase. Changes in the blood levels of the hormones that are responsible for the menstrual cycle also cause physical and emotional changes in the female. A knowledge of these phenomena and the female system is necessary to complete your understanding of the reproductive system.

I—OVERVIEW OF THE FEMALE REPRODUCTIVE SYSTEM

Multiple Choice—select the best answer.

1. Which of the following is *not* an accessory organ of reproduction in women?
   a. ovaries
   b. uterus
   c. vagina
   d. vulva

2. The term that refers to the external female genitalia is:
   a. vagina.
   b. vulva.
   c. perineum.
   d. urogenital triangle.

True or False

3. _____ Ova are the female gametes.

4. _____ An episiotomy is associated with the perineum.

Labeling—match each term with its corresponding number on the following frontal section of the female pelvic organs.

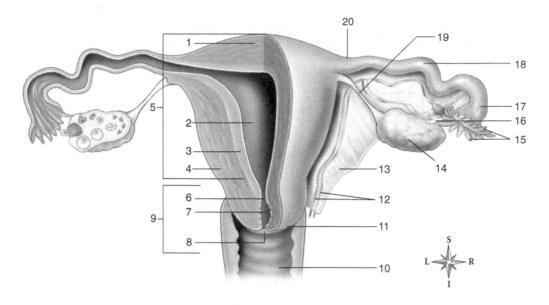

_____ broad ligament	_____ internal os of cervix	_____ ovarian ligament
_____ fundus of uterus	_____ uterine artery and vein	_____ vagina
_____ external os of vaginal cervix	_____ ampulla of uterine tube	_____ ovary
_____ endometrium	_____ isthmus of uterine tube	_____ infundibulopelvic ligament
_____ fimbriae	_____ cervical canal	_____ body of uterus
_____ fornix of vagina	_____ cervix of uterus	_____ infundibulum of uterine
_____ myometrium	_____ uterine body cavity	tube

Labeling—match each term with its corresponding number on the following sagittal section of the pelvis showing the female reproductive organs.

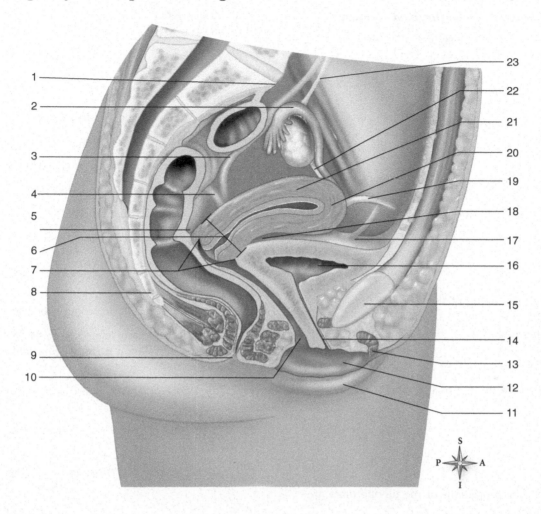

_____ suspensory ligament (of uterine tube)

_____ rectouterine pouch (of Douglas)

_____ labium majus

_____ uterine tube

_____ uterosacral ligament

_____ cervix

_____ fornix of vagina

_____ urethra

_____ coccyx

_____ anus

_____ ovarian ligament

_____ vagina

_____ sacral promontory

_____ ureter

_____ vesicouterine pouch

_____ labium minus

_____ urinary bladder

_____ fundus of uterus

_____ round ligament

_____ clitoris

_____ pubic symphysis

_____ parietal peritoneum

_____ body of uterus

➔ *If you had difficulty with this section, review pages 1058-1060.*

II—OVARIES, UTERUS, UTERINE TUBES, AND VAGINA

Multiple Choice—select the best answer.

5. The ovaries are homologous to the male:
   a. prostate.
   b. testes.
   c. vas deferens.
   d. seminal vesicle.

6. Cells of ovarian tissue secrete:
   a. estradiol.
   b. estrone.
   c. progesterone.
   d. all of the above.

7. The bulging upper component of the uterus is the:
   a. cervix.
   b. fundus.
   c. body.
   d. fornix.

8. The innermost lining of the uterus is the:
   a. endometrium.
   b. myometrium.
   c. perimetrium.
   d. parietal peritoneum.

9. The portion of the uterus that opens into the vagina is the:
   a. internal os.
   b. external os.
   c. fornix.
   d. cervix.

10. The fringelike projections of the uterine tubes are called the:
    a. isthmus.
    b. ampulla.
    c. infundibulum.
    d. fimbriae.

Matching—insert the letter of the correct structure in the blank next to the description.

   a. uterine tubes
   b. uterus
   c. vagina

11. _____ isthmus

12. _____ myometrium

13. _____ terminal end of birth canal

14. _____ site of menstruation

15. _____ intermediate portion called the *ampulla*

16. _____ consists of body, fundus, and cervix

17. _____ site of fertilization

18. _____ also known as *oviduct*

19. _____ receptacle for sperm

True or False

20. _____ Ovarian follicles contain oocytes.

21. _____ Retroflexion refers to the normal position of the uterus in relation to the vagina and urinary bladder.

22. _____ The afterbirth is also referred to as the *fornix*.

23. _____ The "G spot" is an "erotic zone" described by Dr. Grafenberg.

➔ *If you had difficulty with this section, review pages 1060-1066.*

III—VULVA

Multiple Choice—select the best answer.

24. The female organ that is homologous to the penile structure in the male is the:
    a. labia minora.
    b. labia majora.
    c. clitoris.
    d. vulva.

25. The area between the labia minora is the:
    a. vulva.
    b. vestibule.
    c. mons pubis.
    d. "G spot."

26. Which of the following is *not* a structure of the vulva?
    a. vagina
    b. labia majora
    c. urinary meatus
    d. clitoris

27. The Bartholin's glands are homologous to the male:
    a. epididymis.
    b. bulbourethral glands.
    c. seminal vesicles.
    d. prostate gland.

28. The external genitals of the female may be referred to collectively as the:
    a. mons pubis.
    b. labia majora.
    c. greater vestibule.
    d. pudendum.

Labeling—match each term with its corresponding number on the following diagram of the external female genitals (genitalia).

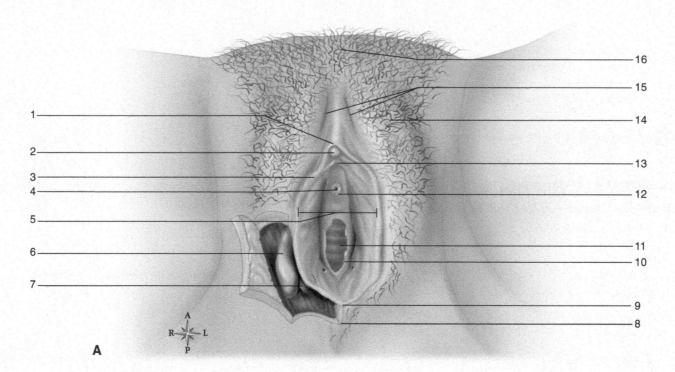

_____ posterior commissure (of labia)

_____ clitoris (glans)

_____ vestibule

_____ mons pubis

_____ labium minus

_____ vestibular bulb

_____ pudendal fissure

_____ opening of lesser vestibular (Skene) gland

_____ external urinary meatus

_____ greater vestibular gland

_____ frenulum (of labia)

_____ labium majus

_____ orifice of vagina

_____ hymen

_____ frenulum (of clitoris)

_____ foreskin (prepuce)

Labeling—match each term with its corresponding number on the following diagram of the vulva.

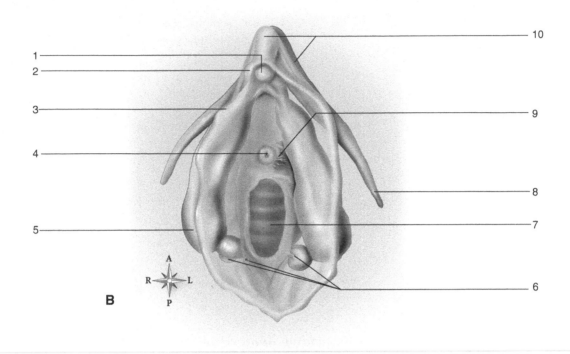

_____ clitoris (glans)
_____ labium minus
_____ external urinary meatus
_____ greater vestibular glands
   and ducts (Bartholin gland)

_____ orifice of vagina
_____ bulb of the vestibule
_____ foreskin (prepuce)
_____ lesser vestibular glands and
   ducts (Skene gland)

_____ crus clitoris
_____ corpus cavernosum

➔ *If you had difficulty with this section, review pages 1066-1068.*

IV—FEMALE REPRODUCTIVE CYCLE

Multiple Choice—select the best answer.

29. Menses occurs on days _____ of a new cycle.
   a. 1 to 5
   b. 1 to 14
   c. 6 to 14
   d. none of the above

30. Ovulation usually occurs on cycle day _____ of a 28-day cycle.
   a. 1
   b. 7
   c. 14
   d. 28

31. Menstrual discharge generally does not clot and is approximately:
   a. 30 to 100 mL.
   b. 100 to 350 mL.
   c. 300 to 550 mL.
   d. 500 to 600 mL.

32. Which of the following hormones triggers ovulation?
   a. estrogen
   b. progesterone
   c. luteinizing hormone (LH)
   d. follicle-stimulating hormone (FSH)

33. The average age at which menopause occurs is:
   a. 40 years.
   b. 45 to 50 years.
   c. 55 to 60 years.
   d. 60 to 65 years.

True or False

34. _____ The time of ovulation can be easily predicted by simply knowing the length of a previous cycle.

35. _____ Cyclical changes in the ovaries result from cyclical changes in the amounts of gonadotropins secreted by the anterior pituitary.

36. _____ Contraceptive pills and implants function by preventing ovulation.

37. _____ The first menstrual flow is known as the *climacteric*.

38. _____ The LH surge occurs at the beginning of the menstrual cycle.

➜ *If you had difficulty with this section, review pages 1069-1076.*

V—BREASTS

True or False

39. _____ The larger the breasts, the greater the amount of glandular tissue present.

40. _____ Milk secretion from the breasts begins about 3 or 4 hours after giving birth.

41. _____ Milk ejection is stimulated by oxytocin.

42. _____ Human milk provides active immunity to the offspring in the form of maternal antibodies.

➜ *If you had difficulty with this section, review pages 1076-1079.*

VI—MECHANISMS OF DISEASE

Matching—choose the correct response.

a. amenorrhea
b. dysmenorrhea
c. exogenous infection
d. dysfunctional uterine bleeding (DUB)
e. myoma
f. vaginitis
g. salpingitis
h. premenstrual syndrome (PMS)
i. pelvic inflammatory disease (PID)
j. Pap smear
k. endometriosis
l. leukorrhea

43. _____ often occurs from STDs or from a "yeast infection"

44. _____ benign tumor of smooth muscle and fibrous connective tissue; also known as a *fibroid tumor*

45. _____ absence of normal menstruation

46. _____ collection of symptoms that regularly occur in many women during the premenstrual phase

47. _____ acute or chronic inflammation caused by pathogens that spread up from vagina (complication of STD organism)

48. _____ uterine tube inflammation

49. _____ results from pathogenic organisms transmitted from another person: i.e., STD

50. _____ painful menstruation

51. _____ whitish discharge

52. _____ results from a hormonal imbalance rather than from an infection or disease condition

53. _____ screening test for cervical cancer

54. _____ characterized by displaced uterine tissue

➜ *If you had difficulty with this section, review pages 1080-1083.*

CROSSWORD PUZZLE

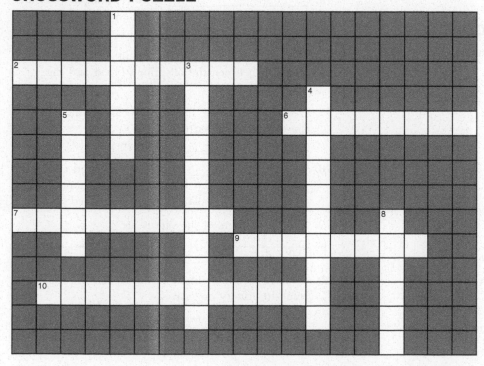

ACROSS
2. Muscle; womb; thing
6. Month; beginning
7. Mountain; groin (2 words)
9. Frenzy; produce
10. Before; bearing; solid or steroid derivative; chemical

DOWN
1. Area or space; little
3. Not; fruitful; state
4. White; flow
5. Sheath
8. Neck

APPLYING WHAT YOU KNOW

55. Prior to having children, Lorena used oral contraceptives to prevent an unwanted pregnancy with her husband. Describe the physiologic mechanism of action of oral contraceptives. After having three children by the age of 35, the couple decided that Lorena would have a tubal ligation. Describe how this procedure prevents pregnancy.

56. Harlean contracted gonorrhea. By the time she made an appointment to see her doctor, it had spread to her abdominal organs. How is this possible when gonorrhea is a disease of the reproductive system?

DID YOU KNOW?

- During menstruation, the sensitivity of a woman's middle finger is reduced.
- During pregnancy, the uterus expands to 500 times its normal size.
- There are an estimated 925,000 daily occurrences of STI transmission and 550,000 daily pregnancies worldwide.

ONE LAST QUICK CHECK

Matching—select the best answer for the descriptions.

a. salpingitis
b. vulva
c. Kegel
d. dysmenorrhea
e. Candida albicans
f. G spot
g. ovary
h. endometriosis
i. climacteric
j. fibroids

57. _____ essential organ of reproduction

58. _____ external reproductive organ

59. _____ yeast infection

60. _____ benign tumors of uterine tissue

61. _____ inflammation of the uterine tube

62. _____ erotic zone

63. _____ exercise to reduce stress incontinence

64. _____ menopause

65. _____ displaced endometrial tissue

66. _____ menstrual cramps

Fill in the blanks.

67. The _____ _____ phase occurs between ovulation and the onset of the menses.

68. _____ stimulates breast alveoli to secrete milk.

69. _____ stimulates breast alveoli to eject milk.

70. Sexual cell division is known as _____.

71. Immediately after ovulation, cells of the ruptured follicle enlarge and become transformed into the _____ _____.

72. A fold of mucous membrane known as the _____ forms a border around the external opening of the vagina, partially closing the orifice.

73. _____ is marked by the passage of 1 full year without menstruation.

74. The _____ occurs on days 1 to 5 of a new cycle.

75. _____ uterine ligaments hold the uterus in its normal position by anchoring it in the pelvic cavity.

76. The _____ permits exchange of materials between the offspring's blood and the maternal blood.

77. Development of the fetus in a location other than the uterus is referred to as an _____ pregnancy.

78. _____ is secreted each month by the corpus luteum to calm uterine contractions for implantation of a fertilized ovum.

79. The three layers of the uterus are _____, _____, and _____.

80. Damage to muscle fibers of the levator ani may result in urinary or fecal _____.

81. _____ is the failure to conceive after 1 year of regular unprotected intercourse.

CHAPTER 47
Growth and Development

Millions of fragile microscopic sperm swim against numerous obstacles to reach the ova and create a new life. At birth, the newborn will fill his lungs with air and cry lustily, signaling to the world that he is ready to begin the cycle of life. This cycle will be marked by ongoing changes, periodic physical growth, and continuous development.

This chapter reviews the more significant events that occur in the normal growth and development of an individual from conception to death. Realizing that each person is unique, we nonetheless can discover amid all the complexities of humanity some constants that are understandable and predictable.

A knowledge of human growth and development is essential in understanding the commonalties that influence individuals as they pass through the cycle of life.

I—A NEW HUMAN LIFE

Multiple Choice—select the best answer.

1. Which of the following processes reduces the number of chromosomes in each daughter cell to half the number present in the parent cell?
   a. mitosis
   b. meiosis
   c. prophase
   d. telophase

2. Forty-six chromosomes per body cell is known as the _____ number of chromosomes.
   a. haploid
   b. diploid
   c. tetrad
   d. both a and c

3. Each primary spermatocyte undergoes meiotic division I to form:
   a. four haploid secondary spermatocytes.
   b. four diploid secondary spermatocytes.
   c. one diploid secondary spermatocyte.
   d. two haploid secondary spermatocytes.

4. A mature follicle ready to burst open from the ovary's surface is a:
   a. graafian follicle.
   b. theca cell.
   c. zygote.
   d. first polar body.

5. Fertilization occurs in the:
   a. ovary.
   b. fallopian tubes.
   c. uterus.
   d. vagina.

6. The phenomenon of "crossing over" takes place during:
   a. meiosis I only.
   b. meiosis II only.
   c. both meiosis I and meiosis II.
   d. both meiosis and mitosis.

True or False

7. _____ Sex cells contain 23 chromosomes and are therefore referred to as *diploid*.

8. _____ The process of "crossing over" allows for almost infinite variety to the genetic makeup of an individual.

9. _____ Completion of meiosis II in the released oocyte requires the head of a sperm cell to enter the oocyte.

10. _____ *Zygote* is the term used to describe the ovulated ovum that is awaiting fertilization.

11. _____ *Insemination* and *fertilization* are synonymous terms.

12. _____ The ovum can live for up to 3 days.

13. _____ During oogenesis, the cytoplasm is not equally divided among daughter cells.

14. _____ Sperm cells can live in the female reproductive tract for up to 3 days.

➡️ *If you had difficulty with this section, review pages 1091-1097.*

II—PRENATAL PERIOD

Multiple Choice—select the best answer.

15. About 3 days after fertilization, the zygote forms into a solid mass of cells called a(n):
    a. morula.
    b. blastocyst.
    c. inner cell mass.
    d. embryo.

16. The outer wall of the blastocyst is referred to as the:
    a. yolk sac.
    b. trophoblast.
    c. chorion.
    d. morula.

17. The "bag of waters" is also called the:
    a. amniotic sac.
    b. yolk sac.
    c. chorion.
    d. placenta.

18. Which of the following is *not* a primary germ layer?
    a. ectoderm
    b. exoderm
    c. endoderm
    d. mesoderm

19. By which month of fetal development are all organ systems formed and functioning?
    a. second
    b. third
    c. fourth
    d. fifth

True or False

20. _____ Placental tissue secretes large amounts of human chorionic gonadotropin (hCG) early in pregnancy.

21. _____ The yolk sac plays a critical role in the nutrition of the developing human offspring.

22. _____ The process by which the primary germ layers develop into many different kinds of tissues is called *organogenesis*.

23. _____ The blastocyst is a hollow ball of cells.

24. _____ Division of the cells of the zygote is called *cleavage*.

Labeling—using the terms provided, label the following parts of the diagram depicting fertilization and implantation.

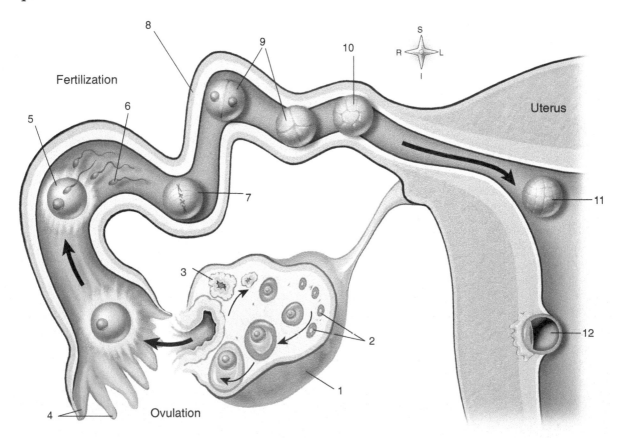

_____ implantation   _____ corpus luteum   _____ fimbriae
_____ developing follicles _____ uterine (fallopian) tube   _____ discharged ovum
_____ morula   _____ blastocyst   _____ first mitosis
_____ spermatozoa   _____ ovary   _____ divided zygote

➔ *If you had difficulty with this section, review pages 1097-1107.*

III—BIRTH, OR PARTURITION, AND THE POSTNATAL PERIOD

Multiple Choice—select the best answer.

25. Stage two of labor is best described as the:
    a. onset of contractions until uterine dilation is complete.
    b. expulsion of the placenta through the vagina.
    c. time of maximum cervical dilation until the baby exits through the vagina.
    d. time after the baby exits through the vagina and the cervix regains normal aperture.

26. Fraternal twins:
    a. are also called *identical twins*.
    b. arise from the same zygote.
    c. arise from two different sperm and two different ova.
    d. arise from a single sperm.

27. The period of infancy lasts approximately from birth to:
    a. 4 weeks.
    b. 6 months.
    c. 12 months.
    d. 18 months.

28. A rare, inherited condition in which an individual appears to age rapidly is:
    a. senescence.
    b. progeria.
    c. preeclampsia.
    d. teratogenia.

29. Birth weight generally triples by:
    a. 6 months.
    b. 12 months.
    c. 18 months.
    d. 24 months.

True or False

30. _____ A cesarean section is a surgical procedure that delivers a newborn through an incision in the abdomen and uterine wall.

31. _____ When a single zygote divides early in its development and forms two separate individuals, it is referred to as *identical twinning*.

32. _____ Stage one of labor usually lasts from a few minutes to an hour.

33. _____ Neonates have both a lumbar and thoracic curve to their spines.

34. _____ Girls experience adolescent growth spurt before boys do.

➔ *If you had difficulty with this section, review pages 1108-1115.*

IV—EFFECTS OF AGING

Multiple Choice—select the best answer.

35. A sound exercise program throughout life could reduce the effects of aging in which of the following body systems?
    a. cardiovascular
    b. skeletal
    c. muscular
    d. all of the above

36. Clouding of the lens of the eye is called:
    a. presbyopia.
    b. myopia.
    c. glaucoma.
    d. cataract.

True or False

37. _____ The number of functioning nephron units in the kidneys decreases by almost 50% between the ages of 30 and 75.

38. _____ Progesterone therapy may be used to relieve some symptoms of menopause.

➔ *If you had difficulty with this section, review pages 1116-1118.*

V—MECHANISMS OF DISEASE

Matching—select the best answer for the descriptions.

a. placenta previa
b. tubal pregnancy
c. preeclampsia
d. spontaneous abortion
e. stillbirth
f. birth defects
g. puerperal fever
h. mastitis
i. teratogen
j. abruptio placentae

39. _____ pregnancy-induced hypertension

40. _____ placenta grows too close to the cervical opening

41. _____ miscarriage

42. _____ common type of ectopic pregnancy

43. _____ breast inflammation

44. _____ congenital abnormalities

45. _____ separation of placenta from uterine wall

46. _____ childbed fever

47. _____ delivery of lifeless infant after 20 weeks

48. _____ disrupts normal histogenesis and organogenesis

➡ *If you had difficulty with this section, review page 1119.*

CROSSWORD PUZZLE

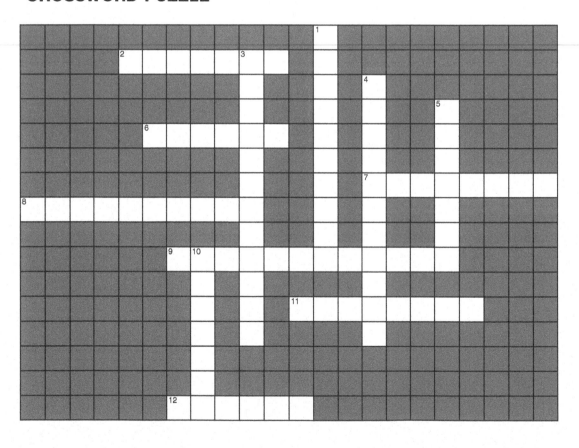

ACROSS
2. Twofold; of or like
6. Mulberry; little
7. Outside; skin
8. Bud; pouch
9. Tissue; produce; process
11. Flat cake
12. Union or yolk

DOWN
1. Grow old; state
3. In; set or place; process
4. Grow up; state
5. Becoming smaller
10. Unable to speak; state

APPLYING WHAT YOU KNOW

49. John is 70 years old. He has always enjoyed food and has a hearty appetite. Lately, however, he has complained that food "just doesn't taste as good anymore." What might be a possible explanation?

50. Gary and Harry were identical twins. Christine gave birth to a baby boy and identified Gary as the father of the child on the birth certificate. Paternity testing later revealed that both twins were the father. How is this possible?

 DID YOU KNOW?

• A 3-week-old embryo is no larger than a sesame seed. A 1-month-old fetus's body is no heavier than an envelope and a sheet of paper. Its hand is no bigger than a teardrop.

• Between the ages of 30 and 70, a nose may lengthen and widen by as much as half an inch and the ears may be a quarter-inch longer because cartilage is one of the few tissues that continues to grow as we age.

ONE LAST QUICK CHECK

Matching—choose the correct term for the appropriate description.

a. placenta
b. gestation
c. antenatal
d. histogenesis
e. C-section
f. endoderm
g. zygote
h. parturition
i. embryonic phase
j. ultrasonogram

51. _____ fertilized ovum

52. _____ inside germ layer

53. _____ before birth

54. _____ length of pregnancy

55. _____ structural "anchor" during pregnancy

56. _____ process of birth

57. _____ surgical procedure in which a newborn is delivered through an incision in the abdomen and uterine wall

58. _____ study of how the primary germ layers develop into many different kinds of tissues

59. _____ fertilization until the end of the eighth week of gestation

60. _____ monitors progress of developing fetus

Multiple Choice—select the best answer.

61. Degenerative changes in the urinary system that accompany old age include which of the following?
    a. decreased capacity of the bladder and the inability to empty or void completely
    b. decrease in the number of nephrons
    c. less blood flow through the kidneys
    d. all of the above

62. Any hardening of the arteries is referred to as which of the following?
    a. angioma
    b. atherosclerosis
    c. angina
    d. arteriosclerosis
    e. all of the above

63. Which of the following is characteristic of the disorder called *presbyopia*?
    a. It is very characteristic of old age.
    b. It causes farsightedness in some individuals.
    c. It is characterized by a lens in the eye becoming hard and losing its elasticity.
    d. All of the above are true.

64. Which of the following events, if any, is *not* characteristic of adolescence?
    a. closure of growth plates
    b. secondary sexual characteristics develop
    c. very rapid growth occurs
    d. all of the above events are characteristic of adolescence

65. Which of the following structures is derived from ectoderm?
    a. lining of the lungs
    b. brain
    c. kidneys
    d. all of the above

Matching—select the best answer from the list of descriptions.

a. older adulthood
b. study of aging
c. Hutchinson-Gilford disease
d. fat accumulation in arteries
e. secondary sexual characteristics

66. _____ atherosclerosis

67. _____ adolescence

68. _____ senescence

69. _____ progeria

70. _____ gerontology

CHAPTER 48
Genetics and Heredity

Look around your classroom and you will notice various combinations of hair color, eye color, body size, skin tone, hair texture, gender, etc. Everyone has unique body features, and this phenomenon alerts us to the marvel of genetics. Independent units, called *genes*, are responsible for the inheritance of biological traits. Genes determine the structure and function of the human body by producing specific regulatory enzymes. Some genes are dominant and some are recessive. Dominant genes produce traits that appear in the offspring, and recessive genes have traits that do not appear in the offspring when they are masked by a dominant gene.

Gene therapy is one of the latest advances of science. This revolutionary branch of medicine combines current technology with genetic research to unlock the secrets of the human body. Daily discoveries into the prevention, diagnosis, treatment, and cure of diseases and disorders are being revealed as a result of genetic therapy. A knowledge of genetics is necessary to understand the basic mechanism by which traits are transmitted from parents to offspring.

I—THE SCIENCE OF GENETICS, CHROMOSOMES AND GENES, GENE EXPRESSION

Multiple Choice—select the best answer.

1. When its genetic codes are being expressed, DNA is in a threadlike form called:
   a. mRNA.
   b. chromosomes.
   c. chromatin.
   d. tRNA.

2. Each DNA molecule can be called either a *chromatin strand* or a:
   a. gene.
   b. genome.
   c. chromosome.
   d. gamete.

3. A person with a genotype expressed as *AA* is said to be:
   a. heterozygous recessive.
   b. heterozygous dominant.
   c. homozygous recessive.
   d. homozygous dominant.

4. Both males and females need at least:
   a. one normal Y chromosome.
   b. two normal X chromosomes.
   c. one normal X chromosome.
   d. two normal Y chromosomes.

5. The entire collection of genetic material in each typical cell of the human body is called the:
   a. genome.
   b. chromosome.
   c. genotype.
   d. phenotype.

6. Mutations are caused:
   a. spontaneously.
   b. by mutagens.
   c. by environmental agents that damage DNA.
   d. all of the above.

7. Red-green color blindness is an example of an X-linked recessive condition. If X is normal, X1 is recessive, and Y is normal, an individual with the genotype XX1 will be a:
   a. normal male.
   b. color-blind male.
   c. normal female and a carrier.
   d. normal female and not a carrier.

8. The scientific study of genetics began in the:
   a. 16th century.
   b. 17th century.
   c. 18th century.
   d. 19th century.

True or False

9. _____ Each of the 23 pairs of chromosomes always appear to be nearly identical to each other.

10. _____ The manner in which genotype is expressed is termed *phenotype.*

11. _____ *Sickle-cell trait* and *sickle-cell anemia* are synonymous terms.

12. _____ Normal males have the sex chromosome combination XX, whereas normal females have the sex chromosome combination XY.

13. _____ X-linked recessive traits appear much more frequently in males than in females.

14. _____ Statistical evidence supports the notion that having sexual intercourse on the day of ovulation increases the probability of conceiving a male.

15. _____ Each cell of the body, except gametes, contains 46 pairs of chromosomes.

16. _____ A person whose genotype is heterozygous for albinism will express the abnormal phenotype of albinism.

➜ *If you had difficulty with this section, review pages 1127-1135.*

II—MEDICAL GENETICS, PREVENTION AND TREATMENT OF GENETIC DISEASES

Multiple Choice—select the best answer.

17. Trisomy and monosomy result from:
    a. an error in meiosis called *disjunction*.
    b. an error in meiosis called *nondisjunction*.
    c. single-gene abnormality.
    d. chromosome breakage.

18. Trisomy 21 is also called:
    a. Klinefelter syndrome.
    b. Down syndrome.
    c. Turner syndrome.
    d. cystic fibrosis.

19. A person with the sex chromosomes XXY is afflicted with:
    a. Klinefelter syndrome.
    b. Down syndrome.
    c. Turner syndrome.
    d. cystic fibrosis.

20. Which of the following is *not* a recessive X-linked genetic disease?
    a. hemophilia
    b. red-green color blindness
    c. sickle-cell anemia
    d. cleft palate

21. Which of the following abnormal genes are linked to some form of cancer?
    a. codominant genes
    b. tumor suppressor genes
    c. oncogenes
    d. recessive genes

22. A grid used to determine the mathematical probability of inheriting genetic traits is called:
    a. a pedigree.
    b. a Punnett square.
    c. amniocentesis.
    d. a chorionic villus sampling.

23. Which of the following genetic diseases can be treated to some degree, if diagnosed early?
    a. PKU
    b. Turner syndrome
    c. Klinefelter syndrome
    d. all of the above

24. In gene replacement therapy:
    a. genetically altered cells are introduced into the body.
    b. genetic disease is treated by inducing an alteration in metabolism.
    c. synthetic hormones are used to relieve symptoms.
    d. genes that specify production of abnormal, disease-causing proteins are replaced by normal, or "therapeutic," genes.

25. Disorders that involve trisomy or monosomy can be detected after a _____ is produced.
    a. genotype
    b. phenotype
    c. karyotype
    d. polytype

26. Cells that display distinct chromosomes during collection via amniocentesis and chorionic villus sampling are in:
    a. prophase.
    b. metaphase.
    c. anaphase.
    d. telophase.

True or False

27. _____ *Congenital disorders* and *inherited disorders* are synonymous terms.

28. _____ Sickle-cell trait is milder than sickle-cell anemia.

29. _____ Parkinson disease is linked to an error in the nuclear DNA.

30. _____ A pedigree is a chart that illustrates genetic relationships in a family over several generations.

31. _____ Xeroderma pigmentosum is characterized by the inability of skin cells to repair genetic damage caused by the (UV) radiation in sunlight.

32. _____ Cystic fibrosis is a blood-clotting disorder.

33. _____ Cleft palate is a recessive X-linked disorder.

34. _____ Chorionic villus sampling is a procedure newer than amniocentesis.

35. _____ "Genes are not there to cause disease."

➜ *If you had difficulty with this section, review pages 1135-1145.*

CROSSWORD PUZZLE

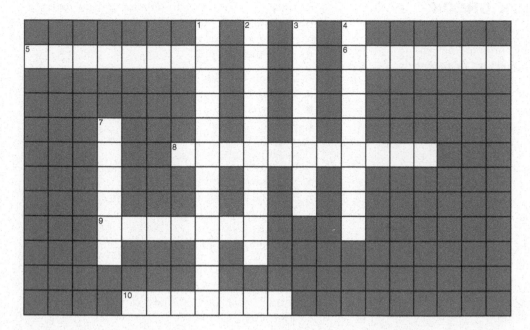

ACROSS
5. Crane's foot pattern
6. Tissue; unit
8. Together; rule; state
9. Change; produce
10. Three; body; state

DOWN
1. Different; union or yoke; characterized by
2. False; produce
3. Produce; relating to
4. Color; substance
7. Produce; entire collection

 APPLYING WHAT YOU KNOW

36. Deb's mother has a dominant gene for dark skin color. Her father has a dominant gene for light skin color. What color will Deb's skin most likely be?

37. Mr. and Mrs. Mihm both carry recessive genes for cystic fibrosis. Using your knowledge of the Punnett square, estimate the probability of one of their offspring inheriting this condition.

 DID YOU KNOW?

• Scientists estimate that they could fill a 1000-volume encyclopedia with the coded instructions in the DNA of a single human cell if the instructions could be translated into English.
• Identical twins do not have identical fingerprints. No two sets of prints are alike, including those of identical twins.

ONE LAST QUICK CHECK

Multiple Choice—select the best answer.

38. Independent assortment of chromosomes ensures:
    a. each offspring from a single set of parents is genetically unique.
    b. at meiosis each gamete receives the same number of chromosomes.
    c. that the sex chromosomes always match.
    d. an equal number of males and females are born.

39. Which of the following statements is *not* true of a pedigree?
    a. It is useful to genetic counselors in predicting the possibility of producing offspring with genetic disorders.
    b. It may allow a person to determine his or her likelihood of developing a genetic disorder later in life.
    c. It indicates the occurrence of those family members affected by a trait, as well as carriers of the trait.
    d. All of the above are true of a pedigree.

40. The genes that cause albinism are:
    a. codominant.
    b. dominant.
    c. recessive.
    d. AA.

41. During meiosis, matching pairs of chromosomes line up and exchange genes from their location to the same location on the other side; a process called:
    a. gene linkage.
    b. crossing over.
    c. cross-linkage.
    d. genetic variation.

42. When a sperm cell unites with an ovum, a _____ is formed.
    a. zygote
    b. chromosome
    c. gamete
    d. none of the above

43. DNA molecules can also be called:
    a. a chromatin strand.
    b. a chromosome.
    c. a and b.
    d. none of the above.

44. Sex-linked traits:
    a. show up more often in females than in males.
    b. are nonsexual traits carried on sex chromosomes.
    c. are the result of genetic mutation.
    d. all of the above.

45. If a person has only X chromosomes, that person is:
    a. missing essential proteins.
    b. abnormal.
    c. female.
    d. male.

46. A karyotype:
    a. can detect trisomy.
    b. is useful for diagnosing a tubal pregnancy.
    c. is frequently used as a tool in gene augmentation therapy.
    d. can detect the presence of oncogenes.

47. Which of the following pairs is mismatched?
    a. osteogenesis imperfecta—dominant
    b. Turner syndrome—trisomy
    c. PKU—recessive
    d. cystic fibrosis—recessive

Completion—using the terms below, complete the following statements.

    a. cystic fibrosis
    b. male
    c. phenylketonuria
    d. carrier
    e. genome
    f. female
    g. dominant
    h. oncogenes
    i. karyotype
    j. Tay-Sachs disease
    k. amniocentesis
    l. hemophilia

48. Abnormal genes called _____ are believed to be related to cancer.

49. Fetal tissue may be collected by a procedure called _____.

50. An abnormal accumulation of phenylalanine results in _____.

51. The entire collection of genetic material in each cell is called the _____.

52. _____ is caused by recessive genes in chromosome pair seven.

53. A _____ is a person who has a recessive gene that is not expressed.

54. Absence of an essential lipid-producing enzyme may result in the recessive condition _____.

55. _____ is a recessive X-linked disorder characterized as a blood-clotting disorder.

56. A gene capable of masking the effects of a recessive gene for the same trait is a _____ gene.

57. A _____ is a more likely candidate for color blindness.

58. A _____ is an arrangement of photographs of chromosomes from a single cell used in genetic counseling.

59. _____ X-linked recessive traits appear less often in this sex.

Fill in the blanks.

60. Each gene in a chromosome contains a genetic code that the cell transcribes to a _____ molecule.

61. The analysis of all mRNA codes actually transcribed from the human genome is known as _____.

62. The shorter segment of a chromosome is called the _____ _____ and the longer segment is called the _____ _____.

63. The most well-known chromosomal disorder is trisomy 21, or _____ _____.

64. To get therapeutic genes to cells that need them, researchers use genetically altered _____ as carriers.

65. An _____ is often used in genomics to show the overall physical structure of a chromosome.

Answer Key

CHAPTER 1
Organization of the Body

Science and Society

1. f, p. 4
2. t, p. 4
3. t, p. 4
4. f, p. 4
5. t, p. 4

Anatomy and Physiology, Language of Science, and Characteristics of Life

6. b, p. 5
7. c, p. 5
8. a, p. 5
9. b, p. 6
10. c, p. 6
11. b, p. 6

Levels of Organization

12. d, p. 7
13. a, p. 7
14. c, p. 8
15. c, p. 8
16. c, p. 8
17. d, p. 7
18. e, p. 8
19. a, p. 8
20. c, p. 8
21. b, p. 8
22. a, p. 9
23. a, p. 9
24. a, p. 9
25. b, p. 9
26. b, p. 9
27. e, p. 9
28. e, p. 9
29. d, p. 9
30. d, p. 9
31. e, p. 9
32. c, p. 9

Anatomical Position, Body Cavities, Body Regions, Anatomical Terms, and Body Planes

33. b, p. 9
34. a, p. 11
35. a, p. 10
36. d, p. 12
37. c, p. 11
38. c, p. 10
39. b, p. 11
40. b, p. 16
41. c, p. 16
42. d, p. 13
43. inferior, p. 14
44. anterior, p. 14
45. lateral, p. 14
46. proximal, p. 15
47. superficial, p. 15
48. equal, p. 16
49. anterior and posterior, p. 16
50. upper and lower, p. 16
51. frontal, p. 16
52. a, p. 10
53. b, p. 11
54. a, p. 11
55. a, p. 11
56. a, p. 10
57. a, p. 10

Applying What You Know

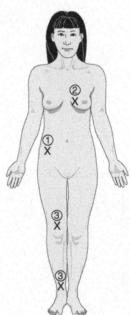

58. #1 on diagram
59. #2 on diagram
60. #3 on diagram

One Last Quick Check

61. d, p. 14
62. d, p. 16
63. a, p. 5
64. b, p. 13
65. d, p. 10
66. d, p. 15
67. d, p. 13
68. a, p. 12
69. c, p. 14
70. b, p. 15
71. eponyms, p. 6
72. bilateral symmetry, p. 9
73. Medullary, p. 15
74. apical, p. 15

75. DNA, p. 17
76. Responsiveness, p. 6
77. f, p. 13
78. f, p. 15
79. f, p. 8
80. t, p. 11

Labeling

Directions and Planes of the Body

1. superior
2. proximal
3. posterior (dorsal)
4. anterior (ventral)
5. inferior
6. sagittal plane
7. frontal plane
8. lateral

Body Cavities

1. cranial
2. spinal
3. thoracic
4. pleural
5. mediastinum
6. diaphragm
7. abdominal
8. abdominopelvic
9. pelvic

CHAPTER 2

Homeostasis

Homeostasis and Homeostatic Control Mechanisms

1. a, p. 24
2. d, p. 26
3. a, p. 27
4. b, p. 28
5. c, p. 30
6. f, p. 31
7. f, p. 27
8. t, p. 27
9. t, p. 28
10. f, p. 27

Mechanisms of Disease

11. b, p. 32
12. e, p. 32
13. a, p. 32
14. d, p. 32
15. c, p. 32
16. f, p. 32
17. h, p. 32
18. i, p. 32
19. g, p. 32
20. j, p. 32
21. Pathophysiology, p. 31
22. homeostasis, p. 31
23. mutated, p. 32
24. parasite, p. 32
25. tumors, p. 33

Applying What You Know

26. Negative feedback control mechanisms will begin to return his blood glucose to normal, and feed forward will assist with anticipatory digestive mechanisms throughout the digestive tract to make digestion occur more smoothly.
27. Different types of pathological organisms, such as viruses and bacteria, may be "infectious cofactors" in the development of certain noninfectious diseases that in the past were not considered to result directly from their presence in the body. Human papillomavirus and cervical cancer are suspected to be often related to this "cofactor theory."

One Last Quick Check

28. a, p. 24
29. a, p. 29
30. d, p. 36
31. a, p. 27
32. c, p. 32
33. homeostatic control mechanism, p. 26
34. Feed forward, p. 30
35. Intrinsic control, p. 30
36. bacteria, p. 32
37. genetic factor, p. 34
38. t, p. 27
39. t, p. 28
40. f, p. 29
41. t, p. 30
42. t, p. 34
43. hypothalamus, p. 27
44. oxytocin, p. 28
45. autoregulation, p. 30
46. Prions, p. 32
47. Young adulthood, p. 31

CHAPTER 3

Chemistry of Life

Units of Matter

1. c, p. 40
2. c, p. 41
3. c, p. 41
4. d, p. 42
5. c, p. 42
6. c, p. 43
7. b, p. 43
8. t, p. 39
9. t, p. 41
10. f, p. 43
11. f, p. 44
12. t, p. 40
13. t, p. 43
14. Oxygen, p. 40
15. Calcium, p. 40
16. Potassium, p. 40
17. Sodium, p. 40
18. Magnesium, p. 40
19. Iron, p. 40
20. Selenium p. 40.

21. electrovalent, p. 43
22. Matter, p. 39
23. hydrogen, p. 44
24. probability distribution, p. 41
25. inert, p. 42

Chemical Reactions

26. synthesis reactions, p. 45
27. Decomposition reactions, p. 46
28. Reversible reactions, p. 46
29. exchange reactions, p. 46
30. synthesis reaction, p. 45

Metabolism

31. a, p. 46
32. d, p. 46
33. b, p. 46
34. c, p. 46
35. e, p. 47

Inorganic Molecules

36. d, p. 47
37. d, p. 47
38. c, p. 48
39. b, p. 48
40. c, p. 50
41. t, p. 49
42. t, p. 49
43. t, p. 48
44. t, p. 47
45. f, p. 47

Applying What You Know

46. (a) basement (b) increasing ventilation or sealing the basement floor
47. Unstable isotopes are used that undergo nuclear breakdown. During this breakdown the radioactive isotopes emit nuclear particles and radiate the area of the tumor.

One Last Quick Check

48. e, p. 41
49. d, p. 42
50. a, p. 42
51. c, p. 44
52. b, p. 39
53. c, p. 40
54. d, p. 41
55. c, p. 46
56. a, p. 42
57. c, p. 44
58. a, p. 40
59. a, p. 46
60. b, p. 45
61. c, p. 42
62. b, p. 41
63. t, p. 39
64. f, p. 39
65. t, p. 41
66. t, p. 42
67. f, p. 41
68. f, p. 42
69. t, p. 39

70. t, p. 40
71. t, p. 41
72. f, p. 46

CHAPTER 4

Biomolecules

Organic Molecules

1. c, p. 56
2. d, p. 56
3. c, p. 63
4. a, p. 63
5. c, pp. 61 and 66
6. b, p. 59
7. c, p. 67
8. d, p. 67
9. a, p. 67
10. f, p. 60
11. t, p. 61
12. f, p. 65
13. t, p. 63
14. t, p. 63
15. t, p. 60
16. nitrogen, p. 61
17. amino acids, p. 63
18. alpha helix, p. 64
19. native state, p. 65
20. RNA, p. 68

Applying What You Know

21. Unsaturated fats can often form a solid mass at higher temperatures. Review page 59 for more information.
22. High blood concentrations of triglycerides (hypertriglyceridemia) and/or cholesterol (hypercholesterolemia) are often linked with death from heart disease and stroke. Joe should be equally concerned with elevated levels in both of these areas to practice preventive medicine.

One Last Quick Check

23. b, p. 57
24. c, p. 58
25. a, p. 63
26. c, p. 58
27. b, p. 57
28. c, p. 58
29. a, p. 63
30. PKU (All others relate to functional groups)
31. salts (All others relate to lipids)
32. calcitriol (All others relate to glycogen)
33. i, p. 63
34. f, p. 63
35. c, p. 63
36. d, p. 64
37. g, p. 65
38. a, p. 66
39. j, p. 65
40. e, p. 68
41. b, p. 60
42. h, p. 71

CHAPTER 5

Anatomy of Cells

Functional Anatomy Of Cells

1. b, p. 78
2. d, p. 86
3. b, p. 83
4. d, p. 86
5. a, p. 83
6. a, p. 87
7. b, p. 87
8. f, p. 80
9. t, p. 81
10. f, p. 86
11. t, p. 86
12. f, p. 85
13. a, p. 87
14. d, p. 80
15. b, p. 85
16. f, p. 83
17. c, p. 82
18. h, p. 87
19. g, p. 86
20. e, p. 82

Cytoskeleton

21. Cytoskeleton, p. 88
22. Microfilaments, p. 88
23. microtubules, p. 88
24. centrosome, p. 88
25. Microvilli, cilia, flagella, p. 90
26. gap junctions, p. 92
27. Desmosomes, p. 92

Applying What You Know

28. (a) CD36 (b) LDL (c) stroke, diabetes, cancer, muscular dystrophy
29. mitochondria

One Last Quick Check

30. b, p. 90
31. c, p. 91
32. b, p. 92
33. b, p. 82
34. b, p. 80
35. e, p. 76
36. d, p. 76
37. b, p. 76
38. a, p. 76
39. c, p. 76
40. composite, p. 77
41. Hydrophilic, p. 80
42. Signal transduction, p. 81
43. Peroxisomes, p. 85
44. nucleus, p. 86
45. integral membrane proteins, p. 80
46. t, p. 78
47. f, p. 90
48. t, p. 88
49. t, p. 83

Labeling

Cell Anatomy

1. Nucleolus
2. Nuclear envelope
3. Nucleus
4. Nuclear pores
5. Plasma membrane
6. Cytoplasm
7. Centrioles
8. Mitochondrion
9. Lysosome
10. Golgi apparatus
11. Free ribosome
12. Microvilli
13. Cilia
14. Smooth endoplasmic reticulum
15. Ribosome
16. Flagellum
17. Rough endoplasmic reticulum
18. Chromatin

CHAPTER 6

Cell Function

Movement of Substances Through Cell Membranes

1. d, p. 106
2. b, p. 100
3. c, p. 108
4. a, p. 102
5. b, p. 104
6. f, p. 99
7. t, p. 118
8. t, p. 108
9. t, p. 101
10. f, p. 101
11. b, p. 117
12. a, p. 102
13. c, p. 117
14. d, pp. 99 and 117
15. e, p. 106

Cell Metabolism

16. b, p. 109
17. d, p. 109
18. a, p. 109
19. d, p. 119
20. b, p. 111
21. b, p. 109
22. t, p. 112
23. t, p. 109
24. f, p. 109
25. t, p. 119
26. t, p. 113
27. f, p. 112
28. b, p. 112
29. c, p. 113
30. a, p. 112

Applying What You Know

31. diffusion
32. shrink

One Last Quick Check

33. a, p. 106
34. b, pp. 99 and 112
35. d, p. 101
36. a, p. 110
37. c, p. 112
38. b, p. 104
39. c, p. 105
40. c, p. 105
41. a, p. 108
42. b, p. 102
43. a, p. 103
44. b, p. 103
45. f, p. 118
46. c, p. 111
47. h, p. 110
48. e, p. 106
49. g, p. 103
50. d, p. 117
51. i, p. 112
52. a, p. 101

Labeling

Cellular Respiration

1. glucose
2. acetyl-CoA
3. citric acid cycle
4. mitochondrion
5. ATP
6. O_2
7. H_2O
8. aerobic
9. anaerobic
10. transition
11. pyruvic acid
12. lactic acid

CHAPTER 7

Cell Growth and Reproduction

Protein Synthesis and Cell Growth

1. d, p. 121
2. a, p. 121
3. b, p. 128
4. b, p. 124
5. c, p. 121
6. d, p. 122
7. a, p. 127
8. e, p. 123
9. a, p. 123
10. c, p. 123
11. d, p. 123
12. f, p. 122
13. b, p. 124

Cell Reproduction

14. enzyme (All others refer to cell reproduction)
15. end phase (All others refer to anaphase)
16. telophase (All others refer to meiosis)
17. mitosis (All others refer to meiosis)
18. interphase (All others are phases of mitosis)
19. a, p. 129
20. b, p. 131
21. b, p. 131
22. d, p. 129
23. c, p. 128
24. telophase, p. 130
25. anaphase, p. 130
26. metaphase, p. 130
27. interphase, p. 129
28. prophase, p. 129

Mechanisms of Disease

29. t, p. 132
30. t, p. 133
31. t, p. 132
32. f, p. 133
33. t, p. 133

Applying What You Know

34. Genes are responsible for all of our healthy attributes or conditions such as sex, hair color, and eyes. Genetic disorders are pathological conditions caused by mistakes, or mutations, in a cell's genetic code. Abnormal genes often cause a specific disease that can be identified just weeks after conception and can many times be treated prior to delivery.
35. When a broken arm is immobilized in a cast for a long period, muscles that move the arm often atrophy. Because the muscles are temporarily out of use, muscle cells decrease in size. Dan's arm will return to normal as he begins to use his arm more and returns to the level of exercise that he had prior to the fracture.

One Last Quick Check

36. a, p. 122
37. a, p. 121
38. d, p. 130
39. d, p. 122
40. c, p. 130
41. b, p. 126
42. c, p. 122
43. a, p. 130
44. a, p. 123
45. c, p. 125
46. uracil (RNA contains the base uracil, not DNA)
47. thymine (All others refer to RNA)
48. interphase (All others refer to translation)
49. prophase (All others refer to anaphase)
50. gene (All others refer to stages of cell division)
51. obligatory base pairing, p. 121
52. proteome, p. 126
53. double helix, p. 121
54. Meiosis, p. 131
55. gametes, p. 131

Labeling
DNA Molecule
1. hydrogen bonds
2. sugar
3. phosphate
4. cytosine
5. guanine
6. adenine
7. thymine

Mitosis
1. prophase
2. metaphase
3. anaphase
4. telophase

CHAPTER 8
Introduction to Tissues
Introduction to Tissues and Extracellular Matrix
1. b, p. 138
2. c, p. 138
3. d, p. 138
4. b, p. 140
5. b, p. 139
6. a, p. 138
7. t, p. 138
8. t, p. 140
9. f, p. 138
10. t, p. 140

Tissue Repair
11. Regeneration, p. 144
12. keloid, p. 145
13. phagocytic, p. 144
14. connective, p. 144
15. nerve, p. 145

Body Membranes
16. a, p. 145
17. b, p. 146
18. f, p. 146
19. t, p. 147

Tumors and Cancer
20. slowly, p. 149
21. are not, p. 149
22. papilloma, p. 149
23. sarcoma, p. 149
24. oncologist, p. 150
25. cytotoxic, p. 150

Applying What You Know
26. Diagnostic tests might include medical imaging, biopsy, and blood tests. Possible treatments might include chemotherapy, laser therapy, radiotherapy, and/or immunotherapy.
27. Joe may have pleurisy (inflammation of the pleura) as a result of the respiratory condition. The pain is caused by irritation and friction as the lungs rub against the walls of the chest cavity. Antibiotics will address the inflammation, and pain medication will reduce the pain until the inflammation subsides and healing takes place.

One Last Quick Check
28. a, p. 145
29. b, p. 146
30. d, p. 148
31. c, p. 146
32. a, p. 145
33. d, p. 148
34. a, p. 148
35. b, p. 146
36. c, p. 146
37. c, p. 146
38. endoderm, p. 139
39. mesoderm, p. 139
40. ectoderm, p. 139
41. histology, p. 138
42. matrix, p. 139
43. keloid, p. 145
44. Muscle, p. 145
45. Regeneration, p. 144
46. Adenoma, p. 149
47. Oncogenes, p. 150
48. c, p. 150
49. b, p. 150
50. a, p. 150
51. i, p. 150
52. e, p. 150
53. g, p. 150
54. j, p. 150
55. d, p. 151
56. h, p. 151
57. f, p. 150

CHAPTER 9
Tissue Types
Epithelial Tissue
1. d, p. 156
2. b, p. 158
3. b, p. 158
4. b, p. 156
5. d, p. 159
6. b, p. 161
7. a, p. 161
8. d, p. 162
9. a, p. 157
10. t, p. 156
11. f, p. 156
12. f, p. 161
13. b, p. 158
14. e, p. 159
15. d, p. 158
16. h, p. 159
17. a, p. 157
18. c, p. 158

Connective Tissue
19. a, p. 159
20. c, p. 162

21. b, p. 163
22. d, p. 165
23. c, p. 165
24. d, p. 167
25. a, p. 168
26. b, p. 168
27. a, p. 169
28. d, p. 165
29. t, p. 163
30. t, p. 168
31. f, p. 168
32. f, p. 169
33. t, p. 166
34. f, p. 168

Muscle Tissue

35. b, p. 171
36. c, p. 171
37. a, p. 172
38. b, p. 171
39. c, p. 170
40. c, p. 170

Nervous Tissue

41. d, p. 172
42. b, p. 172
43. c, p. 172
44. a, p. 172
45. e, p. 172

Applying What You Know

46. Too lean. Holly should be in the 20% to 22% range to be considered normal. Holly's obsession may put her at risk for other disease conditions because of the stress to her body of being "too lean."
47. Singulair and Zyflo are examples of leukotriene-blocking drugs. In asthma, chemicals called *leukotrienes* trigger muscles in the walls of the respiratory tract to contract and constrict the airways. These drugs are often used along with other prescription drugs to prevent or reduce contraction of airway muscles.

One Last Quick Check

48. squamous, p. 157
49. cuboidal, p. 157
50. columnar, p. 157
51. simple squamous, p. 157
52. simple cuboidal, p. 157
53. simple columnar, p. 157
54. stratified squamous, p. 157
55. pseudostratified columnar, p. 157
56. a, p. 160
57. d, p. 160
58. b, p. 162
59. c, p. 163
60. c, p. 165
61. b, p. 170
62. b, p. 162
63. d, p. 156
64. c, p. 156
65. a, p. 162
66. f, p. 165
67. e, p. 169

Labeling

Tissue #1 is simple cuboidal epithelium

1. basement membrane
2. cell nuclei
3. cuboidal epithelial cells
4. lumen of tubule

Tissue #2 is simple columnar epithelial

1. goblet cells
2. columnar epithelial cell

Tissue #3 is pseudostratified columnar ciliated epithelium

1. columnar cell
2. basement membrane
3. cilia

Tissue #4 is stratified squamous (keratinized) epithelium

1. stratified squamous epithelium
2. keratinized layer
3. basal cells
4. dermis
5. basement membrane

Tissue #5 is adipose

1. storage area for fat
2. plasma membrane
3. nucleus of adipose

Tissue #6 is collagenous dense regular fibrous connective

1. fibroblast
2. collagenous fibers

Tissue #7 is compact bone

1. osteon (haversian system)

Tissue #8 is skeletal muscle

1. cross striations of muscle cell
2. nuclei of muscle cell
3. muscle fiber

Tissue #9 is cardiac muscle

1. nucleus
2. intercalated disks

Tissue #10 is nervous

1. nerve cell body
2. axon
3. dendrites

CHAPTER 10

Skin

Structure of the Skin

1. b, p. 181
2. a, p. 181
3. d, p. 183
4. d, p. 183
5. a, p. 183
6. d, p. 186
7. b, p. 181
8. c, p. 187

9. b, p. 188
10. c, p. 189
11. f, p. 181
12. t, p. 187
13. t, p. 189
14. f, p. 186
15. t, p. 187

Functions of the Skin

16. d, p. 192
17. d, p. 192
18. c, p. 193
19. a, p. 192
20. b, p. 194
21. f, p. 192
22. f, p. 192
23. t, p. 194

Appendages of the Skin

24. b, p. 195
25. a, p. 196
26. c, p. 199
27. b, p. 197
28. d, p. 196
29. t, p. 195
30. f, p. 195
31. t, p. 197
32. t, p. 196
33. t, p. 196

Mechanisms of Disease

34. f, p. 199
35. c, p. 199
36. a, p. 200
37. b, p. 200
38. g, p. 200
39. h, p. 200
40. d, p. 200
41. e, p. 200
42. Fever or febrile, p. 201
43. Heat exhaustion, p. 201
44. Heat stroke, p. 201
45. frostbite, p. 202

Burns

46. a, p. 202
47. b, p. 202
48. f, p. 202
49. t, p. 202
50. c, p. 202
51. a, p. 202
52. d, p. 202
53. b, p. 202
54. e, p. 202

Applying What You Know

55. 46, p. 202
56. fingerprints, p. 181
57. It is theorized that adults who had more than two blistering sunburns before the age of 20 have a greater risk of developing melanoma than someone who experienced no burns. Bernie's exposure may have been during his youth or adolescence.

One Last Quick Check

58. a, p. 186
59. d, p. 198
60. b, p. 182
61. d, p. 202
62. b, p. 199
63. c, p. 200 and A & P Connect
64. c, p. 194
65. b, p. 199
66. a, p. 186
67. a, p. 191
68. c, p. 188
69. b, p. 187
70. e, p. 196
71. f, p. 195
72. g, p. 196
73. a, p. 181
74. d, p. 197
75. h, p. 197
76. i, p. 199
77. j, p. 200

Labeling

Skin

1. epidermis
2. dermis
3. hypodermis
4. blood vessels
5. lamellar (Pacini) corpuscle
6. sweat gland
7. subcutaneous adipose tissue
8. reticular layer of dermis
9. papillary layer of dermis
10. arrector pili muscle
11. root of hair
12. hair follicle
13. sebaceous gland
14. sweat gland
15. sweat duct
16. dermal papillae
17. shaft of hair
18. opening of sweat duct
19. sulcus
20. ridges of dermal papillae
21. nerve fibers
22. sweat duct
23. friction ridge
24. sulcus
25. dermoepidermal junction

Rule of Nines

1. 4.5%
2. 4.5%
3. 18%
4. 4.5%
5. 1%
6. 9%
7. 9%
8. 4.5%
9. 4.5%
10. 18%
11. 4.5%

12. 9%
13. 9%

CHAPTER 11
Skeletal Tissues
Types of Bones
1. f, p. 212
2. k, p. 211
3. h, p. 211
4. e, p. 211
5. d, p. 212
6. i, p. 211
7. j, p. 212
8. c, p. 211
9. a, p. 211
10. b, p. 212
11. g, p. 211

Bone Tissue Structure, Bone Marrow, and Regulation of Blood Calcium Levels
12. d, p. 213
13. b, p. 213
14. c, p. 213
15. b, p. 216
16. b, p. 217
17. c, p. 218
18. t, p. 213
19. f, p. 216
20. t, p. 216
21. t, p. 218
22. f, p. 210
23. f, p. 217

Bone Development, Remodeling, and Repair
24. b, p. 220
25. d, p. 220
26. a, p. 220
27. b, p. 223
28. b, p. 224
29. t, p. 220
30. f, p. 219
31. f, p. 217
32. t, p. 224
33. t, p. 221

Cartilage
34. b, p. 225
35. c, p. 225
36. b, p. 227
37. f, p. 225
38. t, p. 226
39. t, p. 226

Mechanisms of Disease
40. Chondrosarcoma, p. 227
41. Osteosarcoma, p. 227
42. Osteoporosis, p. 227
43. Paget's disease, p. 228
44. Osteomyelitis, p. 228

Applying What You Know
45. (a) Osteoporosis (b) DXA—dual energy x-ray absorptiometry scan or bone density (RA) imagery of the wrist (c) hormonal therapy (HRT), bone-building nonhormonal drugs such as Fosamax or Miacalcin, vitamin (D) and mineral (calcium) therapy, and weight-bearing exercises.
46. The bones are responsible for the majority of our blood cell formation. Her disease condition might be inhibiting the production of blood cells.
47. Epiphyseal cartilage is present only while a child is still growing. It becomes bone in adulthood. It is particularly vulnerable to fractures in childhood and preadolescence.

One Last Quick Check
48. support, protection, movement, mineral storage, and hematopoiesis, p. 210
49. medullary cavity, p. 212
50. articular cartilage, p. 212
51. endosteum, p. 212
52. Hematopoiesis, p. 210.
53. red bone marrow, p. 210
54. periosteum, p. 212
55. long, short, flat, irregular, and sesamoid, p. 210
56. calcium, p. 210
57. Hyaline, p. 225
58. d, p. 213
59. b, p. 211
60. e, p. 211
61. a, p. 212
62. c, p. 225
63. i, p. 216
64. f, p. 213
65. j, p. 213
66. g, p. 225
67. h, p. 213

Labeling
Long Bone
1. epiphysis
2. diaphysis
3. epiphysis
4. periosteum
5. yellow marrow
6. endosteum
7. medullary cavity
8. compact bone
9. red marrow cavities
10. epiphyseal line
11. spongy bone
12. articular cartilage

Cross-Section of Cancellous and Compact Bone
1. osteons (haversian systems)
2. periosteum (inner layer)
3. periosteum (outer layer)
4. trabeculae
5. compact bone
6. cancellous (spongy) bone
7. medullary (marrow) cavity

8. transverse (Volkmann) canals
9. central (haversian) canals
10. endosteum

CHAPTER 12

Axial Skeleton

Divisions of the Skeleton

1. a, p. 255
2. a, p. 234
3. b, p. 234
4. a, p. 255
5. b, p. 234
6. b, p. 234
7. a, p. 234
8. b, p. 234
9. a, p. 236
10. b, p. 234

The Skull

11. c, p. 248
12. d, p. 248
13. a, p. 249
14. c, p. 236
15. a, p. 249
16. b, p. 250
17. f, p. 236
18. t, p. 252
19. t, p. 250
20. f, p. 253
21. t, p. 242
22. d, p. 248
23. b, p. 246
24. b, p. 250
25. c, p. 250
26. d, p. 248

Vertebral Column

27. c, p. 254
28. d, p. 258
29. b, p. 255
30. a, p. 258
31. c, p. 254

Sternum and Ribs

32. e, p. 258
33. c, p. 258
34. a, p. 258
35. d, p. 258
36. f, p. 258
37. b, p. 258
38. g, p. 258

Mechanisms of Disease

39. b, p. 260
40. d, p. 260
41. b, pp. 248 and 260
42. c, p. 260
43. f, p. 260
44. t, p. 260

Applying What You Know

45. Sinuses are normally filled with air to give a light sensation to our skull. When filled with mucus, the head begins to feel heavy and the pressure of the once-empty spaces causes pain.
46. If the cribriform plate is damaged as a result of trauma to the nose, it is possible for potentially infectious material to pass directly from the nasal cavity into the cranial fossa. If fragments of a fractured nasal bone are pushed through the cribriform plate, they may tear the coverings of the brain or enter the substance of the brain itself.

One Last Quick Check

47. coxal (All others refer to the spine)
48. maxilla (All others refer to the cranial bones)
49. vomer (All others refer to the ossicles or bones of the middle ear)
50. ulna (All others refer to the coxal bone)
51. nasal (All others refer to cranial bones)
52. anvil (All others refer to the cervical vertebra)
53. c, p. 243
54. g, p. 258
55. a, p. 242
56. b, d, p. 244
57. f, p. 245
58. h, p. 243
59. i, e, p. 248
60. vertebral foramen, p. 255
61. manubrium, p. 258
62. occipital, p. 249
63. sphenoid, p. 244
64. t, p. 236
65. f, p. 248
66. t, p. 251

Labeling

Anterior View of Skull

1. glabella
2. ethmoid bone
3. sphenoid bone
4. nasal bone
5. vomer
6. mental foramen of mandible
7. mandible
8. maxilla
9. perpendicular plate of ethmoid bone
10. optic foramen of sphenoid bone
11. parietal bone
12. frontal bone

Floor of Cranial Cavity

1. crista galli
2. cribriform plate
3. superior orbital fissure
4. optic foramen
5. foramen ovale
6. foramen lacerum
7. foramen spinosum
8. internal acoustic meatus
9. jugular foramen
10. foramen magnum

11. occipital bone
12. parietal bone
13. petrous portion of the temporal bone
14. temporal bone
15. sella turcica
16. greater wing
17. lesser wing
18. sphenoid bone
19. ethmoid bone
20. frontal bone

Skull Viewed from Below

1. incisive foramen
2. zygomatic process of maxilla
3. zygomatic arch
4. temporal bone
5. styloid process
6. foramen ovale
7. carotid canal
8. mastoid process
9. stylomastoid foramen
10. mastoid foramen
11. parietal bone
12. foramen magnum
13. occipital bone
14. occipital condyle
15. jugular foramen
16. foramen lacerum
17. vomer
18. lateral pterygoid plate of sphenoid
19. zygomatic process of temporal bone
20. medial pterygoid plate of sphenoid
21. temporal process of zygomatic bone
22. horizontal plate of palatine bone
23. palatine process of maxilla
24. hard palate

Skull Viewed from the Right Side

1. squamous suture
2. parietal bone
3. lambdoid suture
4. temporal bone
5. occipital bone
6. external acoustic meatus
7. condyloid process of mandible
8. mastoid process of temporal bone
9. styloid process
10. pterygoid process of sphenoid bone
11. coronoid process of mandible
12. mandible
13. mental foramen of mandible
14. maxilla
15. zygomatic bone
16. nasal bone
17. lacrimal bone
18. ethmoid bone
19. sphenoid bone
20. frontal bone
21. coronal suture

Bones of the Left Orbit

1. optic canal of sphenoid bone
2. superior orbital fissure of sphenoid bone

3. ethmoid bone
4. lacrimal bone
5. maxilla
6. inferior orbital fissure
7. infraorbital foramen
8. zygomatic bone
9. sphenoid bone
10. frontal bone
11. supraorbital foramen of the frontal bone
12. supraorbital margin of the frontal bone

The Vertebral Column

1. thoracic curvature
2. intervertebral foramina
3. sacral curvature
4. atlas
5. axis
6. cervical curvature
7. lumbar curvature
8. coccyx
9. sacrum
10. lumbar vertebrae
11. thoracic vertebrae
12. cervical vertebrae

Vertebrae Atlas

1. transverse process
2. transverse foramen
3. anterior arch
4. facet for dens of axis
5. vertebral foramen
6. superior articular facet for occipital condyle
7. posterior arch

Cervical Vertebra

1. spinous process
2. lamina
3. pedicle
4. transverse foramen
5. transverse process
6. superior articular facet
7. vertebral foramen

Lumbar Vertebra

1. spinous process
2. lamina
3. transverse process
4. pedicle
5. superior articular facet
6. vertebral foramen

Axis

1. spinous process
2. transverse process
3. transverse foramen
4. dens
5. superior articular facet
6. vertebral foramen

Thoracic Vertebra

1. spinous process
2. lamina
3. transverse process

4. pedicle
5. superior articular facet
6. inferior articular facet
7. vertebral foramen

Thoracic Cage

1. costosternal articulation
2. true ribs
3. false ribs
4. floating ribs
5. costal cartilage
6. xiphoid process
7. body
8. manubrium
9. sternum
10. clavicle

CHAPTER 13

Appendicular Skeleton

The Appendicular Skeleton/Upper Extremity

1. b, p. 265
2. d, p. 266
3. d, p. 265
4. a, p. 266
5. d, p. 269
6. b, p. 265
7. t, p. 266
8. f, pp. 266 and 269
9. t, p. 266
10. f, p. 269

The Appendicular Skeleton/Lower Extremity

11. b, p. 270
12. a, p. 272
13. a, p. 270
14. c, p. 275
15. b, p. 270
16. f, p. 270
17. f, p. 274
18. f, p. 275
19. f, p. 276
20. f, p. 272

Skeletal Differences in Men and Women

21. b, p. 277
22. a, p. 278
23. a, p. 278
24. a, p. 277
25. b, p. 278

Applying What You Know

26. Bill could have possibly injured his humerus and his ulna.
27. (a) High heels cause a forward thrust to the body, which forces an undue amount of weight on the heads of the metatarsals. (b) Metatarsals, tarsals, and phalanges.

One Last Quick Check

28. axial (All others refer to the appendicular skeleton)
29. ribs (All others refer to the shoulder girdle)
30. ethmoid (All others refer to the hand and wrist)
31. talus (All others refer to the upper extremities)

32. acetabulum (All others refer to a part of the femur)
33. a, d, h, j, p. 271
34. e, p. 272
35. c, p. 268
36. f, p. 272
37. g, p. 265
38. i, p. 272
39. carpal, p. 268
40. calcaneus, p. 276
41. talus, p. 276
42. patella, p. 272
43. tibia, p. 274
44. t, p. 279
45. f, p. 279
46. t, p. 265
47. f, p. 270
48. f, p. 279

Labeling

Scapula Anterior View

1. superior angle
2. superior border
3. coracoid process
4. acromion
5. supraglenoid tubercle
6. glenoid cavity
7. infraglenoid tubercle
8. lateral (axillary) border
9. inferior angle
10. medial (vertebral) border
11. costal surface

Posterior View

1. acromion
2. coracoid process
3. spine
4. superior border
5. medial angle
6. medial (vertebral) border
7. inferior angle
8. posterior (dorsal) surface
9. lateral (axillary) border
10. glenoid cavity

Lateral View

1. coracoid process
2. glenoid cavity
3. infraglenoid tubercle
4. lateral (axillary) border
5. inferior angle

Bones of the Arm Anterior View

1. greater tubercle
2. lesser tubercle
3. intertubercular groove
4. deltoid tuberosity
5. humerus
6. lateral epicondyle
7. capitulum
8. trochlea
9. medial epicondyle
10. coronoid fossa
11. head

12. trochlear notch
13. head of radius
14. radial tuberosity
15. radius
16. styloid process of radius
17. styloid process of ulna
18. ulna
19. coronoid process
20. olecranon process

Posterior View

1. head
2. anatomical neck
3. surgical neck
4. humerus
5. olecranon fossa
6. medial epicondyle
7. trochlea
8. lateral epicondyle
9. greater tubercle
10. coronoid process
11. ulna
12. styloid process of ulna
13. styloid process of radius
14. radius
15. radial tuberosity
16. neck
17. head of radius
18. olecranon process

Bones of the Hand and Wrist

1. trapezoid
2. trapezium
3. scaphoid
4. radius
5. ulna
6. lunate
7. triquetrum
8. capitate
9. pisiform
10. hamate
11. distal phalanx
12. middle phalanx
13. proximal phalanx
14. metacarpal bone
15. hamate
16. capitate
17. pisiform
18. triquetrum
19. lunate
20. ulna
21. radius
22. scaphoid
23. trapezium
24. trapezoid

Coxal Bone

1. ilium
2. anterior superior iliac spine
3. anterior inferior iliac spine
4. margin of acetabulum
5. acetabulum
6. obturator foramen
7. pubis
8. ischial tuberosity
9. ischium
10. ischial spine
11. posterior inferior iliac spine
12. posterior superior iliac spine
13. iliac crest

Bones of the Thigh and Leg

1. greater trochanter
2. lateral epicondyle
3. medial epicondyle
4. femur
5. lesser trochanter
6. intertrochanteric line
7. neck
8. head
9. lateral condyle
10. head of fibula
11. fibula
12. lateral malleolus
13. medial malleolus
14. tibia
15. crest
16. tibial tuberosity
17. medial condyle
18. intercondylar eminence

Foot

1. phalanges
2. metatarsal bones
3. tarsal bones
4. cuneiform bones
5. navicular bone
6. talus
7. calcaneus
8. cuboid

CHAPTER 14

Articulations

Classification of Joints

1. b, p. 284
2. a, p. 284
3. a, p. 284
4. c, p. 286
5. c, p. 286
6. d, p. 286
7. c, p. 288
8. d, p. 287
9. t, p. 286
10. f, p. 287
11. t, p. 288
12. t, p. 284
13. f, p. 286
14. f, p. 284
15. f, p. 287
16. t, p. 289
17. a, p. 286
18. a, p. 285

19. b, p. 289
20. c, p. 284
21. c, p. 284
22. a, p. 284
23. b, p. 288
24. c, p. 284
25. b, p. 286
26. b, p. 286
27. a, p. 284
28. b, p. 286
29. d, p. 287
30. c, p. 289
31. b, p. 288
32. e, p. 287
33. d, p. 287
34. c, pp. 288 and 289
35. a, p. 289
36. a, p. 289
37. f, p. 288

Representative Synovial Joints

38. c, p. 289
39. b, p. 293
40. b, p. 293
41. a, p. 294
42. d, p. 298
43. c, p. 298
44. b, p. 294
45. c, p. 306

Movement at Synovial Joints

46. e, p. 298
47. c, p. 299
48. f, p. 299
49. g, p. 299
50. b, p. 299
51. d, p. 299
52. a, p. 299
53. h, p. 299
54. i, p. 299
55. j, p. 299

Mechanisms of Disease

56. Arthroscopy, p. 307
57. osteoarthritis or degenerative joint disease, p. 306
58. arthritis, p. 308
59. gouty arthritis, p. 308
60. sprain, p. 307

Applying What You Know

61. (a) Nodular swelling, joint pain, tenderness, aching, stiffness, and limited motion. Systemic symptoms may also include fever, anemia, weight loss, profound fatigue, and possible pericarditis. (b) Small joints of the hand, wrist, and feet progressing often to the larger joints.
62. (a) Gouty arthritis. (b) Swelling, tenderness, and pain, typically in the joints of the fingers, wrists, elbows, ankles, and knees. (c) Allopurinol (Zyloprim) is the drug of choice to treat this disease.

One Last Quick Check

63. diarthroses, p. 284
64. synarthrotic, p. 284

65. diarthrotic, p. 287
66. ligaments, p. 287
67. articular cartilage, p. 287
68. least movable, p. 289
69. largest, p. 293
70. two, p. 287
71. mobility, p. 288
72. pivot, p. 299
73. t, p. 287
74. f, p. 285
75. f, p. 306
76. t, p. 290
77. t, p. 299
78. t, p. 299
79. f, p. 299
80. f, p. 299
81. f, p. 308
82. t, p. 294

Labeling

Synovial Joint

1. bone
2. periosteum
3. blood vessel
4. nerve
5. articular cartilage
6. joint cavity
7. joint capsule
8. articular cartilage
9. synovial membrane

Shoulder Joint

1. coracoid process of scapula
2. glenoid cavity
3. superior transverse ligament of scapula
4. articular cartilage of glenoid cavity
5. scapula
6. glenoidal lip (labrum)
7. humerus
8. head of humerus
9. articular cartilage of humerus
10. bursa
11. tendon of long head of biceps brachii muscle
12. synovial cavity

Hip Joint

1. acetabular labrum
2. head
3. articular capsule
4. greater trochanter
5. femur
6. lesser trochanter
7. articular capsule
8. transverse acetabular ligament
9. ligamentum teres
10. articular cavity
11. ilium

Knee Joint Anterior View

1. lateral condyle of femur
2. lateral meniscus
3. fibular collateral (lateral) ligament

4. transverse ligament of knee
5. fibula
6. tibia
7. tibial tuberosity
8. tibial collateral (medial) ligament
9. medial meniscus
10. anterior cruciate ligament (ACL)
11. medial condyle of femur
12. posterior cruciate ligament (PCL)
13. femur

Knee Joint Posterior View

1. femur
2. ligament of Wrisberg
3. medial condyle
4. medial meniscus
5. tibial collateral (medial) ligament
6. posterior cruciate ligament
7. tibia
8. fibula
9. fibular collateral (lateral) ligament
10. lateral meniscus
11. lateral condyle
12. anterior cruciate ligament

Vertebrae

1. lamina
2. anterior longitudinal ligament
3. body of vertebra
4. intervertebral disk
5. posterior longitudinal ligament
6. ligamentum flavum
7. intervertebral foramen
8. supraspinous ligament
9. interspinous ligament
10. spinous process

CHAPTER 15
Axial Muscle
Skeletal Muscle Structure

1. c, p. 314
2. d, p. 317
3. a, p. 314
4. a, p. 318
5. d, p. 318
6. a, p. 319
7. f, p. 317
8. t, p. 318
9. t, p. 318
10. f, p. 319
11. t, p. 319

How Muscles Are Named

12. c, p. 322
13. a, p. 321
14. f, p. 322
15. e, p. 322
16. g, p. 322
17. b, p. 321
18. d, p. 322

Important Skeletal Muscles: Muscles of the Head and Neck

19. b, p. 325
20. e, p. 325
21. a, p. 325
22. c, p. 324
23. f, p. 326
24. d, p. 325

Trunk Muscles

25. t, p. 329
26. t, p. 329
27. f, p. 332
28. t, p. 327
29. t, p. 332
30. t, p. 328

Applying What You Know

31. External intercostals, internal intercostals, diaphragm, and rectus abdominis
32. (1) Optimum angle of pull (2) Flexed at the elbow

One Last Quick Check

33. b, p. 326
34. c, p. 327
35. d, p. 327
36. a, p. 326
37. e, p. 329
38. j, p. 329
39. g, p. 329
40. f, p. 332
41. h, p. 332
42. i, p. 324
43. perimysium, p. 314
44. Convergent, p. 317
45. agonist, p. 318
46. belly, p. 318
47. pull (P), p. 318
48. inspiration, p. 327
49. perineum, p. 332
50. lever, p. 318
51. shape, p. 322
52. masseter and temporalis, p. 325

Labeling
Facial Muscles Lateral View

1. epicranial aponeurosis
2. temporalis
3. occipitofrontalis (occipital portion)
4. masseter
5. sternocleidomastoid
6. depressor anguli oris
7. orbicularis oris
8. buccinators
9. zygomaticus major
10. orbicularis oculi
11. corrugator supercilii
12. occipitofrontalis (frontal portion)

Muscles of the Thorax

1. external intercostals
2. diaphragm

3. central tendon of diaphragm
4. internal intercostals

Muscles of the Trunk and Abdominal Wall

1. linea alba
2. rectus abdominis
3. external oblique
4. internal ligament
5. internal oblique
6. transverse abdominis
7. rectus abdominis

CHAPTER 16

Appendicular Muscles

Upper Limb Muscles

1. a, p. 342
2. c, p. 338
3. a, p. 343
4. d, p. 343
5. f, p. 345
6. t, p. 347
7. t, p. 341
8. t, p. 340
9. f, p. 343

Lower Limb Muscles

10. d, p. 355
11. a, p. 355
12. c, p. 353
13. d, p. 356
14. a, p. 355
15. t, p. 356
16. f, p. 349
17. f, p. 355

Applying What You Know

18. (a) Carpal tunnel syndrome. (b) The wrist, hand, and fingers are affected due to tenosynovitis. Pain may radiate to the forearm and shoulder. (c) Injections of antiinflammatory agents or surgical removal of tissue pressing on median nerve.
19. deltoid area
20. Review the list of Tables (16-1, 16-2, 16-3, 16-4, 16-5, 16-6, 16-7) provided in the chapter that show the muscles involved with the shoulders, elbows, wrists and hips, knees and ankles.

One Last Quick Check

21. b, p. 339
22. e, p. 339
23. a, b, p. 356
24. a, p. 343
25. c, e, p. 349
26. f, p. 356
27. a, p. 349
28. a, d, p. 340
29. b, e, p. 349
30. b, p. 343
31. c, a, b, p. 340
32. b, p. 356
33. a, d, p. 349

34. extrinsic foot muscles, p. 356
35. Achilles, p. 356
36. supraspinatus, p. 341
37. infraspinatus, p. 341
38. teres minor, p. 341
39. subscapularis, p. 341
40. deltoid, p. 353

Labeling

Muscles Acting on the Shoulder Girdle

1. trapezius
2. seventh cervical vertebra
3. rhomboid major
4. rhomboid minor
5. levator scapulae
6. pectoralis minor (cut)
7. subscapularis
8. latissimus dorsi
9. serratus anterior
10. latissimus dorsi (cut)
11. pectoralis minor
12. teres major
13. teres minor
14. subscapularis

Rotator Cuff Muscles

1. clavicle
2. acromion process
3. infraspinatus
4. greater tubercle
5. teres minor
6. intertubercular (bicipital) groove
7. humerus
8. subscapularis
9. lesser tubercle
10. supraspinatus
11. coracoid process

Muscles That Move the Upper Arm

1. deltoid (cut)
2. coracobrachialis
3. pectoralis major
4. serratus anterior
5. deltoid
6. thoracolumbar fascia
7. latissimus dorsi
8. teres major
9. infraspinatus
10. rhomboideus major
11. teres minor
12. rhomboideus minor
13. supraspinatus
14. levator scapulae

Muscles of the Upper Arm

1. triceps brachii
2. brachioradialis
3. brachialis
4. biceps brachii (long head)
5. pectoralis major
6. deltoid
7. clavicle

8. biceps brachii
9. radius
10. pronator teres
11. ulna
12. brachialis
13. triceps brachii
14. teres major
15. coracobrachialis

Muscles That Act on the Forearm

1. coracoid process
2. supraglenoid tuberosity
3. biceps brachii (long head)
4. biceps brachii (short head)
5. radial tuberosity
6. olecranon process of ulna
7. triceps brachii (medial head)
8. triceps brachii: lateral (short head)
9. triceps brachii (long head)
10. posterior surface of humerus; lateral intermuscular septum
11. infraglenoid tubercle
12. coracoid process
13. coracobrachialis
14. medial surface of humerus
15. medial epicondyle of humerus
16. pronator teres
17. lateral surface of radius
18. coronoid process of ulna
19. brachialis
20. humerus (distal half)

Muscles of the Forearm

1. pronator teres
2. palmaris longus
3. flexor policis brevis (superficial)
4. opponens policis (deep)
5. flexor digiti minimi
6. abductor digiti minimi
7. flexor carpi ulnaris
8. flexor carpi radialis
9. palmar interosseus
10. pronator quadratus
11. flexor digitorum profundus
12. supinator
13. brachioradialis
14. flexor digitorum superficialis
15. extensor carpi ulnaris (cut)
16. extensor pollicis brevis
17. extensor pollicis longus
18. abductor pollicis longus
19. extensor carpi radialis brevis
20. extensor carpi radialis longus
21. supinator (deep)

Muscles of the Thigh

1. tensor fasciae latae
2. iliotibial tract
3. vastus lateralis
4. vastus medialis
5. rectus femoris
6. sartorius
7. gracilis

8. iliopsoas
9. adductor brevis
10. adductor longus
11. adductor magnus
12. fibula
13. tibia
14. pectineus

Muscles of the Lower Leg

1. soleus
2. extensor digitorum longus
3. fibularis peroneous brevis
4. tibialis anterior
5. tibia
6. gastrocncmius
7. calcaneal tendon (Achilles tendon)
8. calcaneus

CHAPTER 17

Muscle Contraction

Function of Skeletal Muscle Tissue

1. b, p. 362
2. a, p. 362
3. a, p. 364
4. d, p. 362
5. c, p. 366
6. a, p. 364
7. c, p. 362
8. a, p. 366
9. c, p. 368
10. b, p. 366
11. t, p. 366
12. f, p. 362
13. f, p. 364
14. t, p. 366
15. t, p. 364
16. t, p. 371
17. f, p. 362
18. f, p. 373
19. t, p. 371
20. t, p. 371

Function of Skeletal Muscle Organs

21. d, p. 374
22. d, p. 375
23. a, p. 374
24. d, p. 380
25. a, p. 377
26. c, p. 378
27. c, p. 378
28. f, p. 375
29. t, p. 379
30. t, p. 374
31. f, p. 377

Function of Cardiac and Smooth Muscle Tissue

32. c, p. 381
33. b, p. 381
34. b, p. 381
35. c, p. 381
36. a, p. 381

37. c, p. 381
38. a, p. 381
39. b, p. 381
40. a, p. 381
41. c, p. 381

Mechanisms of Disease

42. myalgia, p. 384
43. myoglobin, p. 385
44. poliomyelitis, p. 385
45. muscular dystrophy, p. 385
46. myasthenia gravis, p. 385

Applying What You Know

47. Linda may have more slow and intermediate fibers than fast fibers. The former are conducive to long races rather than short ones.
48. Muscles in a dead body may be stiff because individual muscle fibers have run out of the ATP required to "turn off" a muscle contraction.

One Last Quick Check

49. a, p. 380
50. b, p. 380
51. b, p. 378
52. d, p. 369
53. a, p. 381
54. d, p. 375
55. f, p. 370
56. t, p. 374
57. t, p. 375
58. t, p. 375
59. t, p. 385
60. t, p. 382
61. t, p. 381
62. t, p. 378
63. f, p. 384

Labeling

Structure of Skeletal Muscle

1. tendon
2. bone
3. muscle fiber (muscle cell)
4. sarcoplasmic reticulum
5. Z disk
6. thin filament
7. thick filament
8. sarcomere
9. myofibril
10. T tubule
11. fascicle
12. endomysium
13. perimysium
14. epimysium
15. muscle
16. fascia

Neuromuscular Junction and Skeletal Muscle Cell

1. motor neuron fiber
2. Schwann cell
3. sarcoplasm
4. acetylcholine (Ach) receptor sites
5. synaptic cleft
6. motor endplate
7. synaptic vesicles (containing Ach)
8. myelin sheath
9. sarcomere
10. sarcolemma
11. mitochondria
12. T tubule
13. sarcoplasmic reticulum
14. triad
15. myofibril

Motor Unit

1. myelin sheath
2. Schwann cell
3. neuromuscular junction
4. nucleus
5. muscle fibers
6. myofibrils
7. motor neuron

Cardiac Muscle Fiber

1. intercalated disks
2. sarcomere
3. sarcolemma
4. myofibril
5. mitochondrion
6. sarcoplasmic reticulum
7. T tubule
8. diad
9. nucleus

CHAPTER 18

Nervous System Cells

Organization of the Nervous System

1. c, p. 393
2. f, p. 394
3. a, p. 394
4. h, p. 395
5. g, p. 394
6. b, p. 395
7. d, p. 394
8. e, p. 395

Glia, Neurons, and Reflex Arc

9. b, p. 396
10. a, p. 396
11. d, p. 398
12. a, p. 395
13. c, p. 397
14. d, p. 398
15. a, p. 395
16. c, p. 398
17. c, p. 399
18. b, p. 399
19. a, p. 401
20. c, p. 402
21. d, p. 402

Nerves and Tracts

22. c, p. 404
23. b, p. 404

24. b, p. 404
25. d, p. 404
26. c, p. 404

Repair of Nerve Fibers

27. t, p. 404
28. t, p. 404
29. f, p. 406

Mechanisms of Disease

30. Multiple sclerosis, p. 407
31. Glioma, p. 407
32. glioblastoma multiforme, p. 407
33. neurofibromatosis, p. 407
34. glia, p. 407

Applying What You Know

35. (a) Multiple sclerosis. (b) CNS. (c) Myelin loss and demyelination of the white matter in the CNS. (d) No known cure. (e) Cause is thought to be related to autoimmunity and viral infections.
36. CNS damage is most often permanent. Because the damage is suspected to involve the spinal cord—which is part of the CNS—the prognosis for repair is not good.

One Last Quick Check

37. skeletal, p. 394
38. afferent, p. 394
39. parasympathetic, p. 395
40. oligodendrocytes, p. 397
41. Schwann cells, p. 397
42. nodes of Ranvier, p. 398
43. mitochondria, p. 399
44. white, p. 398
45. interneurons, p. 402
46. do not, p. 403
47. a, p. 399
48. b, p. 395
49. b, p. 395
50. a, p. 402
51. a, p. 401
52. b, p. 397
53. b, p. 396
54. a, p. 401
55. b, p. 398
56. a, p. 400

Labeling

Typical Neuron

1. telodendria
2. synaptic knobs
3. node of Ranvier
4. axon collateral
5. myelin sheath
6. Schwann cell
7. axon
8. axon hillock
9. nucleus
10. cell body (soma)
11. mitochondrion
12. Golgi apparatus
13. dendrite

Myelinated Axon

1. node of Ranvier
2. neurilemma (sheath of Schwann cell)
3. neurofibrils, microfilaments, and microtubules
4. plasma membrane of axon
5. myelin sheath
6. nucleus of Schwann cell

Classification of Neurons

1. multipolar neuron
2. bipolar neuron
3. (pseudo) unipolar neuron

Reflex Arc

1. gray matter
2. interneuron
3. sensory neuron axon
4. cell body
5. spinal nerve
6. motor neuron axon
7. white matter
8. dendrite
9. synapse

CHAPTER 19
Nerve Signaling
Electrical Nature of Neurons

1. a, p. 413
2. b, p. 413
3. b, p. 413
4. a, p. 414
5. t, p. 413
6. f, p. 414
7. f, p. 414

Action Potential

8. b, p. 417
9. b, p. 415
10. c, p. 418
11. b, p. 418
12. t, p. 415
13. f, p. 417
14. t, p. 418
15. t, p. 419

Synaptic Transmission

16. c, p. 419
17. b, p. 419
18. a, p. 422
19. f, p. 419
20. t, p. 423
21. t, p. 421

Neurotransmitters

22. d, p. 424
23. b, p. 425
24. c, p. 425
25. c, p. 428
26. d, p. 425
27. f, p. 428
28. t, p. 428

Neural Networks

29. reticular theory, p. 429
30. health, p. 429
31. neurotrophins, p. 429
32. convergence, p. 430
33. divergence, p. 430

Mechanisms of Disease

34. t, p. 431
35. t, p. 431
36. f, p. 431
37. f, p. 431
38. t, p. 431

Applying What You Know

39. Marcaine, procaine, and similar drugs produce anesthesia by inhibiting the opening of the sodium channels and thus blocking the initiation and conduction of nerve impulses.
40. Cocaine, which is often used in medical practice as a local anesthetic, produces a temporary feeling of well-being in cocaine abusers by similarly blocking the uptake of dopamine. Unfortunately, cocaine and similar drugs can also adversely affect blood flow and heart function when taken in large amounts—leading to death in some individuals.

One Last Quick Check

41. presynaptic, p. 420
42. neurotransmitter, p. 425
43. communicate, p. 424
44. specifically, p. 424
45. pain, p. 429
46. nerve impulse, p. 415
47. saltatory conduction, p. 418
48. polarized, p. 413
49. nerve impulse, p. 413
50. resting membrane potential, p. 413
51. hyperpolarization, p. 315
52. a synaptic knob, p. 419
53. a synaptic cleft, p. 419
54. the plasma membrane of a postsynaptic neuron, p. 419
55. structural, p. 424
56. acetylcholinesterase, p. 425
57. dopamine, epinephrine, or norepinephrine, p. 425
58. inhibitory neurotransmitters, p. 424
59. t, p. 424
60. t, p. 429

Labeling

Chemical Synapse

1. motor neuron cell body
2. axon of presynaptic neuron
3. axon of motor neuron
4. synaptic knobs
5. action potential
6. voltage-gated Ca^{++} channels
7. synaptic cleft
8. stimulus-gated Na^+ channels
9. neurotransmitters
10. synaptic knob
11. voltage-gated Na^+ channels
12. voltage-gated K^+ channels

CHAPTER 20
Central Nervous System

Coverings of the Brain and Spinal Cord

1. a, p. 437
2. c, p. 437
3. b, p. 439
4. c, p. 437

Cerebrospinal Fluid

5. c, p. 439
6. a, p. 439
7. d, p. 440
8. d, p. 439
9. t, p. 439
10. f, p. 440

The Spinal Cord

11. b, p. 444
12. d, p. 444
13. a, p. 444
14. c, p. 444
15. b, p. 444
16. d, p. 444
17. c, p. 444
18. a, p. 444
19. e, p. 444

The Brain

20. b, p. 445
21. d, p. 447
22. a, p. 449
23. b, p. 453
24. d, p. 454
25. c, p. 454
26. b, p. 460
27. a, p. 456
28. b, p. 461
29. a, p. 459
30. t, p. 449
31. f, p. 460
32. f, p. 449
33. t, p. 454
34. t, p. 456

Somatic Sensory and Motor Pathways

35. c, p. 465
36. c, p. 466
37. a, p. 468
38. t, p. 466
39. f, p. 467

Mechanisms of Disease

40. d, p. 470
41. b, p. 469
42. a, p. 469
43. c, p. 470

Applying What You Know

44. hydrocephalus
45. (a) dementia (b) Alzheimer disease

One Last Quick Check

46. e, p. 446
47. d, p. 447
48. a, p. 452
49. d, p. 453
50. e, p. 460
51. b, p. 457
52. c, p. 457
53. d, p. 451
54. c, p. 454
55. d, p. 443
56. d, p. 453

Labeling

Coverings of the Brain

1. superior sagittal sinus (of dura)
2. periosteum
3. subdural space
4. skull
5. falx cerebri
6. pia mater
7. muscle
8. skin
9. subarachnoid space
10. arachnoid mater
11. dura mater
12. periosteum
13. one functional layer

Fluid Spaces of the Brain

1. cerebral hemisphere
2. anterior horn of lateral ventricle
3. interventricular foramen
4. third ventricle
5. inferior horn of lateral ventricle
6. fourth ventricle
7. pons
8. central canal of spinal cord
9. cerebellum
10. cerebral aqueduct
11. posterior horn of lateral ventricle

Flow of Cerebrospinal Fluid and the Layers of the Brain

1. arachnoid villus
2. choroid plexus of lateral ventricle
3. superior sagittal sinus
4. interventricular foramen
5. choroid plexus of third ventricle
6. cerebral aqueduct
7. choroid plexus of fourth ventricle
8. median foramen
9. central canal of spinal cord
10. dura mater
11. cisterna magna
12. lateral foramen
13. cerebral cortex
14. subarachnoid space
15. arachnoid layer
16. falx cerebri (dura mater)
17. pia mater

Spinal Cord

1. cervical enlargement
2. lumbar enlargement
3. end of spinal cord
4. cauda equina
5. filum terminale
6. lateral column
7. posterior column
8. anterior column
9. gray commissure
10. gray matter
11. posterior median sulcus
12. central canal
13. dorsal (posterior) nerve root
14. dorsal root ganglion
15. spinal nerve
16. ventral (anterior) nerve root
17. lateral column
18. posterior column
19. anterior column
20. white columns (funiculi)
21. anterior median fissure

Spinal Cord Tracts

1. tectospinal
2. vestibulospinal
3. reticulospinal
4. anterior corticospinal
5. rubrospinal
6. lateral corticospinal
7. fasciculus gracilis
8. fasciculus cuneatus
9. posterior spinocerebellar
10. lateral spinothalamic
11. anterior spinocerebellar
12. spinotectal
13. anterior spinothalamic

Left Hemisphere of Cerebrum

1. central sulcus
2. superior frontal gyrus
3. frontal lobe
4. lateral fissure
5. temporal lobe
6. occipital lobe
7. parietooccipital sulcus
8. parietal lobe
9. postcentral gyrus

Cerebral Cortex

1. precentral gyrus
2. premotor area
3. prefrontal area
4. motor speech (Broca) area
5. transverse gyrus
6. auditory association area
7. primary auditory area
8. sensory speech (Wernicke) area
9. visual cortex
10. visual association area

11. somatic sensory association area
12. primary taste area
13. postcentral gyrus

CHAPTER 21
Peripheral Nervous System
Spinal Nerves

1. a, p. 480
2. c, p. 481
3. a, pp. 481-482
4. b, p. 483
5. a, p. 486
6. t, p. 481
7. t, p. 480
8. f, p. 488
9. f, p. 489
10. t, p. 485

Cranial Nerves

11. g, p. 490
12. a, p. 490
13. j, p. 493
14. h, p. 493
15. b, p. 490
16. e, p. 490
17. i, p. 493
18. c, p. 490
19. d, p. 490
20. f, p. 490
21. l, p. 493
22. k, p. 493

Somatic Motor Nervous System

23. b, p. 495
24. a, p. 497
25. a, p. 495

Applying What You Know

26. The two nerves that might possibly be involved are cranial nerve IX (glossopharyngeal) and cranial nerve X (vagus). Both nerves are mixed, meaning that they contain axons of sensory and motor neurons.
27. (a) Herpes zoster, or shingles. (b) Varicella zoster virus, or chickenpox. (c) It attacks a dermatome (T-4) and symptoms occur in that region. (d) His immunologic protective mechanism may have become diminished due to the stress.

One Last Quick Check

28. a, p. 489
29. d, p. 494
30. a, p. 494
31. c, p. 490
32. vestibulocochlear, p. 493
33. trigeminal, p. 492
34. diabetes mellitus, p. 480
35. voluntary, p. 495
36. skeletal, p. 495
37. phrenic and phrenic, p. 485
38. a, p. 480
39. b, p. 487
40. a, p. 494

41. b, p. 488
42. b, p. 480
43. a, p. 489
44. b, p. 480
45. b, p. 482
46. b, p. 489
47. a, p. 494

Labeling
Spinal Nerves

1. cervical vertebrae
2. brachial plexus
3. thoracic vertebrae
4. lumbar vertebrae
5. sacrum
6. coccyx
7. filum terminale
8. coccygeal nerve
9. sacral nerves
10. sacral plexus
11. lumbar nerves
12. lumbar plexus
13. cauda equina
14. dura mater
15. thoracic nerves
16. cervical nerves
17. cervical plexus

Cranial Nerves

1. trochlear nerve
2. optic nerve
3. oculomotor nerve
4. abducens nerve
5. facial nerve
6. vestibulocochlear nerve
7. vagus nerve
8. accessory nerve
9. hypoglossal nerve
10. glossopharyngeal nerve
11. trigeminal nerve
12. olfactory nerve

Patellar Reflex

1. gray matter
2. spinal cord
3. motor neuron
4. quadriceps muscle (effector)
5. patellar tendon
6. patella
7. stretch receptor
8. sensory neuron
9. dorsal root ganglion

CHAPTER 22
Autonomic Nervous System
Structures of the Autonomic Nervous System

1. c, p. 505
2. d, p. 507
3. b, p. 509
4. a, p. 514

5. b, p. 515
6. t, p. 505
7. t, pp. 504-505
8. t, p. 506
9. f, p. 516
10. t, p. 507
11. autonomic nerves, ganglia, and plexuses, p. 505
12. Preganglionic, p. 505
13. collateral, p. 507
14. ramus, p. 507
15. norepinephrine, p. 509
16. short and then long, p. 507
17. adrenergic, p. 509
18. characteristics of the receptor, p. 509
19. nicotinic, p. 510
20. quickly, p. 511

Functions of the Autonomic Nervous System

21. t, p. 512
22. f, p. 512
23. t, p. 512
24. t. p. 515
25. f, p. 516

Applying What You Know

26. (1) Sympathetic (2a) Muscular—skeletal muscles faster (2b) Circulatory—stronger heartbeat, dilated blood vessels (2c) Respiratory—dilated bronchi (2d) Digestive—increased blood sugar levels (3) Dysfunction of the sympathetic effectors and perhaps even the ANS itself.
27. Biofeedback

One Last Quick Check

28. d, p. 504
29. e, p. 505
30. f, p. 505
31. b, p. 504
32. a, p. 504
33. c, p. 504
34. c, p. 505
35. b, p. 507
36. b, p. 507
37. d, p. 507
38. b, p. 514
39. a, p. 514
40. a, p. 514
41. b, p. 514
42. a, p. 514
43. b, p. 514
44. a, p. 514
45. a, p. 514
46. b, p. 514
47. b, p. 514

Labeling

Autonomic Conduction Path

1. axon of somatic motor neuron
2. collateral ganglion
3. postganglionic neuron's axon
4. sympathetic ganglion
5. axon of preganglionic sympathetic neuron

CHAPTER 23
Physiology of Sensation
Sensory Receptors

1. b, p. 520
2. d, p. 522
3. a, p. 526
4. b, p. 527
5. a, p. 526
6. f, p. 522
7. t, p. 522
8. f, p. 522
9. t, p. 527
10. t, p. 522

Sense of Pain

11. nociceptor, p. 523
12. somatic, p. 523
13. visceral, p. 523
14. neuropathy, p. 524
15. fibromyalgia, p. 525

Sense of Temperature, Touch, and Proprioception

16. d, p. 525
17. g, p. 525
18. e, pp. 527 and 528
19. j, p. 525
20. a, p. 526
21. c, p. 526
22. i, p. 526
23. b, p. 526
24. f, p. 523
25. h, p. 525

Applying What You Know

26. Brain tissue is unique and lacks the type of nociceptors that transmit sensation of pain. The brain is, therefore, incapable of sensing painful stimuli.
27. Thermoreceptors are cold or warm. They are also not spread uniformly across the skin. Doctors use this technique to determine the extent and degree of numbness or sensitivity.

One Last Quick Check

28. encapsulated nerve endings, p. 522
29. referred pain, p. 524
30. internal organs, p. 522
31. touch, temperature, and pain, p. 520
32. nociceptors, p. 522
33. Ruffini's, p. 526
34. proprioceptors, p. 522
35. Free nerve endings, p. 522
36. adaptation, p. 521
37. d, p. 522
38. c, p. 522
39. e, p. 522
40. f, p. 522
41. a, p. 522
42. b, p. 522
43. t, p. 521
44. f, p. 521

45. t, p. 521
46. f, p. 521
47. t, p. 526

CHAPTER 24

Sense Organs

The Sense of Smell and the Sense of Taste

1. b, p. 533
2. d, p. 533
3. c, p. 536
4. b, p. 536
5. t, p. 534
6. f, p. 533
7. t, p. 534
8. f, pp. 534-535

The Ear: Sense of Hearing and Balance

9. a, p. 537
10. c, p. 538
11. d, p. 538
12. d, p. 540
13. b, p. 540
14. b, p. 541
15. d, p. 540
16. t, p. 538
17. f, p. 537
18. t, p. 540
19. t, p. 540
20. f, p. 541

Vision: The Eye

21. c, p. 544
22. a, p. 544
23. a, p. 546
24. d, p. 546
25. d, p. 547
26. a, p. 544
27. c, p. 543
28. a, p. 548
29. c, p. 548
30. a, p. 544
31. f, p. 543
32. f, p. 544
33. t, p. 555
34. t, p. 544
35. f, p. 550
36. t, p. 550
37. t, p. 546
38. t, p. 548
39. f, p. 548
40. f, p. 550

Mechanisms of Disease

41. c, p. 553
42. a, p. 553
43. d, p. 553
44. e, p. 554
45. b, p. 553
46. f, p. 554
47. c, p. 554
48. e, p. 554

49. f, p. 555
50. a, p. 555
51. j, p. 554
52. b, p. 555
53. h, p. 554
54. g, p. 555
55. i, p. 555
56. d, p. 555

Applying What You Know

57. The eustachian tube connects the throat to the middle ear and provides a perfect pathway for the spread of infection.
58. (a) Legally blind (b) 20/200 (c) myopia (d) concave contact lenses or glasses

One Last Quick Check

59. a, p. 538
60. b, p. 539
61. a, p. 536
62. c, p. 542
63. b, p. 544
64. b, p. 535
65. d, p. 546
66. b, p. 545
67. d, p. 534
68. a, p. 537
69. t, p. 537
70. f, p. 555
71. t, p. 554
72. f, p. 541
73. t, p. 554
74. t, p. 545
75. t, p. 546
76. t, p. 533
77. t, p. 526 (review of previous chapter material)
78. t, p. 540

Labeling

Midsagittal Section of the Nasal Area

1. olfactory bulb
2. fibers of olfactory nerve
3. cribriform plate of ethmoid bone
4. olfactory tract
5. olfactory recess
6. nasopharynx
7. palate
8. nasal cavity
9. frontal bone

The Ear

1. malleus
2. incus
3. stapes
4. auditory ossicles
5. auditory tube
6. round window
7. vestibule
8. cochlea
9. cochlear nerve
10. vestibular nerve
11. vestibulocochlear (acoustic) nerve
12. facial nerve
13. oval window

14. semicircular canals
15. inner ear
16. tympanic membrane
17. middle ear
18. temporal bone
19. external acoustic meatus
20. auricle (pinna)
21. external ear

The Eye

1. pupil
2. lens
3. lacrimal caruncle
4. optic disk
5. optic nerve
6. central artery and vein
7. fovea centralis
8. macula
9. posterior cavity
10. sclera
11. choroid
12. retina
13. ciliary body
14. lower lid
15. iris
16. anterior chamber
17. cornea

Extrinsic Muscles of the Right Eye

1. superior oblique
2. medial rectus
3. superior rectus
4. optic nerve
5. levator palpebrae superioris (cut)
6. lateral rectus
7. inferior oblique
8. trochlea

Lacrimal Apparatus

1. lacrimal caruncle
2. lacrimal canals
3. lacrimal sac
4. nasolacrimal duct
5. puncta
6. lacrimal ducts
7. lacrimal gland

CHAPTER 25

Endocrine Regulation

The Endocrine System and Hormones

1. a, p. 562
2. c, p. 563
3. d, p. 564
4. c, p. 563
5. a, p. 564
6. d, p. 564
7. c, p. 564
8. a, p. 568
9. c, pp. 569 and 570
10. b, p. 567
11. t, p. 563
12. t, p. 564
13. f, p. 567
14. f, p. 574
15. t, p. 571
16. b, p. 570
17. a, p. 570
18. a, p. 570
19. a, p. 570
20. a, p. 570
21. b, p. 570
22. b, p. 570
23. b, pp. 569 and 570

Eicosanoids

24. b, p. 572
25. c, p. 573
26. Paracrine, p. 573
27. Autocrine, p. 573
28. seminal vesicles, p. 573
29. immunity, p. 574
30. peristalsis, p. 574

Applying What You Know

31. Prostaglandin F (PGF)
32. In the presence of an injury, prostaglandins may be synthesized and released into surrounding tissue fluid. They may serve as an inflammatory agent and may cause swelling, redness, and pain. Aspirin is a COX inhibitor that reduces the effect of prostaglandins in the body.

One Last Quick Check

33. endocrine reflexes, p. 570
34. kidneys, p. 567
35. antagonism, p. 567
36. endocytosis, p. 569
37. amount, p. 569
38. signal—transduction, p. 563
39. hyposecretion, p. 575
40. second messenger, p. 568
41. calcium, p. 569
42. pituitary, p. 570
43. d, p. 574
44. e, p. 574
45. a, p. 573
46. b, p. 572
47. c, p. 573
48. a, p. 563
49. c, p. 564
50. d, p. 564
51. b, p. 567
52. a, p. 567

Labeling

Endocrine Glands

1. pineal
2. parathyroids
3. testes (male)
4. ovaries (female)
5. pancreas (islets)
6. adrenals
7. thymus
8. thyroid

9. pituitary
10. hypothalamus

Target Cell Concept

1. target
2. receptors
3. nontarget cells
4. hormone
5. capillary

CHAPTER 26

Endocrine Glands

Pituitary Gland

1. b, p. 580
2. a, p. 583
3. d, p. 585
4. c, p. 582
5. b, p. 585
6. a, p. 583
7. d, p. 581
8. c, p. 583
9. e, p. 583
10. h, p. 582
11. g, p. 586
12. f, p. 582
13. i, p. 582
14. b, p. 586

Pineal, Thyroid, and Parathyroid Glands

15. b, p. 588
16. b, p. 588
17. b, p. 587
18. b, p. 591
19. c, p. 590
20. t, p. 589
21. f, p. 589
22. t, p. 590
23. t, p. 587
24. f, p. 587

Adrenal Glands

25. b, p. 594
26. d, p. 595
27. a, p. 593
28. t, p. 592
29. f, p. 595
30. t, p. 594

Pancreatic Islets

31. c, p. 596
32. a, p. 596
33. t, p. 596
34. f, p. 597
35. b, p. 596
36. c, p. 596
37. a, p. 596
38. d, p. 596

Gonads and Other Endocrine Glands and Tissues

39. a, p. 598
40. b, p. 598

41. c, p. 598
42. f, p. 598
43. f, p. 600
44. t, p. 599

Mechanisms of Disease

45. e, p. 601
46. h, p. 601
47. a, p. 601
48. c, p. 601
49. f, p. 602
50. g, p. 602
51. b, p. 602
52. d, p. 602

Applying What You Know

53. (a) hCG is high during early pregnancy (b) placenta (c) It forms on the lining of the uterus as an interface between the circulatory systems of the mother and the developing child. It is a temporary endocrine gland.
54. (a) diabetes mellitus (b) inadequate amount or abnormal type of insulin (c) insulin

One Last Quick Check

55. a, p. 592
56. c, p. 586
57. d, p. 590
58. c, p. 582
59. d, p. 580
60. d, pp. 585 and 586
61. b, p. 598
62. d, p. 595
63. d, p. 595
64. b, p. 594
65. j, p. 602
66. g, p. 587
67. h, p. 602
68. i, p. 587
69. b, p. 601
70. f, p. 599
71. a, p. 601
72. d, p. 587
73. e, p. 601
74. c, p. 593

Labeling

Location and Structure of Pituitary Gland

1. optic chiasma
2. infundibulum
3. pituitary diaphragm
4. pituitary gland (hypophysis)
5. nasal cavity
6. brainstem
7. hypothalamus
8. pineal gland
9. thalamus
10. pars anterior
11. pars intermedia
12. adenohypophysis
13. sella turcica (of sphenoid bone)
14. neurohypophysis
15. infundibulum

16. mammillary body
17. third ventricle
18. optic chiasma

Structure of Thyroid and Parathyroid Glands

1. epiglottis
2. hyoid bone
3. larynx (thyroid cartilage)
4. superior parathyroid glands
5. thyroid gland
6. inferior parathyroid glands
7. trachea

CHAPTER 27

Blood

Composition of Blood, Plasma, and Red Blood Cells

1. a, p. 612
2. a, p. 613
3. c, p. 613
4. b, p. 611
5. d, p. 616
6. t, p. 613
7. f, p. 615
8. t, p. 615
9. f, p. 617
10. f, p. 618
11. t, p. 612
12. t, p. 613
13. f, p. 614
14. t, p. 614
15. f, p. 615

Blood Types

16. b, p. 618
17. a, p. 619
18. d, p. 620
19. Type AB, p. 619
20. antigen, p. 619
21. antibodies, p. 620

White Blood Cells and Platelets

22. d, p. 621
23. i, p. 622
24. b, p. 622
25. c, p. 622
26. f, p. 622
27. h, p. 622
28. j, p. 624
29. g, p. 624
30. a, p. 622
31. e, p. 622

Hemostasis

32. b, p. 625
33. d, p. 628
34. c, p. 628

Mechanisms of Disease

35. Polycythemia, p. 630
36. Aplastic anemia, p. 630

37. pernicious anemia, p. 630
38. sickle cell anemia, p. 630
39. Leukopenia, p. 630
40. thrombus, p. 631
41. embolus, p. 631
42. Hemophilia, p. 631

Applying What You Know

43. Theoretically, infused red blood cells and elevation of hemoglobin levels after transfusion should increase oxygen consumption and muscle performance during exercise. In practice, however, the advantage appears to be minimal.
44. No. If Mrs. Shearer were a negative Rh factor and her husband were a positive Rh factor, it would set up the strong possibility of erythroblastosis fetalis.
45. Both procedures assist the clotting process.

One Last Quick Check

46. b, pp. 630 and 631
47. b, p. 615
48. a, p. 622
49. a, p. 613
50. d, p. 613
51. a, p. 622
52. a, p. 631
53. d, p. 620
54. c, p. 615
55. b, p. 625
56. d, p. 622
57. f, p. 630
58. h, p. 618
59. a, p. 622
60. g, p. 630
61. c, pp. 624 and 625
62. b, p. 622
63. e, p. 620
64. i, p. 613
65. j, p. 622
66. l, p. 622
67. k, p. 613
68. m, p. 622

Diagrams

Blood Typing

Recipient's blood		Reactions with donor's blood			
RBC antigens	Plasma antibodies	Donor type O	Donor type A	Donor type B	Donor type AB
None (Type O)	Anti-A Anti-B				
A (Type A)	Anti-B				
B (Type B)	Anti-A				
AB (Type AB)	(none)				

 Normal blood 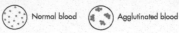 Agglutinated blood

Human Blood Cells

BODY CELL		FUNCTION
Erythrocyte		Oxygen and carbon dioxide transport
Neutrophil		Immune defense (phagocytosis)
Eosinophil		Defense against parasites
Basophil		Inflammatory response and heparin secretion
B lymphocyte		Antibody production (precursor of plasma cells)
T lymphocyte		Cellular immune response
Monocyte		Immune defenses (phagocytosis)
Thrombocyte		Blood clotting

CHAPTER 28

The Heart

Heart

1. b, p. 642
2. c, p. 642
3. a, p. 643
4. a, p. 644
5. d, p. 645
6. d, p. 648
7. c, p. 648
8. d, p. 643
9. d, p. 644
10. b, p. 649
11. Trace the Blood Flow, p. 647: right atrium (1) tricuspid valve (2) right ventricle (3) pulmonary semilunar valve (4) pulmonary arteries (5) pulmonary veins (6) left atrium (7) left atrioventricular (mitral) valve (8) left ventricle (9) aortic semilunar valve (10) aorta (11)
12. CPR (cardiopulmonary resuscitation), p. 638
13. troponins and C-reactive protein, p. 643
14. autorhythmic, p. 643
15. chordae tendineae, p. 644

The Heart as a Pump

16. b, p. 653
17. b, p. 649
18. a, p. 653
19. b, p. 653
20. a, p. 655
21. t, p. 654
22. f, p. 649
23. f, p. 653
24. t, p. 655
25. t, p. 655

26. Subendocardial branches, p. 649
27. ectopic pacemakers, p. 650
28. cardiac cycle, p. 654
29. residual volume, p. 655
30. heart murmur, p. 656

Mechanisms of Disease

31. e, p. 657
32. g, p. 658
33. i, p. 659
34. h, p. 658
35. a, p. 656
36. k, p. 660
37. b, p. 656
38. f, p. 659
39. c, p. 657
40. d, p. 657
41. j, p. 659
42. l, p. 660

Applying What You Know

43. Congestive heart failure. Left-sided heart failure often leads to right-sided heart failure. The combination of both problems may require a transplant or implant or may lead to death.
44. Coronary bypass surgery.
45. Cardiac enzymes usually increase over the next few hours following a heart attack. These elevations suggest that Mr. Wertz may have had a myocardial infarction with resulting heart muscle damage.

One Last Quick Check

46. c, p. 647
47. d, p. 656
48. c, p. 642
49. d, p. 644
50. b, p. 657
51. septum, p. 643
52. veins, p. 643
53. coronary arteries, p. 647
54. myocardial infarction, p. 657
55. coronary sinus, p. 649
56. depolarization, p. 653
57. depolarization, p. 653
58. repolarizing, p. 653
59. repolarization, p. 653
60. myocardial infarction, p. 653
61. t, p. 655
62. t, p. 656
63. t, p. 657
64. t, p. 657
65. f, p. 659

Labeling

Heart

1. aorta
2. superior vena cava
3. right atrium
4. left AV (mitral) valve
5. right AV (tricuspid) valve
6. chordae tendineae
7. right ventricle

8. interventricular septum
9. papillary muscle
10. left ventricle
11. right ventricle
12. pulmonary veins
13. right atrium
14. openings to coronary arteries
15. pulmonary trunk
16. aortic semilunar valve
17. left atrium

ECG Strip Recording

1. atrial depolarization
2. ventricular depolarization (and atrial repolarization)
3. ventricular repolarization

CHAPTER 29
Blood Vessels
Blood Vessel Types

1. d, p. 666
2. c, p. 666
3. e, p. 670
4. g, p. 670
5. f, p. 667
6. b, p. 666
7. a, p. 666
8. t, p. 669
9. f, p. 670
10. t, p. 669
11. f, p. 669

Circulation Routes and Major Blood Vessels

12. d, p. 670
13. c, p. 670
14. b, p. 671
15. d, p. 686
16. d, p. 685
17. systemic circulation, p. 670
18. cerebral arterial circle (of Willis), p. 675
19. veins, p. 681
20. hepatic portal circulation, p. 685
21. ascites, p. 686
22. veins, p. 681

Fetal Circulation

23. b, p. 688
24. b, p. 689
25. a, p. 689
26. (a) umbilical arteries, p. 688; (b) umbilical vein, p. 688
27. ductus arteriosus, p. 691
28. t, p. 688
29. t, p. 691

Mechanisms of Disease

30. i, p. 692
31. b, p. 692
32. d, p. 692
33. e, p. 692
34. a, p. 692
35. c, p. 692
36. f, p. 693

37. g, p. 694
38. j, p. 694
39. h, p. 693
40. l, p. 692
41. k, p. 692

Applying What You Know

42. The foramen ovale is an opening in the septum between the right and left atria. The foramen ovale normally becomes functionally closed soon after a newborn takes the first breath and full circulation through the lungs becomes established. Complete structural closure usually requires 9 months or more. If closure does not occur, surgical closure may be required if symptoms become apparent.

43. (a) Varicose veins (b) Rochelle should elevate her feet as much as possible to assist the return flow of venous blood. She should also consider elastic supportive stockings when she stands, which will provide support as blood is attempting to return to the heart.

One Last Quick Check

44. b, p. 693
45. c, p. 675
46. b, p. 670
47. b, p. 669
48. a, p. 681
49. t, p. 675
50. t, p. 666
51. t, p. 670
52. f, p. 675
53. f, p. 666
54. g, p. 675
55. a, p. 690
56. i, p. 688
57. c, p. 689
58. f, p. 692
59. b, p. 694
60. h, p. 671
61. d, p. 692
62. e, p. 670
63. j, p. 666

Labeling
Blood Vessels

1. valve
2. endothelium (tunica intima)
3. basement membrane (tunica intima)
4. smooth muscle (tunica media)
5. fibrous connective (tunica externa)
6. endothelium (tunica intima)
7. basement membrane (tunica intima)
8. internal elastic membrane
9. smooth muscle (tunica media)
10. fibrous connective tissue (tunica externa)
11. internal elastic membrane

Veins

1. right brachiocephalic
2. right subclavian
3. superior vena cava
4. right pulmonary
5. small cardiac

6. inferior vena cava
7. hepatic
8. hepatic portal
9. superior mesenteric
10. median cubital (basilic)
11. common iliac
12. external iliac
13. femoral
14. great saphenous
15. small saphenous
16. fibular
17. anterior tibial
18. posterior tibial
19. venous dorsal arch
20. digital
21. popliteal
22. femoral
23. digital
24. internal iliac
25. common iliac
26. inferior mesenteric
27. splenic
28. long thoracic
29. basilic
30. great cardiac
31. cephalic
32. axillary
33. left subclavian
34. left brachiocephalic
35. internal jugular
36. external jugular
37. facial
38. angular
39. occipital

Arteries

1. right common carotid
2. right subclavian
3. brachiocephalic
4. right coronary
5. axillary
6. brachial
7. superior mesenteric
8. abdominal aorta
9. common iliac
10. internal iliac (hypogastric)
11. external iliac
12. deep medial circumflex femoral
13. descending branch of lateral circumflex femoral
14. deep artery of thigh
15. popliteal
16. anterior tibial
17. peroneal
18. posterior tibial
19. arcuate
20. dorsal pedis
21. femoral
22. perforating arteries
23. digital
24. superficial palmar arch
25. deep palmar arch
26. ulnar

27. radial
28. inferior mesenteric
29. celiac
30. renal
31. splenic
32. aorta
33. left coronary
34. pulmonary
35. arch of aorta
36. left subclavian
37. left common carotid
38. external carotid
39. internal carotid
40. facial
41. occipital

Fetal Circulation

1. aortic arch
2. abdominal aorta
3. common iliac arteries
4. internal iliac arteries
5. umbilical arteries
6. fetal umbilicus
7. umbilical cord
8. fetal side of placenta
9. maternal side of placenta
10. umbilical vein
11. hepatic portal vein
12. ductus venosus
13. inferior vena cava
14. foramen ovale
15. superior vena cava
16. ascending aorta
17. pulmonary trunk
18. ductus arteriosus

Hepatic Portal Circulation

1. inferior vena cava
2. stomach
3. gastric vein
4. spleen
5. pancreatic vein
6. splenic vein
7. gastroepiploic vein
8. descending colon
9. inferior mesenteric vein
10. small intestine
11. appendix
12. ascending colon
13. superior mesenteric vein
14. pancreas
15. duodenum
16. hepatic portal vein
17. liver
18. hepatic veins

CHAPTER 30

Circulation of Blood

Hemodynamics and Arterial Blood Pressure

1. d, p. 700
2. a, p. 700

3. b, p. 701
4. a, p. 702
5. d, p. 703
6. t, p. 702
7. t, p. 704
8. f, p. 703
9. t, p. 703
10. f, p. 706
11. c, p. 706
12. a, p. 706
13. i, p. 701
14. b, p. 701
15. e, p. 708
16. h, p. 708
17. g, p. 711
18. j, p. 703
19. f, p. 708
20. d, p. 706

Venous Return to the Heart

21. stress-relaxation effect, p. 711
22. circulation, p. 712
23. Capillary exchange, p. 713
24. Osmotic pressure, p. 713
25. reabsorbed, p. 713
26. Renin-angiotensin aldosterone system, p. 714
27. Atrial natriuretic, p. 714
28. Hypertension, p. 714

Blood Pressure

29. b, p. 715
30. a, p. 716
31. d, p. 716
32. Sphygmomanometer, p. 714
33. artery, p. 717
34. arterial, p. 720

Mechanisms of Disease

35. septic shock, p. 721
36. Cardiogenic shock, p. 721
37. anaphylaxis; anaphylactic shock, p. 721
38. Neurogenic shock, p. 721
39. low blood volume, p. 721
40. toxic shock syndrome, p. 721

Applying What You Know

41. (a) Hypovolemic shock (b) The body might respond by increasing the heart rate, decreasing the urine output, and decreasing available fluids to the tissues.
42. Ventricular fibrillation is an immediately life-threatening condition. Unless ventricular fibrillation is corrected immediately by defibrillation or another method, death may occur within minutes. Automatic external defibrillators (AED) can be used by nearly anyone and are becoming available in many public areas for emergency use until medical help can arrive.

One Last Quick Check

43. c, p. 703
44. d, p. 703
45. d, p. 706
46. c, p. 720
47. b, p. 706

48. a, p. 721
49. c, p. 721
50. a, p. 711
51. b, p. 702
52. a, p. 718
53. volume, p. 701
54. inotropic, p. 703
55. stronger, p. 703
56. ejection fraction, p. 703
57. afterload, p. 703
58. epinephrine, p. 705
59. skeletal, p. 708
60. brachial artery, p. 715
61. Korotkoff sounds, p. 715
62. (a) arteries (b) capillaries, p. 718

Labeling
Pulse Points

1. Superficial temporal artery
2. Facial artery
3. Carotid artery
4. Brachial artery
5. Radial artery
6. Femoral artery
7. Popliteal artery
8. Posterior tibial artery
9. Dorsalis pedis artery

CHAPTER 31
Lymphatic System
Lymphatic Vessels, Lymph, and Circulation of Lymph

1. c, p. 729
2. b, p. 730
3. a, p. 731
4. d, p. 731
5. c, p. 732
6. b, p. 733
7. a, p. 732
8. t, p. 729
9. f, p. 729
10. t, p. 730
11. t, p. 731
12. t, p. 732
13. t, p. 731
14. t, p. 733

Lymph Nodes

15. b, p. 735
16. d, p. 734
17. a, p. 737
18. c, p. 737
19. f, p. 734
20. t, p. 734

Lymphatic Drainage of the Breast

21. a, p. 739
22. c, p. 738

Tonsils, Thymus, and Spleen

23. a, p. 744
24. c, p. 740

25. c, p. 739
26. f, p. 740
27. f, p. 742
28. t, p. 742

Mechanisms of Disease

29. Lymphoma, p. 744
30. acute otitis media, p. 744
31. blood poisoning, p. 744
32. filarial, p. 743
33. Hodgkin and non-Hodgkin, p. 744

Applying What You Know

34. (a) Yes (b) Yes (c) The spleen destroys old blood cells and platelets. Preventing this will allow Ms. Langston to preserve her own supply and avoid anemia.
35. Baby Wilson had no means of producing T cells, thus making him susceptible to several diseases. Isolation was a means of controlling his exposure to these diseases.

One Last Quick Check

36. b, p. 739
37. c, p. 742
38. c, p. 742
39. a, p. 739
40. c, p. 742
41. a, p. 740
42. a, p. 739
43. t, p. 731
44. t, p. 732
45. t, p. 733
46. f, p. 734
47. t, p. 743
48. f, p. 738
49. f, p. 740
50. f, p. 742

Labeling

Principal Organs of the Lymphatic System

1. tonsils
2. cervical lymph node
3. right lymphatic duct
4. superficial cubital (supratrochlear) lymph nodes
5. aggregated lymphoid nodules (Peyer patches) in intestinal wall
6. red bone marrow
7. inguinal lymph node
8. cisterna chyli
9. spleen
10. thoracic duct
11. axillary lymph node
12. thymus gland
13. entrance of thoracic duct into subclavian vein

Lymph Node

1. afferent lymph vessel
2. capsule
3. efferent lymph vessel
4. hilum
5. medullary cords
6. cortical nodules
7. sinuses
8. germinal center

Lymphatic Drainage of Breast

1. supraclavicular nodes
2. interpectoral (Rotter) nodes
3. midaxillary nodes
4. lateral axillary (brachial) nodes
5. subscapular nodes
6. anterior axillary (pectoral) nodes
7. parasternal nodes
8. subclavicular nodes

CHAPTER 32

Innate Immunity

Innate Immunity

1. d, p. 751
2. c, p. 752
3. a, p. 757
4. a, p. 756
5. b, p. 756
6. f, p. 750
7. t, p. 752
8. f, p. 757
9. f, p. 759
10. t, p. 757
11. a, p. 750
12. i, p. 759
13. b, p. 751
14. e, p. 759
15. j, p. 754
16. h, p. 750
17. g, p. 757
18. f, pp. 750-751
19. d, p. 750
20. c, p. 758

Applying What You Know

21. (1) No. (2) Phagocytes have a very short life span, and thus dead cells tend to "pile up" at the inflammation site, forming most of the white substance called *pus*.

One Last Quick Check

22. inflammation, p. 753
23. nonspecific immunity, p. 751
24. cytokines, p. 751
25. lymphocytes, p. 757
26. self-tolerance, p. 750
27. f, p. 754
28. t, p. 756
29. f, p. 750
30. t, p. 752
31. t, p. 750

CHAPTER 33

Adaptive Immunity

Adaptive Immunity

1. b, p. 763
2. b, p. 763
3. d, p. 763
4. a, p. 766

5. b, p. 770
6. b, p. 767
7. c, p. 766
8. b, p. 771
9. b, p. 768
10. b, p. 772
11. immunoglobulin, p. 766
12. IgM, p. 767
13. cowpox virus, p. 770
14. attenuated, p. 770
15. Active immunity, p. 775
16. tumor markers, p. 774
17. PSA, p. 774
18. adaptive immune, p. 773
19. natural passive, p. 767
20. artificial active, p. 767

Mechanisms of Disease

21. c, p. 779
22. a, p. 779
23. b, p. 780
24. e, p. 778
25. d, p. 778

Applying What You Know

26. (a) Passive acquired immunity (b) active artificial immunity (c) Active immunity usually lasts longer than passive.
27. (a) AIDS (b) azidothymidine (AZT) and ritonavir (Norvir)

One Last Quick Check

28. a, p. 771
29. d, p. 780
30. d, p. 766
31. b, p. 768
32. d, p. 769
33. c, p. 767
34. allergy, p. 778
35. antihistamines, p. 778
36. specific immunity, p. 751 (previous chapter review)
37. lymphotoxin, p. 773
38. f, p. 780
39. t, p. 780
40. t, p. 778
41. f, p. 779
42. f, p. 779
43. humoral, p. 763
44. immunoblobins, p. 766
45. cytolysis, p. 768
46. cytokines, p. 772
47. active, p. 770

Labeling

T Cell Development

1. stem cell
2. T cell
3. sensitized T cell
4. memory cell
5. effector T cell

CHAPTER 34
Stress

Selye's Concept of Stress

1. b, p. 788
2. b, p. 788
3. b, p. 789
4. b, p. 788
5. d, p. 788
6. f, p. 790
7. f, p. 795
8. t, p. 788
9. f, p. 788
10. t, p. 792
11. c, p. 790
12. e, p. 790
13. d, p. 788
14. f, p. 786
15. b, p. 790
16. a, p. 788

Some Current Concepts about Stress

17. c, p. 792
18. d, p. 791
19. b, p. 793
20. t, p. 790
21. f, p. 793
22. f, p. 793
23. t, p. 792
24. f, p. 788
25. t, p. 791

Applying What You Know

26. (a) Stress (b) See Figure 34-6, p. 791 (c) Immune diseases, decreased quality of life, ulcers, hypertension, chemical dependency, impaired relationships, and loss of contact with reality.
27. (a) Sympathetic (b) No, digestion decreases under the influence of the sympathetic nervous system.

One Last Quick Check

28. general adaptation syndrome, p. 786
29. exhaustion, p. 790
30. corticotropin-releasing hormone, p. 790
31. fight or flight reaction, p. 792
32. Psychophysiology, p. 793
33. f, p. 795
34. t, p. 786
35. t, p. 793
36. f, p. 793
37. t, p. 788
38. t, p. 792

Stress-Related Diseases and Conditions (possible answers for Fill in the Blanks questions 39-48)

TARGET ORGAN OR SYSTEM	DISEASE OR CONDITION
Cardiovascular system	Coronary artery disease Hypertension Stroke Disturbances of heart rhythm
Muscles	Tension headaches Muscle contraction backache
Connective tissue	Rheumatoid arthritis (autoimmune disease) Related inflammatory diseases of connective tissue
Pulmonary system	Asthma (hypersensitivity reaction) Hay fever (hypersensitivity reaction) Changes in breathing patterns
Immune system	Immunosuppression or immune deficiency Autoimmune diseases
Gastrointestinal system	Ulcer Irritable bowel syndrome Diarrhea Nausea and vomiting Ulcerative colitis
Genitourinary system	Diuresis Impotence (erectile dysfunction) Loss of libido (sexual desire)
Skin	Eczema Neurodermatitis Acne
Endocrine system	Diabetes mellitus Amenorrhea
Central nervous system	Fatigue and lethargy Type A behavior Overeating Depression Insomnia

CHAPTER 35

Respiratory Tract

Upper Respiratory Tract

1. a, p. 801
2. c, p. 800
3. d, p. 802
4. c, p. 804
5. a, p. 806
6. f, p. 802
7. f, p. 805
8. t, p. 805
9. f, p. 807
10. t, p. 807

Lower Respiratory Tract

11. a, p. 807
12. b, p. 811
13. c, p. 812
14. d, p. 816

15. f, p. 807
16. f, p. 807
17. t, p. 810
18. f, p. 812
19. f, p. 812
20. t, p. 815
21. f, p. 816
22. t, p. 815
23. t, p. 811
24. f, p. 814

Mechanisms of Disease

25. d, p. 819
26. g, p. 819
27. b, p. 818
28. a, p. 818
29. c, p. 818
30. f, p. 817
31. e, p. 817
32. h, p. 817

Applying What You Know

33. (a) epiglottitis (b) *Haemophilus influenzae* type B (c) yes
34. During the day Mr. Gorski's cilia are paralyzed because of his heavy smoking. They use the time when Mr. Gorski is asleep to sweep accumulations of mucus and bacteria toward the pharynx. When Mr. Gorski awakens, these collections are waiting to be eliminated.

One Last Quick Check

35. a, p. 804
36. b, p. 805
37. a, p. 804
38. a, p. 802
39. a, p. 802
40. b, p. 805
41. b, p. 818
42. c, pp. 805-806
43. a, p. 817
44. b, p. 817
45. a, p. 802
46. air distributor, p. 800
47. gas exchanger, p. 800
48. filters, p. 800
49. warms, p. 800
50. humidifies, p. 800
51. nose, p. 801
52. pharynx, p. 801
53. larynx, p. 801
54. trachea, p. 801
55. bronchi, p. 801
56. lungs, p. 801
57. alveoli, pp. 809-810
58. Exchange, p. 815
59. respiratory membrane, p. 815
60. surface, p. 815

Labeling

Respiratory System

1. upper respiratory tract
2. lower respiratory tract
3. bronchioles
4. bronchioles
5. capillary
6. alveolar sac
7. alveoli
8. alveolar duct
9. left and right primary bronchi
10. trachea
11. larynx
12. laryngopharynx
13. oropharynx
14. nasopharynx
15. pharynx
16. nasal cavity

Divisions of the Pharynx and Nearby Structures

1. lingual tonsil
2. hyoid bone
3. vocal cords
4. trachea
5. esophagus
6. laryngopharynx

7. epiglottis
8. oropharynx
9. palatine tonsil
10. uvula
11. soft palate
12. nasopharynx
13. opening of the auditory (eustachian) tube
14. pharyngeal tonsil (adenoids)

Paranasal Sinuses

1. sphenoid sinus
2. maxillary sinus
3. lacrimal sac
4. ethmoid air cells
5. superior nasal concha of ethmoid
6. middle nasal concha of ethmoid
7. inferior concha
8. oral cavity
9. maxillary sinus
10. sphenoid sinus
11. frontal sinus
12. ethmoid air cells
13. frontal sinus

Lobes and Fissures of the Lungs

1. first rib
2. right superior lobe
3. right primary bronchus
4. horizontal fissure
5. right middle lobe
6. oblique fissure
7. seventh rib
8. right inferior lobe
9. sternum (xiphoid process)
10. left inferior lobe
11. oblique fissure
12. body of sternum
13. left primary bronchus
14. left superior lobe
15. sternum (manubrium)
16. trachea

CHAPTER 36

Ventilation

Respiratory Physiology/Ventilation

1. b, p. 827
2. c, p. 827
3. b, p. 828
4. c, p. 831
5. d, p. 834
6. d, p. 836
7. d, p. 826
8. d, p. 834
9. a, p. 825
10. d, p. 826
11. t, p. 826
12. f, p. 834
13. t, p. 831
14. t, p. 838
15. t, p. 831

16. compliance, p. 828
17. transpulmonary pressure, p. 830
18. total minute volume, p. 835
19. respiratory cycle, p. 828
20. medullary rhythmicity area, p. 838

Mechanisms of Disease

21. COPD (chronic obstructive pulmonary disease), p. 842
22. Bronchitis, p. 843
23. Emphysema, p. 843
24. Asthma, p. 843
25. Sudden infant death syndrome (SIDS), p. 842

Applying What You Know

26. (a) obstructive pulmonary disorders (b) COPD, which may include bronchitis, emphysema, and asthma (c) They obstruct inspiration and expiration. The primary difficulty is in emptying their lungs adequately, which creates a buildup of CO_2 in the lungs.
27. The "diving reflex" was responsible for this phenomenon. It is a protective response of the body to cold water immersion that slows the metabolism and tissue requirements to enable survival.

One Last Quick Check

28. d, p. 825
29. b, p. 828
30. d, p. 834
31. d, p. 831
32. d, p. 834
33. b, p. 839
34. t, p. 835
35. f, p. 832
36. f, p. 836
37. t, p. 836
38. e, p. 831
39. c, p. 831
40. a, p. 835
41. f, p. 834
42. d, p. 837
43. b, p. 832
44. i, p. 836
45. j, p. 838
46. g, p. 841
47. h, p. 838

Labeling

Pulmonary Volumes

1. total lung capacity (TLC)
2. inspiratory reserve volume (IRV)
3. tidal volume (TV)
4. expiratory reserve volume (ERV)
5. residual volume (RV)
6. vital capacity (VC)

Respiratory Centers of Brainstem

1. limbic system (emotional responses)
2. PRG
3. apneustic center
4. pons
5. central chemoreceptors

6. DRG
7. VRG
8. medullary rhythmicity area
9. medulla
10. respiratory muscles
11. stretch receptors in lungs and thorax
12. aortic chemoreceptors and baroreceptors
13. carotid chemoreceptors and baroreceptors
14. cortex (voluntary control)

CHAPTER 37
Gas Exchange and Transport
Pulmonary Gas Exchange

1. a, p. 849
2. d, p. 850
3. c, p. 849
4. a, p. 851
5. t, p. 849
6. f, p. 851
7. t, p. 849

Blood Transportation of Gases/Systemic Gas Exchange

8. d, pp. 853-854
9. b, p. 854
10. d, p. 855
11. c, pp. 853-854
12. t, p. 853
13. f, p. 854
14. f, p. 856
15. t, p. 857

Applying What You Know

16. Emphysema is an abnormal condition characterized by the trapping of air in the alveoli of the lung. This causes the alveoli to rupture and fuse to other alveoli. This decrease in the number of functioning alveoli in the lungs compromises the ability of the lungs to exchange the necessary volume of air, and the person may experience progressive difficulty in breathing as the disease progresses.
17. Carbon monoxide is an odorless, invisible, gas that binds to Hb more than 200 times more strongly than oxygen. As more and more carbon monoxide is formed, less and less oxygen is carried by your blood, which becomes a life-threatening situation.

One Last Quick Check

18. c, p. 854
19. c, p. 853
20. a, p. 857
21. b, p. 851
22. d, p. 851
23. a, p. 850
24. (1) plasma (2) hemoglobin, p. 854
25. carbaminohemoglobin, p. 854
26. carbonic acid, p. 854
27. Carbon dioxide, p. 852

CHAPTER 38
Upper Digestive Tract

Overview of the Digestive System

1. c, p. 862
2. b, p. 862
3. t, p. 861
4. f, p. 863
5. a, p. 861
6. a, p. 861
7. a, p. 861
8. b, p. 861
9. b, p. 861
10. b, p. 861
11. b, p. 861
12. b, p. 861
13. a, p. 861
14. a, p. 861

Mouth and Pharynx

15. d, p. 864
16. b, p. 866
17. c, p. 867
18. d, p. 867
19. b, p. 869
20. t, p. 867
21. f, p. 864
22. f, p. 868
23. t, p. 869
24. f, p. 864

Esophagus and Stomach

25. b, p. 869
26. d, p. 872
27. c, p. 873
28. t, p. 872
29. t, p. 872
30. t, p. 872

Mechanisms of Disease

31. Sjögren syndrome, p. 874
32. dental caries, p. 874
33. Gingivitis, p. 874
34. leukoplakia, p. 874
35. cleft lip; cleft palate, p. 875
36. heartburn, p. 875
37. anorexia, p. 876
38. *Helicobacter pylori*, p. 877

Applying What You Know

39. (a) mumps (b) inflammation of the testes (c) reduced fertility
40. pylorospasm

One Last Quick Check

41. d, p. 868
42. a, p. 868
43. c, p. 868
44. d, p. 868
45. d, p. 874
46. a, p. 867
47. c, p. 873
48. b, p. 868
49. c, p. 869
50. t, p. 865
51. t, p. 863
52. t, p. 870
53. t, p. 864
54. t, pp. 860-861
55. f, p. 872

Labeling

Digestive Organs

1. parotid gland
2. submandibular salivary gland
3. pharynx
4. esophagus
5. diaphragm
6. transverse colon
7. hepatic flexure of colon
8. ascending colon
9. ileum
10. cecum
11. vermiform appendix
12. rectum
13. anal canal
14. sigmoid colon
15. descending colon
16. splenic flexure of colon
17. spleen
18. stomach
19. liver
20. trachea
21. larynx
22. sublingual salivary gland
23. tongue
24. common hepatic duct
25. cystic duct
26. gallbladder
27. duodenum
28. pancreas
29. stomach
30. spleen
31. liver

Tooth

1. crown
2. neck
3. root
4. bone
5. cementum
6. periodontal membrane
7. periodontal ligament
8. root canal
9. gingiva (gum)
10. pulp cavity with nerves and vessels
11. dentin
12. enamel
13. cusp

Stomach

1. esophagus
2. gastroesophageal opening
3. lower esophageal sphincter (LES)
4. cardia

5. lesser curvature
6. pylorus
7. pyloric sphincter
8. duodenal bulb
9. duodenum
10. rugae
11. greater curvature
12. mucosa
13. submucosa
14. oblique muscle layer
15. circular muscle layer
16. longitudinal muscle layer
17. muscularis
18. serosa
19. body of stomach
20. fundus

CHAPTER 39

Lower Digestive Tract

Small Intestine, Large Intestine, Appendix, and Peritoneum

1. c, p. 883
2. b, p. 884
3. a, p. 887
4. b, p. 888
5. f, p. 886
6. f, p. 887
7. t, pp. 886-887
8. t, p. 888
9. t, p. 883
10. t, p. 885

Liver, Gallbladder, and Pancreas

11. b, p. 890
12. d, p. 890
13. b, p. 891
14. a, pp. 891-892
15. c, p. 891
16. t, p. 889
17. f, p. 891
18. t, p. 893
19. t, p. 893
20. t, p. 884

Mechanisms of Disease

21. d, p. 896
22. g, p. 895
23. f, p. 895
24. e, p. 895
25. i, p. 895
26. a, p. 895
27. h, p. 896
28. b, p. 896
29. c, p. 896
30. j, p. 893

Applying What You Know

31. (a) cholelithiasis (b) jaundice (c) obstruction of the bile flow into the duodenum (d) cholecystectomy or ultrasound lithotripsy.

32. (a) appendicitis (b) The opening between the appendix and the cecum is often completely obliterated in elderly persons, which explains the low incidence of appendicitis.

One Last Quick Check

33. c, p. 885
34. a, p. 891
35. b, p. 884
36. d, p. 893
37. c, p. 888
38. f, p. 886
39. f, p. 886
40. t, p. 888
41. t, p. 887
42. f, p. 887

Labeling

Wall of Small Intestine

1. mesentery
2. serosa
3. muscularis
4. longitudinal muscle
5. circular muscle
6. submucosa
7. mucosa
8. plica (fold)

Divisions of Large Intestine

1. superior mesenteric artery
2. hepatic (right colic) flexure
3. ascending colon
4. cecum
5. rectum
6. superior rectal artery and vein
7. sigmoid colon
8. sigmoid artery and vein
9. descending colon
10. inferior mesenteric artery and vein
11. splenic (left colic) flexure
12. transverse colon

Liver

1. inferior vena cava
2. right lobe
3. gallbladder
4. round ligament
5. falciform ligament
6. left lobe
7. right lobe proper
8. common hepatic duct
9. hepatic portal vein
10. inferior vena cava
11. caudate lobe
12. falciform ligament
13. hepatic artery
14. left lobe
15. quadrate lobe
16. gallbladder

Common Bile Duct and Its Tributaries

1. corpus (body) of gallbladder
2. neck of gallbladder

3. cystic dust
4. liver
5. minor duodenal papilla
6. accessory pancreatic duct
7. major duodenal papilla
8. duodenum
9. sphincter muscles
10. pancreas
11. superior mesenteric artery and vein
12. pancreatic duct
13. common bile duct
14. common hepatic duct
15. right and left hepatic ducts

CHAPTER 40

Digestion and Absorption

Digestion

1. b, p. 904
2. a, p. 904
3. b, p. 910
4. a, p. 910
5. b, p. 910
6. b, p. 907
7. c, p. 910
8. f, p. 905
9. f, p. 906
10. t, p. 908
11. f, p. 908
12. t, p. 912
13. f, p. 907
14. t, p. 910

Secretion and Control of Digestive Gland Secretion

15. b, p. 914
16. b, p. 914
17. d, p. 916
18. d, p. 918
19. t, p. 915
20. t, p. 918
21. f, p. 918
22. t, p. 906

Absorption and Elimination

23. b, p. 921
24. b, p. 923
25. c, p. 922
26. f, p. 920
27. t, p. 920
28. f, p. 923
29. f, p. 922
30. t, p. 912

Applying What You Know

31. Diarrhea may occur as a result of increased motility of the small intestine. Chyme moves through too rapidly, decreasing absorption of water. The large volume of material arriving in the large intestine exceeds the absorption ability of the large intestine and a watery stool results.
32. Replacement of fluids should focus on large amounts of cool, diluted, or isotonic fluids.

One Last Quick Check

33. a, p. 916
34. c, p. 906
35. a, p. 913
36. d, p. 904
37. c, p. 910
38. c, p. 910
39. a, p. 914
40. b, p. 913
41. d, p. 909
42. c, pp. 910 and 912
43. b, p. 907
44. a, p. 916
45. d, p. 904
46. c, p. 904
47. f, p. 923
48. t, p. 904
49. t, p. 920
50. t, p. 905
51. t, p. 916
52. f, p. 909

Diagrams

Chemical Digestion

DIGESTIVE JUICES AND ENZYMES	SUBSTANCE DIGESTED (OR HYDROLYZED)	RESULTING PRODUCT*
Saliva		
Amylase (ptyalin)	Starch (polysaccharide)	Maltose (disaccharide)
Gastric juice		
Protease (pepsin)[†] plus hydrochloric acid	Proteins	Partially digested proteins
Pancreatic Juice		
Proteases (e.g., trypsin)[‡]	Proteins (intact or partially digested)	Peptides and **amino acids**
Lipases	Fats emulsified by bile	**Fatty acids, monoglycerides, and glycerol**
Amylase	Starch	Maltose
Nucleases	Nucleic acids (DNA, RNA)	Nucleotides
Intestinal Enzymes[§]		
Peptidases	Peptides	**Amino acids**
Sucrase	Sucrose (cane sugar)	**Glucose** and **fructose**[‖] (monosaccharides)
Lactase	Lactose (milk sugar)	**Glucose** and **galactose** (monosaccharides)
Maltase	Maltose (malt sugar)	**Glucose**
Nucleotidases and phosphatases	Nucleotides	Nucleosides

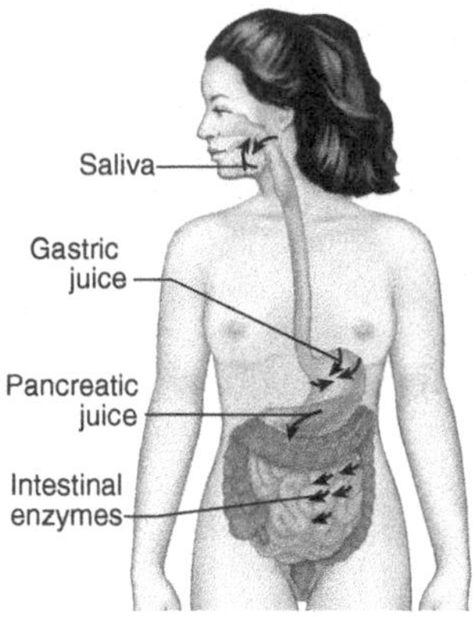

*Substances in **boldface type** are end products of digestion (that is, completely digested nutrients ready for absorption).

[†]Secreted in inactive form (pepsinogen); activated by low pH (hydrochloric acid).

[‡]Secreted in inactive form (trypsinogen); activated by enterokinase, an enzyme in the intestinal brush border.

[§]Brush-border enzymes.

[‖]Glucose is also called *dextrose*; fructose is also called *levulose*.

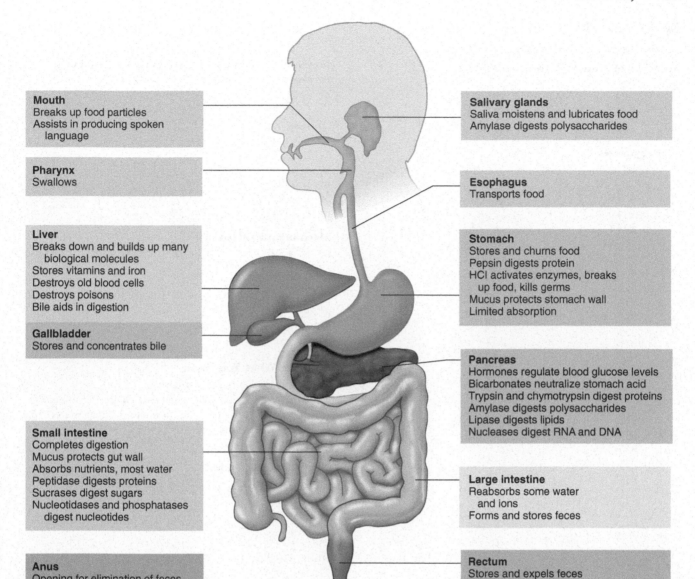

Mouth
Breaks up food particles
Assists in producing spoken
language

Pharynx
Swallows

Liver
Breaks down and builds up many
biological molecules
Stores vitamins and iron
Destroys old blood cells
Destroys poisons
Bile aids in digestion

Gallbladder
Stores and concentrates bile

Small intestine
Completes digestion
Mucus protects gut wall
Absorbs nutrients, most water
Peptidase digests proteins
Sucrases digest sugars
Nucleotidases and phosphatases
digest nucleotides

Anus
Opening for elimination of feces

Salivary glands
Saliva moistens and lubricates food
Amylase digests polysaccharides

Esophagus
Transports food

Stomach
Stores and churns food
Pepsin digests protein
HCl activates enzymes, breaks
up food, kills germs
Mucus protects stomach wall
Limited absorption

Pancreas
Hormones regulate blood glucose levels
Bicarbonates neutralize stomach acid
Trypsin and chymotrypsin digest proteins
Amylase digests polysaccharides
Lipase digests lipids
Nucleases digest RNA and DNA

Large intestine
Reabsorbs some water
and ions
Forms and stores feces

Rectum
Stores and expels feces

CHAPTER 41

Nutrition and Metabolism

Overview of Nutrition and Metabolism

1. a, p. 932
2. d, p. 931
3. t, p. 932
4. f, p. 932

Carbohydrates

5. a, p. 933
6. b, p. 933
7. c, p. 933
8. a, p. 934
9. a, p. 934
10. b, p. 934
11. d, p. 940
12. b, p. 940
13. t, p. 934
14. t, p. 934
15. f, p. 934
16. f, p. 939
17. t, p. 941
18. t, p. 939
19. f, p. 943
20. t, p. 941
21. t, p. 942
22. f, p. 942
23. f, p. 933
24. t, p. 935
25. t, p. 935
26. f, p. 936
27. f, p. 941

Lipids

28. a, p. 944
29. c, p. 944
30. a, p. 944
31. c, p. 946
32. d, p. 944
33. f, p. 945
34. t, p. 945
35. t, p. 946
36. t, p. 944
37. t, p. 945

Proteins

38. b, p. 947
39. b, p. 947
40. d, p. 948
41. f, p. 947
42. t, p. 947
43. t, p. 948
44. f, pp. 947-948
45. t, p. 947

Vitamins and Minerals

46. b, pp. 948 amd 950
47. a, p. 950
48. c, p. 951
49. f, p. 948
50. t, p. 950

51. t, p. 959
52. f, p. 948

Metabolic Rate and Mechanisms for Regulating Food Intake

53. b, p. 952
54. c, p. 953
55. c, p. 955
56. b, p. 956
57. f, p. 954
58. t, p. 956
59. t, p. 955
60. f, p. 954
61. f, p. 952

Mechanisms of Disease

62. b, p. 958
63. c, p. 959
64. a, p. 957
65. f, p. 959
66. d, p. 958
67. c, p. 958
68. g, p. 959

Applying What You Know

69. weight loss and anorexia nervosa
70. Iron would be the first mineral of choice. It is found in meat, eggs, vegetables, and legumes. Copper sources that might also help the anemia would be seafood, organ meats, and legumes.

One Last Quick Check

71. b, p. 935
72. a, p. 940
73. c, p. 942
74. c, p. 955
75. b, p. 955
76. d, p. 933
77. a, p. 933
78. bile (All others refer to carbohydrate metabolism)
79. amino acids (All others refer to fat metabolism)
80. M (All others refer to vitamins)
81. iron (All others refer to protein metabolism)
82. insulin (All others tend to increase blood glucose)
83. folic acid (All others are minerals)
84. ascorbic acid (All others refer to the B-complex vitamins)
85. a, p. 933
86. c, p. 946
87. d, p. 950
88. e, p. 951
89. a, p. 934
90. c, p. 951
91. a, p. 934
92. b, p. 945
93. b, p. 944

CHAPTER 42

Urinary System

Anatomy of the Urinary System

1. d, p. 966
2. c, p. 968

3. c, p. 968
4. b, p. 971
5. d, p. 972
6. c, p. 976
7. c, p. 978
8. a, p. 976
9. f, p. 968
10. f, p. 968
11. t, p. 971
12. t, p. 974
13. f, p. 968
14. t, p. 971
15. f, p. 968

Physiology of the Urinary System

16. b, p. 978
17. a, p. 978
18. d, p. 978
19. a, p. 980
20. c, p. 981
21. d, p. 985
22. c, p. 990
23. d, p. 989
24. c, pp. 981 and 985
25. t, p. 981
26. f, p. 979
27. t, p. 982
28. t, p. 978
29. f, p. 979
30. f, p. 979
31. t, p. 980
32. f, p. 978
33. f, p. 987
34. f, p. 988
35. t, p. 979

Mechanisms of Disease

36. i, p. 990
37. c, p. 990
38. f, p. 992
39. g, p. 990
40. k, p. 991
41. a, p. 991
42. h, p. 991
43. j, p. 992
44. b, p. 990
45. d, p. 991
46. e, p. 991
47. l, p. 991

Applying What You Know

48. Hemorrhage causes a drop in blood pressure, which decreases the urine output and can eventually lead to kidney failure.
49. Stage I—often asymptomatic because healthy nephrons compensate for the ones destroyed by disease. Stage 2—renal insufficiency; BUN increases, polyuria and dehydration may occur. Stage 3—uremia; high BUN, loss of kidney function, oliguria, edema, hypertension, and eventual death if an artificial kidney or transplant not available.

One Last Quick Check

50. b, p. 992
51. d, p. 993
52. a, p. 984
53. c, p. 989
54. c, p. 980
55. b, p. 971
56. c, p. 969
57. b, p. 972
58. a, p. 968
59. b, p. 969
60. e, p. 990
61. c, p. 990
62. f, p. 991
63. d, p. 971
64. j, p. 990
65. h, p. 990
66. a, p. 971
67. g, p. 991
68. i, p. 970
69. b, pp. 970-971
70. k, p. 991

Labeling

Kidney

1. interlobular arteries
2. renal column
3. renal sinus
4. hilum
5. renal pelvis
6. renal papilla of pyramid
7. ureter
8. medulla
9. medullary pyramid
10. major calyces
11. minor calyces
12. cortex
13. capsule (fibrous)

Nephron

1. proximal convoluted tubule (PCT)
2. renal corpuscle
3. distal convoluted tubule (DCT)
4. arcuate artery and vein
5. papilla of renal pyramid
6. thin ascending limb of Henle loop (tALH)
7. Henle loop
8. descending limb of Henle loop
9. thick ascending limb of Henle loop (TAL)
10. vasae rectae
11. collecting duct (CD)
12. peritubular capillaries
13. juxtamedullary nephron
14. interlobular artery and vein
15. afferent arteriole
16. efferent arteriole
17. cortical nephron

Male Urinary Bladder

1. ureter
2. opening of ureter

3. rugae
4. prostate gland
5. external urinary sphincter
6. bulbourethral gland
7. prostatic urethra
8. internal urethral sphincter
9. opening of ureter
10. trigone
11. smooth muscle (detrusor)
12. cut edge of peritoneum

CHAPTER 43
Fluid and Electrolyte Balance
Overview of Fluid and Electrolyte Balance

1. c, p. 1001
2. c, p. 1001
3. a, p. 1001
4. b, p. 1001
5. d, p. 1003
6. d, p. 1004
7. c, p. 1000
8. f, p. 1001
9. t, p. 1001
10. t, p. 1003
11. f, p. 1000
12. t, p. 1004
13. f, p. 1003
14. t, p. 1002

Mechanisms That Maintain Homeostasis of Total Fluid Volume

15. d, p. 1005
16. c, p. 1005
17. f, p. 1005
18. t, p. 1007

Regulation of Water and Electrolyte Levels in Plasma, Interstitial Fluid, and Intracellular Fluid

19. a, p. 1007
20. c, p. 1008
21. c, p. 1007
22. c, p. 1011
23. t, p. 1009
24. f, p. 1010
25. t, pp. 1010-1011
26. t, p. 1011

Regulation of Sodium and Potassium Levels in Body Fluids

27. f, p. 1011
28. t, p. 1012
29. t, p. 1012
30. f, p. 1008
31. t, p. 1012

Mechanisms of Disease

32. a, p. 1014
33. d, p. 1015
34. e, p. 1014
35. b, p. 1014

36. c, p. 1014
37. t, p. 1014
38. f, p. 1015
39. t, p. 1014
40. f, p. 1015

Applying What You Know

41. Ms. Titus could not accurately measure water intake created by foods or catabolism, nor could she measure output created by lungs, skin, or the intestines.
42. Jack's body contained more water. Obese people have a lower water content than slender people.

One Last Quick Check

43. inside, p. 1001
44. extracellular, p. 1001.
45. extracellular, p. 1001
46. lower, p. 1001
47. more, p. 1000
48. decreases, p. 1001
49. a, p. 1001
50. d, p. 1001
51. c, p. 1003
52. e, p. 1003
53. d, p. 1007
54. c, p. 1005
55. b, p. 1008
56. d, p. 1003
57. a, p. 1009
58. a, p. 1002
59. d, p. 1012
60. t, p. 1002
61. t, p. 1008
62. t, p. 1005

CHAPTER 44
Acid-Base Balance
Mechanisms That Control pH of Body Fluids

1. c, p. 1020
2. a, p. 1020
3. b, p. 1021
4. d, p. 1021
5. c, p. 1020
6. a, p. 1021
7. c, p. 1021
8. t, p. 1020
9. f, p. 1021
10. t, p. 1021
11. f, p. 1020
12. t, p. 1021
13. t, p. 1025

Buffer Mechanisms for Controlling pH of Body Fluids

14. a, p. 1024
15. c, p. 1024
16. t, p. 1024
17. f, p. 1025
18. f, p. 1023
19. f, p. 1025
20. t, p. 1022

Respiratory and Urinary Mechanisms of pH Control

21. d, p. 1025
22. b, p. 1026
23. b, p. 1027
24. a, p. 1027
25. c, p. 1029
26. t, p. 1027
27. f, p. 1027
28. t, p. 1029
29. f, p. 1024
30. t, p. 1027

Mechanisms of Disease

31. f, p. 1030
32. e, p. 1030
33. a, p. 1030
34. b, p. 1030
35. g, p. 1026
36. c, p. 1031
37. d, p. 1031

Applying What You Know

38. Normal saline contains chloride ions, which replace bicarbonate ions and thus relieve the bicarbonate excess that occurs during severe vomiting.
39. Most citrus fruits, although acid tasting, are fully oxidized with the help of buffers during metabolism and have little effect on acid-base balance. Cranberry juice is one of the few exceptions.

One Last Quick Check

40. a, pp. 1025-1026
41. c, p. 1030
42. a, p. 1030
43. d, p. 1020
44. a, p. 1030
45. d, p. 1031
46. d, p. 1024
47. a, p. 1022
48. g, p. 1020
49. c, p. 1027
50. h, p. 1021
51. e, p. 1031
52. f, p. 1031
53. a, p. 1030
54. b, p. 1030
55. d, p. 1025

CHAPTER 45
Male Reproductive System
Male Reproductive Organs

1. a, p. 1039
2. b, p. 1039
3. c, p. 1039
4. d, p. 1040
5. c, p. 1043
6. a, p. 1043
7. a, p. 1043
8. c, p. 1044
9. t, p. 1043

10. f, p. 1043
11. f, p. 1039
12. t, p. 1044
13. f, p. 1040
14. f, p. 1039
15. t, p. 1043

Reproductive Ducts and Accessory Reproductive Glands

16. b, p. 1045
17. c, p. 1047
18. a, p. 1047
19. c, p. 1048
20. b, p. 1048
21. t, p. 1045
22. t, p. 1047
23. t, p. 1047
24. f, p. 1048

Supporting Structures, Seminal Fluid, and Male Fertility

25. c, p. 1047
26. b, p. 1048
27. b, p. 1050
28. c, p. 1050
29. f, p. 1049
30. t, p. 1049
31. f, p. 1050

Mechanisms of Disease

32. oligospermia, p. 1051
33. 2 months, p. 1051
34. cryptorchidism, p. 1051
35. benign prostatic hypertrophy, p. 1052
36. Phimosis, p. 1052
37. impotence; erectile dysfunction, p. 1052
38. hydrocele, p. 1052
39. inguinal hernia, p. 1052

Applying What You Know

40. (a) cryptorchidism (b) easily detected by palpation of the scrotum (c) surgery or testosterone injections (d) may cause permanent sterility if not treated (e) early detection results in normal testicular and sexual development.
41. (a) hydrocele or inguinal hernia (b) inguinal hernia (c) Swelling of the scrotum occurs when the intestine pushes through the weak area of the abdominal wall, which separates the abdominopelvic cavity from the scrotum. (d) external supports or surgical repair

One Last Quick Check

42. b, p. 1048
43. c, p. 1049
44. b, p. 1039
45. c, p. 1041
46. a, p. 1041
47. d, p. 1048
48. d, p. 1044
49. d, p. 1044
50. c, p. 1043
51. c, p. 1043
52. a, p. 1044
53. b, pp. 1045-1046

54. h, p. 1049
55. g, p. 1048
56. a, p. 1045
57. f, p. 1047
58. c, p. 1046
59. i, p. 1047
60. e, p. 1049
61. d, p. 1052
62. j, p. 1049

Labeling

Male Pelvis—Sagittal Section

1. seminal vesicle
2. ejaculatory duct
3. prostate gland
4. rectum
5. bulbourethral (Cowper) gland
6. anus
7. epididymis
8. testis
9. scrotum
10. foreskin (prepuce)
11. penis
12. urethra
13. vas (ductus) deferens
14. pubic symphysis
15. urinary bladder
16. ureter

Tubules of Testis and Epididymis

1. nerves and blood vessels in the spermatic cord
2. vas (ductus) deferens
3. septum
4. lobule
5. tunica albuginea
6. testis
7. seminiferous tubules
8. epididymis

Penis

1. bladder
2. prostate
3. bulb
4. deep artery
5. foreskin (prepuce)
6. external urinary meatus
7. glans penis
8. corpus spongiosum
9. urethra
10. corpus cavernosum
11. opening of bulbourethral gland
12. crus penis
13. bulbourethral gland
14. openings of ejaculatory ducts

CHAPTER 46

Female Reproductive System

Overview of the Female Reproductive System

1. a, p. 1058
2. b, p. 1059

3. t, pp. 1058-1059
4. t, p. 1060

Ovaries, Uterus, Uterine Tubes, and Vagina

5. b, p. 1060
6. d, p. 1062
7. b, p. 1062
8. a, p. 1063
9. b, p. 1064
10. d, p. 1065
11. a, p. 1065
12. b, p. 1063
13. c, p. 1066
14. b, p. 1064
15. a, p. 1065
16. b, p. 1062
17. a, p. 1065
18. a, p. 1064
19. c, p. 1066
20. t, p. 1061
21. f, p. 1063
22. f, p. 1066
23. t, p. 1066

Vulva

24. c, pp. 1067-1068
25. b, p. 1067
26. a, p. 1066
27. b, p. 1068
28. d, p. 1066

Female Reproductive Cycle

29. a, p. 1069
30. c, p. 1069
31. a, p. 1069
32. c, p. 1071
33. b, p. 1075
34. f, p. 1070
35. t, p. 1071
36. t, p. 1075
37. f, p. 1075
38. f, p. 1071

Breasts

39. f, p. 1076
40. f, p. 1078
41. t, p. 1078
42. f, p. 1079

Mechanisms of Disease

43. f, p. 1082
44. e, p. 1082
45. a, p. 1080
46. h, p. 1081
47. i, p. 1081
48. g, p. 1081
49. c, p. 1081
50. b, p. 1080
51. l, p. 1082
52. d, p. 1080
53. j, p. 1083
54. k, p. 1083

Applying What You Know

55. (a) Contraceptive pills contain synthetic progesterone-like compounds such as progestin, sometimes combined with synthetic estrogens. By sustaining a high blood concentration of these substances, contraceptive pills prevent the monthly development of a follicle. With no ovum to be expelled, ovulation does not occur, and therefore pregnancy cannot occur. (b) Tubal ligation involves tying a piece of suture material around each uterine tube in two places, then cutting the tube between these two points. Sperm and eggs are thus prevented from meeting. This procedure is a surgical sterilization.

56. The uterine tubes are not attached to the ovaries, and infections can exit at this area and enter the abdominal cavity.

One Last Quick Check

57. g, p. 1058
58. b, p. 1059
59. e, p. 1082
60. j, p. 1082
61. a, p. 1064
62. f, p. 1066
63. c, p. 1066
64. i, p. 1069
65. h, p. 1083
66. d, p. 1080
67. premenstrual or postovulatory, p. 1070
68. Prolactin, p. 1078
69. Oxytocin, p. 1078
70. meiosis, p. 1069
71. corpus luteum, p. 1069
72. hymen, p. 1066
73. Menopause, p. 1079
74. menses or menstrual period, p. 1069
75. Eight, p. 1063
76. placenta, p. 1064
77. ectopic, p. 1061
78. Relaxin, p. 1062
79. endometrium, myometrium, and perimetrium (parietal peritoneum), p. 1063
80. incontinence, p. 1066
81. Infertility, p. 1072

Labeling

Female Pelvic Organs

1. fundus of uterus
2. uterine body cavity
3. endometrium
4. myometrium
5. body of uterus
6. internal os of cervix
7. cervical canal
8. external os of vaginal cervix
9. cervix of uterus
10. vagina
11. fornix of vagina
12. uterine artery and vein
13. broad ligament
14. ovary
15. fimbriae

16. infundibulopelvic ligament
17. infundibulum of uterine tube
18. ampulla of uterine tube
19. ovarian ligament
20. isthmus of uterine tube

Sagittal Section of Female Pelvis

1. sacral promontory
2. uterine tube
3. ureter
4. uterosacral ligament
5. rectouterine pouch (of Douglas)
6. cervix
7. fornix of vagina
8. coccyx
9. anus
10. vagina
11. labium majus
12. labium minus
13. clitoris
14. urethra
15. pubic symphysis
16. urinary bladder
17. parietal peritoneum
18. vesicouterine pouch
19. round ligament
20. fundus of uterus
21. body of uterus
22. ovarian ligament
23. suspensory ligament (of uterine tube)

External Female Genitals (Genitalia)

1. foreskin (prepuce)
2. clitoris (glans)
3. labium minus
4. external urinary meatus
5. vestibule
6. vestibular bulb
7. greater vestibular gland
8. mons pubis
9. pudendal fissure
10. labium majus
11. frenulum (of clitoris)
12. opening of lesser vestibular (Skene) gland
13. orifice of vagina
14. hymen
15. frenulum (of labia)
16. posterior commissure (of labia)

Vulva

1. clitoris (glans)
2. foreskin (prepuce)
3. labium minus
4. external urinary meatus
5. bulb of the vestibule
6. greater vestibular glands and ducts (Bartholin glands)
7. orifice of vagina
8. crus clitoris
9. lesser vestibular glands and ducts (Skene gland)
10. corpus cavernosum

CHAPTER 47
Growth and Development

A New Human Life

1. b, p. 1091
2. b, p. 1091
3. d, p. 1093
4. a, p. 1093
5. b, p. 1096
6. a, p. 1091
7. f, p. 1091
8. t, p. 1091
9. t, p. 1093
10. f, p. 1093
11. f, p. 1095
12. f, p. 1097
13. t, p. 1093
14. t, p. 1097

Prenatal Period

15. a, p. 1097
16. b, p. 1098
17. a, p. 1098
18. b, p. 1103
19. c, p. 1106
20. t, p. 1099
21. f, p. 1098
22. f, p. 1106
23. t, p. 1097
24. t, p. 1097

Birth, or Parturition, and the Postnatal Period

25. c, p. 1108
26. c, p. 1110
27. d, p. 1111
28. b, p. 1113
29. b, p. 1111
30. t, p. 1109
31. t, p. 1110
32. f, p. 1109
33. f, p. 1112
34. t, p. 1112

Effects of Aging

35. d, p. 1116
36. d, p. 1117
37. t, p. 1116
38. f, p. 1117

Mechanisms of Disease

39. c, p. 1119
40. a, p. 1119
41. d, p. 1119
42. b, p. 1119
43. h, p. 1119
44. f, p. 1119
45. j, p. 1119
46. g, p. 1119
47. e, p. 1119
48. i, p. 1119

Applying What You Know

49. Only about 40% of the taste buds present at age 30 remain at age 75.
50. Identical twins have the same genetic code.

One Last Quick Check

51. g, p. 1093
52. f, p. 1103
53. c, p. 1103
54. b, p. 1102
55. a, p. 1098
56. h, p. 1108
57. e, p. 1109
58. d, p. 1106
59. i, p. 1102
60. j, p. 1103
61. d, p. 1116
62. d, p. 1116
63. d, p. 1117
64. a, p. 1113
65. b, p. 1103
66. d, p. 1116
67. e, p. 1112
68. a, p. 1114
69. c, p. 1113
70. b, p. 1113

Labeling

Fertilization and Implantation

1. ovary
2. developing follicles
3. corpus luteum
4. fimbriae
5. discharged ovum
6. spermatozoa
7. first mitosis
8. uterine (fallopian) tube
9. blastocyst
10. morula
11. blastocyst
12. implantation

CHAPTER 48
Genetics and Heredity

The Science of Genetics, Chromosomes and Genes, Gene Expression

1. c, p. 1127
2. c, p. 1127
3. d, p. 1131
4. c, p. 1133
5. a, p. 1128
6. d, p. 1135
7. c, pp. 1134-1135
8. d, p. 1127
9. f, p. 1130
10. t, p. 1131
11. f, p. 1132

12. f, p. 1133
13. t, p. 1134
14. t, p. 1133
15. f, p. 1130
16. f, p. 1132

Medical Genetics; Prevention and Treatment of Genetic Diseases

17. b, p. 1136
18. b, pp. 1139-1140
19. a, p. 1140
20. c, p. 1132
21. c, p. 1141
22. b, pp. 1141-1142
23. d, pp. 1137; 1140-1141
24. d, p. 1143
25. c, p. 1142
26. b, p. 1142
27. f, p. 1136
28. t, p. 1138
29. f, p. 1138
30. t, p. 1141
31. t, p. 1141
32. f, p. 1145
33. t, p. 1136
34. t, p. 1142
35. t, p. 1136

Applying What You Know

36. In a form of dominance called *codominance*, the effect will be equal, causing "light brown" skin to occur.
37. One in four, or 25%

One Last Quick Check

38. a, p. 1130
39. d, p. 1141
40. c, p. 1131
41. b, p. 1130
42. a, p. 1130
43. c, p. 1127
44. b, p. 1134
45. c, p. 1133
46. a, p. 1142
47. b, p. 1141
48. h, p. 1141
49. k, p. 1142
50. c, p. 1137
51. e, p. 1128
52. a, p. 1137
53. d, p. 1147
54. j, p. 1139
55. l, p. 1138
56. g, p. 1131
57. b, pp. 1134-1135
58. i, p. 1142
59. f, p. 1134
60. RNA, p. 1127
61. transcriptomics, p. 1129
62. p-arm and q-arm, p. 1130.
63. Down syndrome, p. 1140
64. viruses, p. 1143
65. ideogram, p. 1130

Solutions to Crossword Puzzles

CHAPTER 1

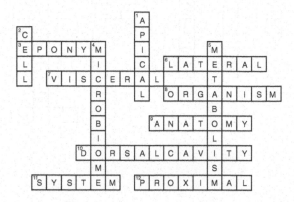

CHAPTER 2

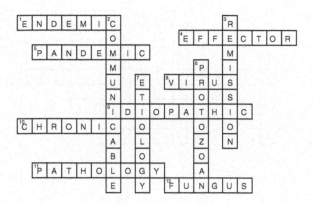

CHAPTER 3

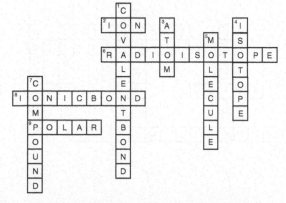

CHAPTER 4

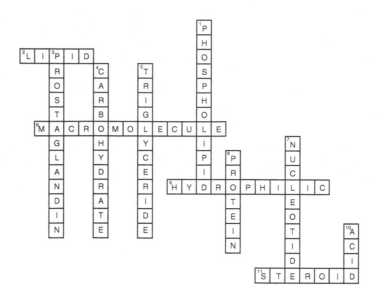

CHAPTER 5

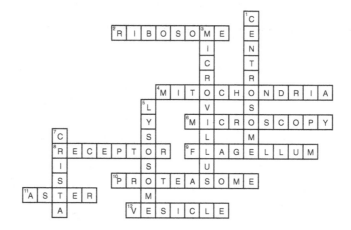

CHAPTER 6

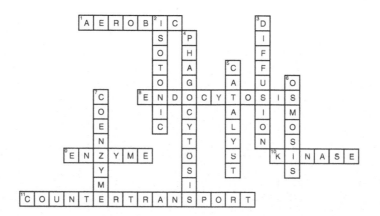

CHAPTER 7

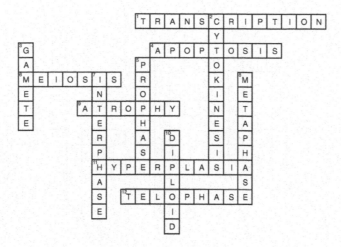

CHAPTER 8

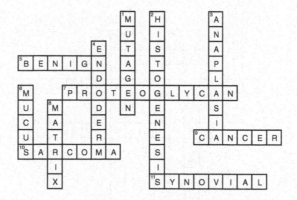

CHAPTER 9

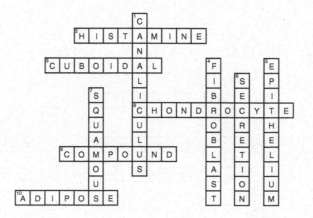

CHAPTER 10

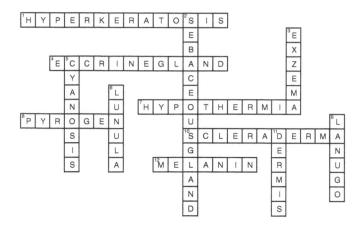

Across: HYPERKERATOSIS, ECCRINEGLAND, HYPOTHERMIA, PYROGEN, SCLERADERMA, MELANIN
Down: SEBACEOUS, CYANOSIS, EXZEMA, LUUULA, SUDORIFEROUSGLAND, DERMIS, LANUGO

CHAPTER 11

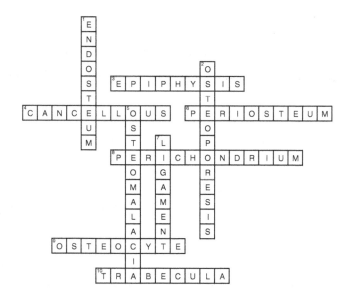

Across: EPIPHYSIS, CANCELLOUS, PERIOSTEUM, PERICHONDRIUM, OSTEOCYTE, TRABECULA
Down: ENDOSTEUM, OSTEOPOROSIS, CALCIUM, OSTEOMALACIA, LIGAMENT

CHAPTER 12

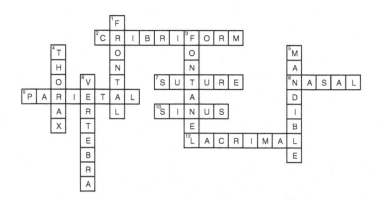

Across: CRIBRIFORM, SUTURE, NASAL, PARIETAL, SINUS, LACRIMAL
Down: FRONTAL, THORAX, VERTEBRA, CONCHA, MANDIBLE

CHAPTER 13

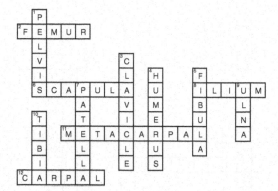

CHAPTER 14

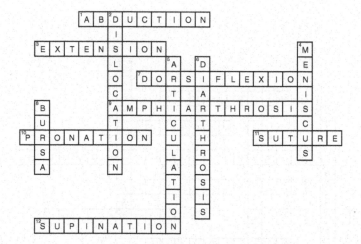

CHAPTER 15

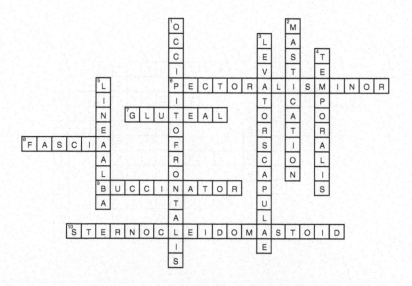

CHAPTER 16

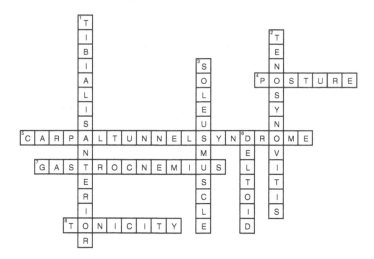

CHAPTER 17

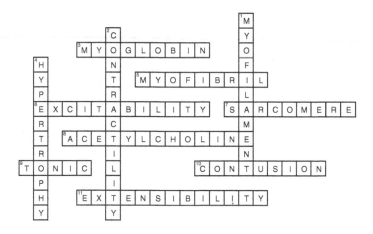

CHAPTER 18

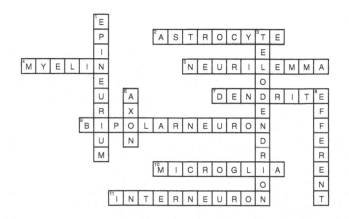

CHAPTER 19

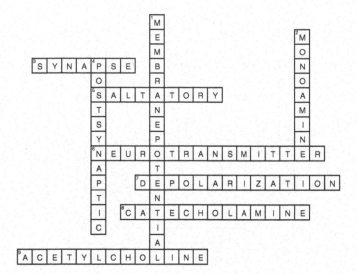

CHAPTER 20

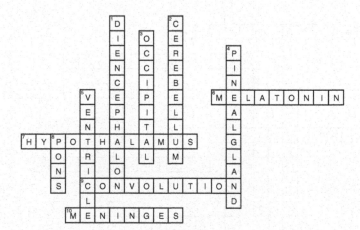

CHAPTER 21

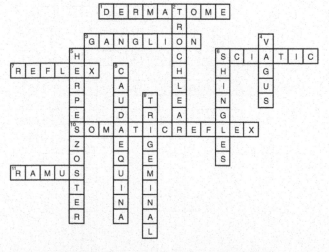

CHAPTER 22

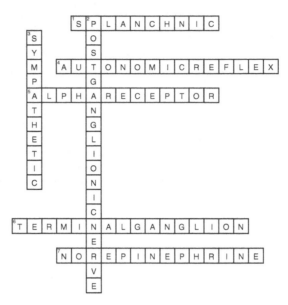

Across:
1. SPLANCHNIC
4. AUTONOMICREFLEX
6 (Across). ALPHARECEPTOR
6. TERMINALGANGLION
7. NOREPINEPHRINE

Down:
2. POSTGANGLIONICNERVE
3. SYMPATHETIC

CHAPTER 23

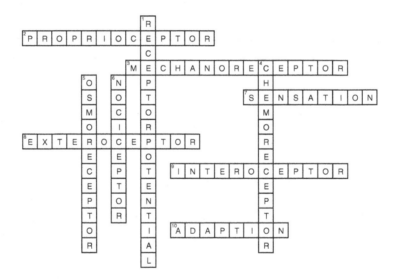

2. PROPRIOCEPTOR
3. MECHANORECEPTOR
7. SENSATION
8. EXTEROCEPTOR
9. INTEROCEPTOR
10. ADAPTION
1. RECEPTORPOTENTIAL
4. CHEMORECEPTOR
5. OSMORECEPTOR
6. NOCICEPTOR

CHAPTER 24

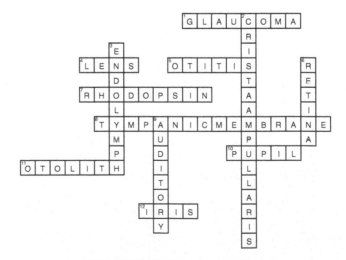

1. GLAUCOMA
4. LENS
5. OTITIS
7. RHODOPSIN
8. TYMPANICMEMBRANE
10. PUPIL
11. OTOLITH
12. IRIS
2. CRISTAA
3. EDOLYMPH
6. RETINA
9. AUDITORY
10. PUPILLARIS

CHAPTER 25

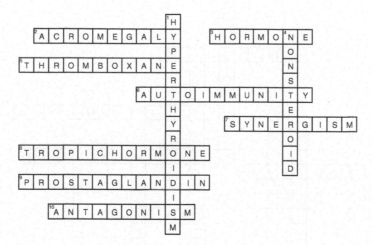

Across:
2. ACROMEGALY
3. HORMONE
5. THROMBOXANE
6. AUTOIMMUNITY
7. SYNERGISM
8. TROPICHORMONE
9. PROSTAGLANDIN
10. ANTAGONISM

Down:
1. HYPERTHYROIDISM
4. NONSTEROID

CHAPTER 26

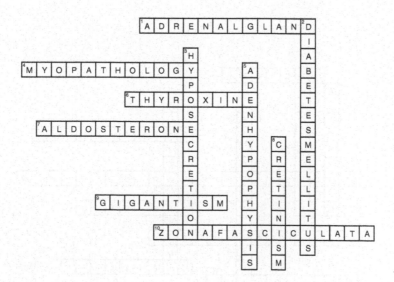

1. ADRENALGLAND
2. DIABETESMELLITUS
3. HYPOSECRETION
4. MYOPATHOLOGY
5. ADENHYPOPHYSIS
6. THYROXINE
7. ALDOSTERONE
8. CRETINISM
9. GIGANTISM
10. ZONAFASCICULATA

CHAPTER 27

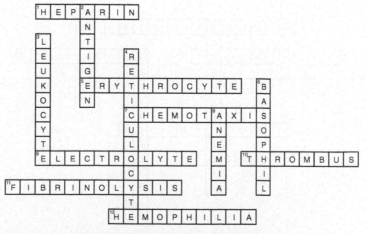

1. HEPARIN
2. ANTIGEN
3. LEUKOCYTE
4. RETICULOCYTE
5. ERYTHROCYTE
6. BASOPHIL
7. CHEMOTAXIS
8. ANEMIA
9. ELECTROLYTE
10. THROMBUS
11. FIBRINOLYSIS
12. HEMOPHILIA

CHAPTER 28

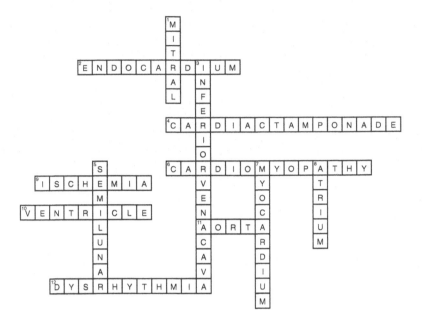

CHAPTER 29

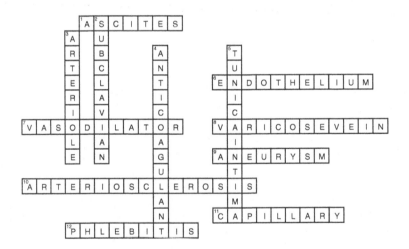

CHAPTER 30

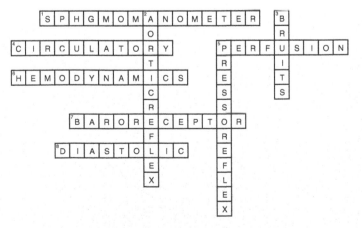

CHAPTER 31

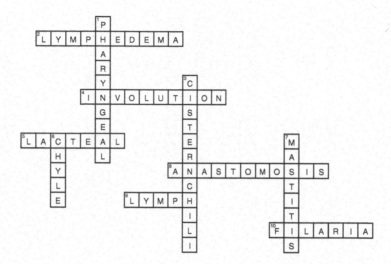

CHAPTER 32

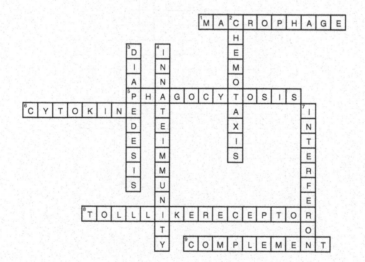

CHAPTER 33

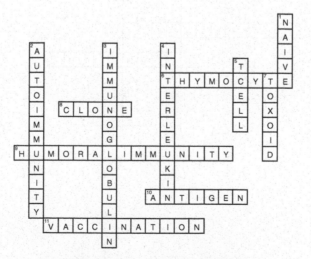

CHAPTER 34

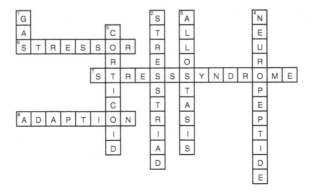

CHAPTER 35

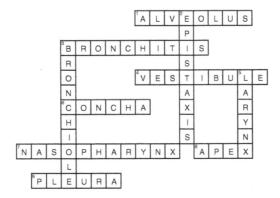

CHAPTER 36

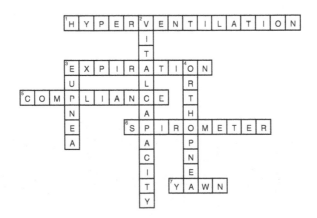

CHAPTER 37

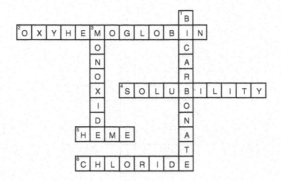

Across: OXYHEMOGLOBIN, SOLUBILITY, HEME, CHLORIDE
Down: BICARBONATE, MONOXIDE

CHAPTER 38

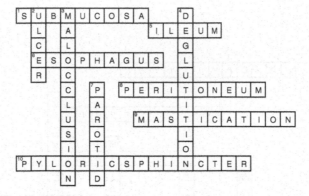

Across: SUBMUCOSA, ILEUM, ESOPHAGUS, PERITONEUM, MASTICATION, PYLORICSPHINCTER
Down: SLCCRCCLUSI, BALCCLUSI, DGLUITIO, PAROTID

CHAPTER 39

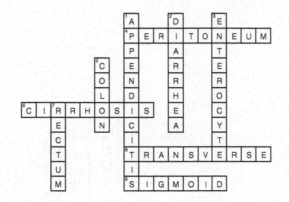

Across: PERITONEUM, CIRRHOSIS, TRANSVERSE, SIGMOID
Down: APPENDICITIS, DARRHEA, ETEROCYT, COLON, RECTUM

CHAPTER 40

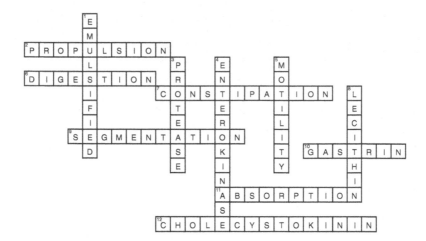

CHAPTER 41

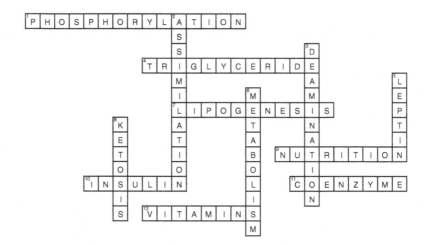

CHAPTER 42

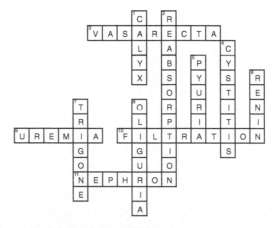

CHAPTER 43

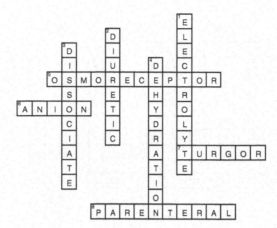

CHAPTER 44

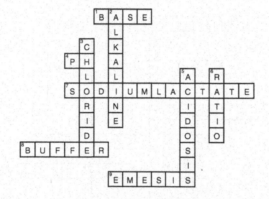

CHAPTER 45

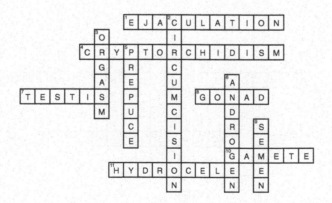

CHAPTER 46

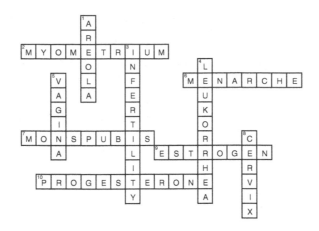

CHAPTER 47

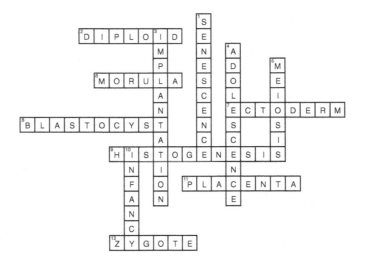

CHAPTER 48

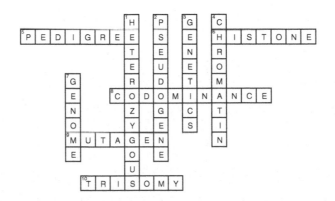